Reinventing Hippocrates

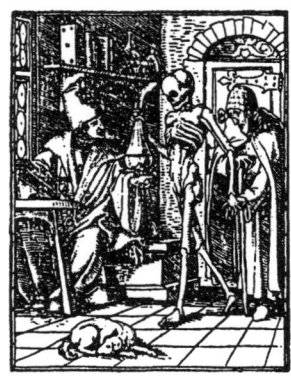

The History of Medicine in Context

Series Editors: Andrew Cunningham and Ole Peter Grell

Department of History and Philosophy of Science
University of Cambridge

Department of History
The Open University

Titles in this series include:

The Making of the Dentiste, *c. 1650–1760*
Roger King

*'The Battle for Health': A Political History of the
Socialist Medical Association, 1930–51*
John Stewart

*Medicine and Charity in Georgian Bath:
A Social History of the General Infirmary, c. 1739–1830*
Anne Borsay

The Nurse Apprentice, 1860–1977
Ann Bradshaw

*The Return of Epidemics:
Health and Society in Peru during the Twentieth Century*
Marcos Cueto

Reinventing Hippocrates

Edited by

DAVID CANTOR

Ashgate

Aldershot • Burlington USA • Singapore • Sydney

© The editor and contributors, 2002

All rights reserved. No part of this publication may be reproduced, stored in a retrieval system, or transmitted in any form or by any means, electronic, mechanical, photo-copying, recording, or otherwise without the prior permission of the publisher.

The author has asserted his moral right under the Copyright, Designs and Patents Act, 1988, to be identified as the author of this work.

Published by
Ashgate Publishing Limited
Gower House
Croft Road
Aldershot
Hants GU11 3HR
England

Ashgate Publishing Company
131 Main Street
Burlington, VT 05401–5600 USA

Ashgate website: http://www.ashgate.com

British Library Cataloguing in Publication Data

Reinventing Hippocrates. – (The History of Medicine in Context)
　1. Hippocrates – Influence　2. Medicine – History – 16th century　3. Medicine – History – 17th century　4. Medicine – Ancient　5. Medicine – Philosophy – History – 16th century　6. Medicine – Philosophy – History – 17th century
I. Cantor, David
610.9031

Library of Congress Cataloging-in-Publication Data

Reinventing Hippocrates / edited by David Cantor.
　　p.　cm. – (The history of medicine in context)
　Includes bibliographical references.
　ISBN 0-7546-0528-0 (alk. paper)
　1. Hippocrates.　2. Medicine, Greek and Roman.　3. Medicine, Ancient.
I. Cantor, David.　II. Series

R126.H8 R35 2001
610–dc21   2001022834

ISBN 0 7546 0528 0

Printed on acid-free paper

Typeset in Times by N²productions
Printed and bound in Great Britain by MPG Books Ltd, Bodmin, Cornwall

Contents

List of Figures	vii
Acknowledgements	viii
Notes on Contributors	ix

1 Introduction: The Uses and Meanings of Hippocrates   1
   David Cantor

PART I   Renaissance Constructions of Hippocratism

2 The Power of Paternity: The Father of Medicine Meets the Prince of Physicians   21
   Helen King

3 Hippocrates and the Construction of 'Progress' in Sixteenth- and Seventeenth-century Medicine   37
   Thomas Rütten

4 The Chemical Hippocrates: Paracelsian and Hippocratic Theory in Petrus Severinus' Medical Philosophy   59
   Jole Shackelford

PART II   The Transformations of Hippocratism in Seventeenth- and Eighteenth-century Britain

5 The Transformation of Hippocrates in Seventeenth-century Britain   91
   Andrew Cunningham

6 Hippocrates and the Politics of Medical Knowledge in Early Modern England   116
   Robert L. Martensen

7 Hippocrates, Bacon, and Medical Meteorology at the Royal Society, 1700–1750   136
   Andrea Rusnock

PART III   Hippocratism in Eighteenth- and Nineteenth-century France and North America

8 Hippocrates and the Montpellier Vitalists in the French Medical Enlightenment   157
   Elizabeth A. Williams

9 The Rhetoric of Hippocrates at the Paris School   178
   Ann F. La Berge

10 Making History in American Medical Culture: The Antebellum
   Competition for Hippocrates   200
   John Harley Warner

PART IV Twentieth-century Hippocratic Revivals

11 Hippocrates American Style: Representing Professional Morality
   in Early Twentieth-century America   239
   Susan E. Lederer

12 Hippocrates, Holism and Humanism in Interwar France   257
   George Weisz

13 The Name and the Word: Neo-Hippocratism and Language in
   Interwar Britain   280
   David Cantor

14 A Model for the New Physician: Hippocrates in Interwar Germany   302
   Carsten Timmermann

Index   325

List of Figures

11.1	The front page of Sinclair Lewis's 'The Hippocratic Oath'	250
12.1	Hippocratic titles by decade	258

Acknowledgements

This book has its origins in a conference organised at the College of Physicians of Philadelphia. I would like to thank the College and the Barra Foundation for their generous financial support of the meeting. Thanks also go to Tom Horrocks and to Monique Bourque for ensuring that it ran smoothly and successfully.

David Cantor

Notes on Contributors

David Cantor is a 'Special Expert' at the National Cancer Institute, Bethesda, Maryland where he is working on a history of cancer prevention and control in the United States. He has previously published works on the histories of cancer and the rheumatic diseases.

Andrew Cunningham has taught history of medicine and history of science at Cambridge University for over 20 years. He is the author of three books: on the history of anatomy; the history of natural philosophy; and the history of crises in sixteenth-century Europe. Currently he holds a Wellcome Trust Senior Research Fellowship.

Helen King is Reader in the History of Classical Medicine at the University of Reading. She is the author of *Hippocrates' Woman: Reading the Female Body in Ancient Greece* (Routledge, 1998) and, with Sander Gilman, Roy Porter, George Rousseau and Elaine Showalter, co-author of *Hysteria Beyond Freud* (University of California, 1993).

Ann La Berge is Associate Professor of STS at Virginia Tech. Her research interests are in nineteenth-century French medicine and public health. Her most recent book (co-edited with Caroline Hannaway) is *Constructing Paris Medicine* (1998). She is currently working on medical microscopy in nineteenth-century France.

Susan E. Lederer teaches in the Section of the History of Medicine at Yale University School of Medicine. A historian of twentieth-century American medicine, she has published on the history of human and animal experimentation, medical ethics, and is currently writing a history of blood transfusion and organ transplantation in the United States.

Robert L. Martensen serves as Professor and Chair of the Department of History and Philosophy of Medicine at the University of Kansas, where he has been since 1995. A practising physician for many years, he earned a doctorate in history of medicine in 1993 at the University of California, San Francisco. His main historical interests include the early modern period in Europe and the Progressive Era in the United States.

Andrea Rusnock teaches in the History Department at the University of Rhode Island. She is the editor of *The Correspondence of James Jurin (1684–1750), Physician and Secretary of the Royal Society* (1996), and she has recently completed a book entitled *Vital Accounts: Measuring Health and Population in Eighteenth-Century England and France*.

Thomas Rütten is a doctor and *Privatdozent* in the Theory and History of Medicine at the University of Münster, Germany, where he wrote both his doctoral dissertation 'Demokrit – lachender Philosoph und sanguinischer Melancholiker' (1992) and his 'Habilitation' thesis 'Geschichten vom hippokratischen Eid' (1995). His research focuses on the reception of Hippocratic writings and the history of his chosen discipline, medical history. He works as a freelance author, literary translator and lecturer.

Jole Shackelford gained a PhD degree at the University of Wisconsin in the History of Science, with an emphasis on history of medicine. His research interest is in early modern European medicine, particularly the social and intellectual responses to the chemical, medical, and religious ideas of the Paracelsians.

Carsten Timmermann is a Wellcome Research Associate at the Centre for the History of Science, Technology and Medicine in Manchester (www.man.ac.uk/chstm/), working on a comparative history of high blood pressure research in the UK and Germany. He studied biochemistry in Berlin, lived in California for two years, and completed MA and PhD programmes in Manchester. He is currently revising his dissertation on 'Weimar Medical Culture' for publication.

John Harley Warner is Professor of the History of Medicine, of American Studies and of History at Yale University. He is author of *The Therapeutic Perspective* (1986) and *Against the Spirit of System* (1998), and co-editor, with Janet Tighe, of *Major Problems in the History of American Medicine and Public Health* (2001).

George Weisz is Professor of the History of Medicine at McGill University. His most recent books are: *The Medical Mandarins: The French Academy of Medicine in the Nineteenth and Twentieth Centuries* (1995) and *Greater Than the Parts: Holism in Biomedicine, 1920–1950* (1998) (editor with Christopher Lawrence). He is currently working on a history of medical specialization in comparative perspective.

Elizabeth A. Williams is Associate Professor in the Department of History at Oklahoma State University. Author of *The Physical and the Moral: Anthropology, Physiology, and Philosophical Medicine in France, 1750–1850* (Cambridge, 1994), she is now completing a study of medical vitalism in Enlightenment Montpellier.

CHAPTER ONE

Introduction: The Uses and Meanings of Hippocrates

David Cantor

The recent enthusiasm for computer games may not seem the most obvious place to begin a book on the father of medicine. But, at the end of the twentieth century, Hippocrates found his way into those imaginary worlds, and in such a bewildering variety of guises! In the late 1990s he was the joint ruler of the Beastmaker Mountain, a medical swordfish, a beast or monster, the member of an Immortal Staff, and the founder of the Hippocrates Circle which manipulated medical technology for the purposes of world domination. His name was adopted by game players in at least three role-playing games; there were starships called Hippocrates in two others, and the Hippocrates Ambulance ran through another. Elsewhere, he appeared in a virtual version of Dante's Hell, provided clues as to the rescue of a kidnap victim, and inspired a group called the healercraft. One game claimed to be based on his insights into personality type; and he was cited in instructions on how to decide when a player should go mad. Such were some of the uses of Hippocrates at the turn of the millennium.[1]

These varied uses of Hippocrates may be historically specific, but they highlight a general problem in the historiography of his legacy. Until recently, most accounts of the Hippocratic tradition tended not to explain variety, but to consider whether or not the various visions and uses of Hippocrates captured something of the original historical figure or his insights.[2] From such a perspective, the historiographical task was to identify the 'true' Hippocrates, and then to assess the authenticity of subsequent depictions of him and his medicine. While such an approach might help to make the obvious point that none of the 'Hippocrateses' in late twentieth-century computer games measured up to current scholarly conceptions of the man and his medicine, that is hardly the point. With few exceptions these games made no pretensions to historical accuracy, and those that did made no claim to rigorous academic scholarship. The reasons why game players or others might wish to portray Hippocrates in a particular way would be unexplored in traditional scholarship, if it ever looked at popular culture as more than a curiosity. It is one of the points of this book that such scholarship also tells us little about the meanings and uses of Hippocrates for the many groups and individuals that *do* assert some claim to historical accuracy, and so also tells us little about the related question of how Hippocrates came to have such a pervasive presence in Western medicine and culture.[3]

There are other reasons why older accounts of Hippocrates created problems for understanding the various ways in which he has been portrayed and used since antiquity. Firstly, they tended to give Hippocrates or his ideas the primary role in influencing subsequent generations. Somehow Hippocrates reached out from death and the distant ancient world to shape the thoughts and actions of later peoples. The emphasis was on the ways in which ideas were transmitted from one generation to another. But these ideas were problematically connected to those people who held them. The interests and agendas that shaped their reading of Hippocrates were often of interest only to the extent that they hindered or facilitated the uptake of his ideas. Secondly, Hippocratic values were often regarded as unproblematic and unchanging – despite a growing literature on diversity and contradiction within the Hippocratic *Corpus*. From such a perspective it was quite possible to measure those who claimed to be Hippocratic against 'true' Hippocratic values. If they failed to live up to such values, then the historian's task was to set out the reasons why they strayed from the path, and to pinpoint those who brought medicine back to the light.[4] There may have been many portrayals of Hippocrates but, in such accounts, only one authentic vision. Thirdly, traditional approaches tended – and still tend – to tell tales of decline and degradation. Thus one recent historian urges a study of the 'corruption of the Hippocratic Corpus',[5] while survivalist accounts discuss the 'simplification' or 'degeneration' of a 'stripped down' Hippocratic medicine in the Horn of Africa, South Asia and Latin America.[6] This emphasis on corruption and simplification tends to downplay the possibility of creative reinventions of Hippocrates and his medicine.[7]

Some of these features are exemplified by Wesley Smith's path-breaking account of the abandonment since the Renaissance of Galenic interpretations of Hippocrates. Smith argues that accounts of Hippocrates and Hippocratic medicine have been shaped by what he calls the 'scientific'[8] interests of doctors and that these accounts have been taken up uncritically by subsequent historians and philologists. He focuses on what he calls the 'errors' or 'aberrations' of past interpretations in order to overcome them.[9] Unlike the contributors to this book, Smith is concerned to recover 'genuine' Hippocratic texts, as well as to show how such allegedly aberrant interpretations came about. His focus on how scientists' progressive attitudes 'infected' medical history also points to differences with many of the contributors to this book.[10] Most would question the notion that science (or any cultural artifact) infects an otherwise healthy body of historical knowledge. Instead, these papers tend to see the cultural and social shaping of historical knowledge – including the papers presented here – as a normal, routine part of knowledge production.

Whilst the papers in this book vary considerably in approach and topic there are a number of themes that unite them. For most, the existence of an historical

Hippocrates is less important than the various ways in which Hippocrates has been used over time. Hippocrates is not so much a 'real' person as a malleable cultural artifact, constantly moulded and remoulded according to need. The identification of 'genuine' Hippocratic texts is less important to most authors than changing historical perceptions of what may be genuine or useful Hippocratic texts. As the following essays show, different writers have chosen quite different and often contradictory messages from the *Corpus* by favouring one or other of the texts – perhaps the *Oath*, perhaps *Epidemics*, perhaps *On Ancient Medicine*. Contributors to this volume tend not to see Hippocrates or his ideas as primary actors, but focus instead on the ways in which Hippocrates and his medicine have been represented or read by particular groups and individuals within particular historical, cultural and social circumstances. The key words of 'constructing', 'shaping', 'using' and 'reading' all evoke active attempts by various groups and individuals to imagine the father of medicine and to bring specific social, cultural and technical resources to such visions. The Hippocratic tradition is, therefore, an 'invented tradition', constantly reinvented over time.[11] It is not passed unproblematically from one generation to another, nor is it a refuge for backward minds – those unable to cope with modernity. On the contrary, the classical world has often provided a fruitful way of way of shaping and making sense of the modern world.[12] Indeed, as Thomas Rütten notes in this collection, key modernist concepts such as 'progress' have sometimes been oriented as much to the past as to the future.

The book also seeks to address some of the ways in which a focus on the invention and reinvention of the past might be achieved. Contributors to this volume attempt to tie the many variants of Hippocrates and Hippocratism into broader concerns about personal, professional, class, regional and national identity. Some invoke pre-existing 'interests' and 'forces' to explain such variants; others focus on the practices of medicine, science and politics to explore the production of 'Hippocrateses'; and others explore the histories of readings that shape and reshape conceptions of Hippocrates. Alongside such causal explanations of the constructions and reconstructions are others that provide interpretative accounts of the variants of Hippocrates. From this perspective, the social mechanisms by which various 'Hippocrateses' have been produced are less a concern than what such variants say about the particular cultures that produce them. As John Harley Warner states in his essay, there is a growing appreciation that cultural heros embody the aspirations of the groups and individuals that create them; they validate their endeavours and reaffirm their perceptions of self.

A focus on the cultural meanings and constructions of Hippocrates has been facilitated by recent scholarship that highlights differences between modern and ancient understandings of Hippocrates and his medicine. For example, although Hippocrates is often portrayed as the founder of modern observational methods, Geoffrey Lloyd has shown that the ancient Greeks had no exact equivalent to our word 'observation':[13] the Greek word *teresis* did not appear until later. Indeed, some ancient observational methods appear to be quite the opposite of those of today. Volker Langholf notes that the verb *skopéomai* used in the *Epidemics* meant to 'consider' in the light of existing rules or theories:[14] the observation of individual cases in the *Epidemics* is in fact not done in order to move from observation to theory, but rather to extend the applicability of existing theories. The authors of the *Epidemics*, according to Langholf, do not consider abstract rules or theories in the light of cases.[15] 'Never', he writes,[16] 'does a question restrict the validity or applicability of any medical theory'; the *Epidemics* shows 'a tendency to present reality in conformity with theory'.[17] Thus, Hippocrates the observer is an invention rather than an original subsequently misrepresented by those who wish him to support their cause.

A similar point can be made about Hippocratic ethics. Today the roots of modern medical ethics are constantly traced to Hippocrates, as if the meaning of the *Oath* is timeless and unproblematic.[18] 'Hippocrates, schmippocrates,'[19] is all that Dr Hibbert in television's *The Simpsons* (1995) has to say to evoke his unethical behaviour in agreeing to the request of some children for an unnecessary surgical operation. But there have been many versions of the Oath, and the original document is probably not from the Hippocratic period.[20] Indeed, the *Oath* and other 'ethical' writings such as *Decorum* and *The Physician* can been seen as quite unethical in modern terms. They can be read to advocate a morality of deceit, teaching physicians the correct way to look in order to fool patients by giving a convincing impression. The notion of a timeless set of Hippocratic ethics is therefore problematised, as is the notion of later corruptions of Hippocrates's 'high' ideals.

Transformations of Hippocrates

This book begins with sixteenth-century transformations of Hippocrates, the time when, according to Vivian Nutton, the modern picture of Hippocrates was formed and the historical figure first took on flesh and blood.[21] Yet transformations of Hippocrates can be traced almost back to the man himself;[22] his younger contemporary, Plato, being perhaps the first, as Langholf puts it, to interpret 'the available information about Hippocrates's method on the basis of his own system of thought'.[23] Galen subsequently adopted this procedure, constructing an image of Hippocratic medicine that was remarkably like his own, and which he bolstered by classifying as 'genuine' those Hippocratic writings that echoed his own ideas.[24] On the basis of such a classification, Galen was able to combine often conflicting Hippocratic writings into a unitary theory of fluids, organs and *pepsis*. It was thus not so much the originality of Galen's work as the immense magnitude of his invention that allowed Galenic medicine to dominate in the West until the sixteenth century. Some Hippocratic works had been part of the Latin medical curriculum since the early Middle Ages,[25] but the Hippocrates known to writers of the late Middle Ages was essentially Galen's Hippocrates, and the abandonment of such a portrayal of Hippocrates was neither inevitable nor sudden.

The story of a gradual abandonment of Galen's Hippocrates reflects a broader tendency within Renaissance scholarship to avoid accounts that portray the sixteenth century as a sudden breach with the medieval or early Renaissance medical past.[26] Humanist scholars started to study Hippocratic texts in the late fifteenth century, a study that represented a greater reliance on the ancient past, but also led to a repudiation of some parts of that past.[27] Crucial to this patchwork process of reclamation and abandonment was the availability of the entire Latin printed edition of the Hippocratic *Corpus* in 1525, and of a complete Greek edition the following year, followed by the appearance of numerous other new translations, editions and commentaries.[28] The fact that readers had to master a much broader range of Hippocratic texts, and in two ancient languages, may help to explain why Hippocrates tended to remain subordinate to Galen until the 1560s.[29] Those who quoted Hippocrates may not have read him or, if they did, they read him through Galen's eyes. Galen portrayed himself as merely an interpreter of Hippocrates, and subsequent generations accepted his claim, seldom distinguishing the two.

From the fifteenth century the dominance of Galen was threatened by the arrival of 'new diseases' for which there was no precedent in his medicine. As Jole Shackelford notes in his contribution, practitioners began to attempt to shape a new medicine that could address such new diseases. One solution to the problem could be found in the classical authors themselves. Pliny, for example, blamed the new diseases of his day on the new foodstuffs imported from areas newly conquered by the Romans.[30] Another solution was to study more deeply the ancient medical texts in the belief that they included a description of every disease. Far from being a dry academic issue, this study had immediate implications for treatment. If Hippocrates or Galen mentioned a particular condition, it followed that the medical treatment was worth attempting: an explanation of the nature of the disease and its mode of transmission could also offer doctors a competitive advantage in the medical marketplace. Faithful translations of drug substances or body parts were valuable because, as John Arrizabalaga, John Henderson and Roger French put it, 'bad texts mean bad medical practice'.[31] 'New diseases' thus became a stimulus to philological study.

A third solution was to dismiss Galenic medicine as no longer relevant. The essays by Shackelford, Helen King, Andrew Cunningham and Robert Martensen all highlight individuals for whom this was an option. But rejecting Galen did not necessarily mean rejecting Hippocrates. Indeed, it was quite possible to argue that to reject Galen and to keep Hippocrates was *consistent* with Galenism. As Helen King suggests in her contribution, if Galen suggested that he was merely the mouthpiece of Hippocrates, then a return to Hippocrates could be portrayed as a Galenic move. As such, it was feasible to represent substantial change as no change at all. Shackelford, for example, notes that the Paracelsian, Petrus Severinus, portrayed himself as the restorer of Hippocrates while at the same time advocating a new chemical medicine.

The nature of the *Corpus* was important to the shift from Galen to Hippocrates. The *Corpus* is not the work of one individual: no text in the 60 or so collected under his name can be unequivocally proclaimed as the work of Hippocrates, and the *Corpus* itself is a hotchpotch from different periods, packed with conflicting theories and other internal inconsistencies.[32] Hippocrates has therefore often been whatever assortment of texts a reader determined upon, mixed and matched to fit his or her own ideas. Such a process of selection allowed Galenic readings of the *Corpus* but, from the sixteenth century, it also allowed practitioners to reject Galen by choosing a different set of works or by reinterpreting particular writings in ways that Galen might have balked at. Thus, it was quite possible for writers to keep Hippocrates while abandoning Galen.

At the same time, however, the reasons why they turned to Hippocrates also began to change. For establishment physicians he increasingly became less a source of substantive explanations of the body and illness, and more a source of method and a model of conduct or morals. These methods and morals would often be regarded as timeless – unchanged, at least in principle, since classical antiquity. While, as we have already noted, such a view is quite mistaken, it illustrates the use of the classical world to assert authority.

As many essays in this book show, by the seventeenth-century Hippocrates had become a symbol of empiricism and practice against Galen who stood for rationalism and theory.[33] But the problem with a Hippocrates who supported experience and observation was that, logically, it could become his downfall. If observation was so important, then the accumulated experience since Hippocrates also had claim to a place in medicine. In this volume, Andrew Cunningham notes the emergence of a theme of improvement which persisted in the following three centuries, often as a means of overturning orthodoxies in the name of an older truth. For example, Thomas Broman has shown how some late eighteenth-century German writers took care not to turn Hippocrates into an unchallengeable canon of sacred work.[34] They argued that the Hippocratic authors were often wrong, and they attacked those whom they believed elevated them to the status of a god, including Galen and Sydenham. For these writers, Hippocrates was the patient observer of bedside medicine, an observer of illness who let Nature speak for herself, who valued an understanding of the semiotics by which Nature's language was translated, and who trusted in Nature's healing powers. In his essay, John Harley Warner suggests that some nineteenth-century American physicians also resisted the elevation of Hippocrates to the level of scriptural authority. In addition, he discusses the nineteenth-century idea that treatments in Hippocrates were not appropriate to the conditions of the USA.

This is not to say that everyone who wanted to improve on Hippocrates also wanted to keep him. Robert Martensen locates the theme of improvement not among Hippocratists but among those who rejected Hippocrates, notably experimentalists associated with the Royal Society. By contrast, Andrea Rusnock notes that the eighteenth-century English physician, Francis Clifton attempted to improve on the Hippocratic method of clinical observation in line with the modern experimental approach of the Royal Society. Similarly, Michael Osborne argues elsewhere that the translator of the Hippocratic *Corpus*, Emile Littré, noted that although the progress of the medical art had improved on Hippocrates, his method and the method of modern medicine did not differ in their essence since both were the experimental method.[35] What counted as the Hippocratic method was thus quite fluid; it could be clinical observation or it could be the experimental method, each of which was in turn malleable. Such fluidity might help provide a solution to one of the problems facing improvers of Hippocrates who also wanted to keep him. One could improve on Hippocrates without contradicting him, simply by redefining what was meant by observation or experiment.

Reading Hippocrates

The essays in this collection document the ways in which physicians and others rummaged through the *Corpus* for writings that fitted their own interpretations of medicine and how they read the same texts in very different ways. Iain Lonie has noted that Hippocrates could be read as an iatromechanist,[36] but Jole Shackelford notes that he could also be read as an iatrochemist. He has been portrayed as the founder of clinical observation, but also of experimental medicine. He has been an advocate of environmental medicine (Rusnock),[37] clinical medicine focused on the individual patient (Cantor, Weisz),[38] and a 'social' medicine focused on the collective (Timmermann).[39] Ancient materials may therefore be creatively adapted to fulfil new objectives – although some 'ancient' material may have had little relation to antiquity.

Not only do the essays document the different ways in which the *Corpus* was read, but they also record the diverse meanings of reading to Hippocratists. An inability to read Hippocrates has been both despised and prized. On the one hand, commentators have validated their own interpretation of Hippocrates and Hippocratic medicine by criticising those who expounded on Hippocrates without ever have read him. An ability to read Hippocrates, especially in the original Greek, has often been a means of defending elite, learned culture. On the other hand, others have made a virtue of the inability to read Hippocrates. Thus John Worth Estes suggests that Samuel Thomson – the nineteenth-century founder of the Thomsonian system of medical botany – may have concealed the extent of his reading of Hippocrates, reflecting an age when writers disowned formal education even if they had it.[40] In this volume, Elizabeth

Williams notes that some eighteenth-century Montpellier physicians saw a sort of natural Hippocratism among the ill-educated, presumably not dependent on their reading of Hippocrates. Also in this volume, David Cantor notes that some twentieth-century British practitioners felt that a reading of Hippocrates was quite unnecessary to Hippocratic medicine. From such a perspective, Hippocratism was something quite natural to some doctors who could intuitively adopt it even without reading a word of the father of medicine.

The centrality of reading the *Corpus* was challenged by growing scepticism about the links between the *Corpus* and the historical Hippocrates. Wesley Smith has documented the complex process by which scholars abandoned the notion of genuine texts, and this abandonment raises questions about what this meant for those who subsequently sought to revive Hippocratism. One response was to assert the notion of a spirit of Hippocrates or his 'Age' which could be found in the *Corpus* or certain parts of it, irrespective of its links to the historical Hippocrates. Another response was simply to ignore the doubts about the link between the historical Hippocrates and the *Corpus*. For example, for many unorthodox practitioners simply assume the genuineness of Hippocratic texts in order to promote the notion of a golden holistic age subsequently corrupted by modern high-tech medicine. Yet another response has been to treat the genuineness or otherwise of the Hippocratic texts as quite irrelevant. For example, many of the game players mentioned above, Hippocrates may be associated with medicine – as is Dr Hippocrates the swordfish. But he is also a complex mix of characteristics derived from fantasy and science-fiction genres, combined with personal imagination. Many doctors have been portrayed as the 'new' Hippocrates, but in role-playing games it is quite possible to *be* Hippocrates. Such games highlight the ways in which the personal, professional and political may converge on the figure of the father of medicine.

If the *Corpus* was significant to the transformations of Hippocrates so too were the scant facts of his 'real' life. His younger contemporaries, Plato and Aristotle, suggest that the historical Hippocrates was born in or around 460 BC on the Greek island of Cos, a member of the Asclepiads who claimed to be descendants of Asclepius. He was short in height, he was willing to charge for teaching medicine, he seems to have been well known before his death, and that is about all they have to say.[41] These meagre details have left ample room for imaginative constructions of his life and works, and tales about them began to appear in the ancient world, notably in the *Vita* and *Pseudepigrapha*.[42] Among the more famous were stories that he burned the library of Cos, that he cured King Perdiccas of lovesickness, that he patriotically refused the gold of the Persian King Artaxerxes, that he cured the Athenian plague, and that he died in Larrissa in Thessaly. But the sources for these accounts emerged several hundred years after his death, perhaps in part as a means of creating authority for the Coan medical school, and were read in different ways. To ancient Greeks, Hippocrates's refusal of barbarian gold was a sign of his patriotism, to later Roman commentators it was a sign of the untrustworthiness of Greek physicians.[43]

For later generations, such stories have also provided a useful means of discussing political order.[44] For example, the story of Hippocrates's refusal of barbarian gold was a staple of many nineteenth-century British accounts of Hippocrates, in which its political message about despotism and tyranny was often linked to the passage in *Airs, Waters and Places* where Hippocrates contrasts Asiatic despotism and Greek freedom. The liberal reformer, William Farr, read in *Airs, Waters and Places* an indictment of the 'very nerve and withering arm' of despotism.[45] For Farr, Hippocrates attributed the unenergetic character of Asiatics to their system of government, the greater part of Asia being governed by despotic kings. 'Independence', he claimed, 'enlarges, and gives energy to, all the faculties; it is the vital breath of the mind; it gives health to a nation.'[46] The point was echoed by others. 'What a noble picture of a free over a slave State!', commented the physician J. Rutherfurd Russell[47] in 1861 of this passage in *Airs, Waters and Places*, concluding with a reference to the Artaxerxes story: 'No wonder that the mind which conceived it should revolt from the idea of serving a tyrant!'[48] For Russell, the modern parallel with Persia was the France of Napoleon III.[49] Francis Adams, the translator of the Hippocratic *Corpus*, saw the invitation itself as an acknowledgement by the Persians of Greek superiority.[50] For the Edinburgh physician, James Warburton Begbie, writing in 1872 the story indicated the reasons why a free Greece averted a Persian invasion, and the pride with which the Coans viewed Hippocrates. According to Begbie, Artaxerxes demanded that the Coans hand over the insolent Hippocrates, but they refused to hand over a man of whom they were proud and to whom they owed so much: 'The firmness of the attitude which these patriots assumed, and the unity by which at that time the different Grecian states asserted their common independence, averted in all probability a Persian invasion.'[51]

If the genuineness of the *Corpus* has been questioned, so too have been the tales about his life. As with the questions about which works were genuine, the process by which belief in the veracity of such tales was abandoned was long and complex, and physicians were often unpersuaded by those who queried their accuracy. For example in 1849 Francis Adams argued that it was not the stories that were false, but the evidence on which they were based. For Adams the stories had to be true for, even if the letters were forgeries 'it would have been preposterous to make them relate to stories of which every person of that age must have been able to detect a falsehood'.[52] Since the Hippocratic correspondence was of a date not much later than the time of Hippocrates, Adams reassured his readers that the main facts to which they alluded were believed to be authentic, and he was cited with approval by other writers such as James Warburton Begbie. For Begbie the critics of such stories were attempting to 'stifle all free and generous sentiments'.[53] This is not the place to trace the scholarly debates about their truth, what these said about those who made the arguments, or the process by which physicians abandoned their belief in their authenticity. Nevertheless, few today would accord them much truth and they survive mainly in fiction. George Weisz notes how they were used by the early twentieth-century French physician, Gaston Baissette in his biography of Hippocrates. They also appear in fictional form in Wilder Penfield's 1960s novel *The Torch*.[54]

The structure of *Reinventing Hippocrates*

The essays in this collection are divided into four Parts which structure the themes discussed above. In Part I – on Renaissance constructions of Hippocrates – Helen King argues that the portrayal of Hippocrates as the Father of Medicine can be traced, in part, to Galen's need to project his own views of medicine back to a conveniently distant past. Since Galen had insisted that Hippocrates was God, and he himself merely his prophet, sixteenth-century medical writers were able to represent a return to Hippocrates as consistent with Galenic medicine, while at the same time distancing themselves from Galen. By hailing Hippocrates as 'Father of Medicine' such writers could, as she puts it, keep the baby (a long and illustrious past that differentiated medicine from other forms of healing) while throwing out the (Galenic) bathwater. Hippocrates was particularly valuable as a father because so little was known about him, thus opening the paradoxical possibility of the Father of Medicine himself being fathered by his sons. At a time when Renaissance writers came to suggest that the father played a more prominent role than the mother in shaping the foetus (corporal and social), commentators were able to shape their own vision of Hippocrates's paternity to reflect contemporary notions of science, knowledge, gender, authority and morality.

Thomas Rütten's account of Renaissance notions of progress also suggest a complex view of the relations between past and present among sixteenth-century writers. Such writers, he claims, looked to the past as a source of progress in two different ways, since progress was both past-oriented and future-oriented. Thus while the historical Hippocrates could be construed as the origin of progress, from the mid-sixteenth century, he increasingly became the ultimate goal of progress. Through an analysis of the writings of Vesalius, Paracelsus, Harvey and others, Rütten suggests that such views must be understood in terms of changing Renaissance attitudes towards history, degeneration, revelation, personal authority and seniority, and a reimagining of Hippocrates that allowed practitioners to credit him with some of the 'progress' that had been achieved since his death. By ascribing new ideas to him, Hippocrates could, therefore, be constantly re-envisaged according to changing notions of what was 'progressive'.

Finally, Jole Shackelford explores the ways in which the reading and reevaluation of Hippocratic texts was implicated in the formation of Paracelsian chemical philosophy in the 1560s. Through a detailed reading of the work of the Danish physician Petrus Severinus, Shackelford revises our understanding of the emergence and significance of Paracelsian interpretations of Hippocrates. In his view, Renaissance discussions of Paracelsus's ideas were implicated in the renewal of Hippocratism much earlier than some historians have suggested. He shows shows that Severinus used particular Hippocratic texts (especially *On Diet*) to clarify and legitimate a medical philosophy based predominantly on Paracelsus's ideas. By anchoring Paracelsian theory in an older Hippocratic tradition, he suggests, Severinus aimed to quiet criticism from those who were hostile to Paracelsus. Like Rütten, Shackelford suggests that ideas that emerged after Hippocrates death could be ascribed to the Father of Medicine. The past had a complex relation to the present in Serverinus's Hippocratism.

If the first three essays emphasise the complexities of sixteenth-century Hippocratism, the following three, in Part II, examine aspects of his transformation in seventeenth- and eighteenth-century Britain. Andrew Cunningham sees the separation of Hippocrates from Galen in seventeenth-century Britain in political terms, involving a transformation of Hippocrates from Galen's interpretation of him as rational and academic to one in which he was portrayed as empirical and practical. He was the collector of case studies, the compiler of medical detail, the inductivist, the early founder of the true methods of natural history whose achievements had been devalued by the rationalist practitioners who followed him. Cunningham argues that this change from a glorification of the rational and academic in medicine to the elevation of the empirical and practical was about class politics especially around the Royal College of Physicians in Restoration London. Focusing on Sydenham's reinvention of Hippocrates, Cunningham shows how such politics surfaced as conflicts between elite and popular social and intellectual forms, the learned and unlearned, the theoretical and manual, the empirical and rational, and Latin and English.

Robert Martensen explores another aspect of the differential use of Hippocrates by British physicians and healers between 1640 and 1740. He argues that Hippocrates was often cited by physicians and others who favoured medical knowledge that was aphoristic and based on superficial observations. By contrast, Hippocrates was rarely cited by physicians and natural philosophers who encouraged the formation of experimental knowledge through anatomical investigation and chemistry. He suggests that the reason why people did or did not choose Hippocrates can be explained in terms of the historical moment, as well as the intellectual, professional and social commitments of practitioners, notably their religious and political affiliations. For Martensen, the value of Hippocrates as an intellectual resource was intimately tied to the prominence of religious dispute in seventeenth-century England and the political unrest that accompanied the Revolution, Protectorate and Restoration.

Finally, Andrea Rusnock's essay explores the relations between Baconianism and Hippocratism in the early eighteenth-century Royal Society. Focusing on medical meteorology, Rusnock argues that writers tended to portray themselves as perfecting and testing the observations of Hippocrates, but in a way that was consistent with the Hippocratic method, conceived in Baconian terms. Rusnock argues that such a focus on method marked a shift from the seventeenth-century interest in Hippocrates as a source of substantive, ontological explanations of disease. She claims that such a shift must be explained in terms of attempts to come to terms with the new diseases and climatic conditions of the New World, a new focus on the health of populations, as well as the political meanings of 'observation' in early eighteenth-century British science and medicine.

Part III explores eighteenth- and nineteenth-century French Hippocratism and its transfer to the United States. Elizabeth Williams explores the divergent images of Hippocrates among late eighteenth- and early nineteenth-century physicians at the Montpellier medical school. She argues that, on the one hand, Hippocrates was used to argue for the simplicity of nature's work in both health and illness, and for the availability of medical truth to the unlearned. On the other hand, Hippocrates was also used to insist on the complexity of disease and, concomitantly, on the indispensability of medical erudition and professional authority. Where the former Hippocrates shared with sick peasants a natural language of health and healing, the latter insisted that the people must not be left to follow the natural process of their degeneration but must be guided by the state and by religion. Williams links such views to the decline of Enlightenment values, the professionalising aspirations of Montpellier physicians, as well as to the particular circumstances of the French Revolution.

Anne La Berge examines the relations between Hippocrates and Paris medicine. She argues that appeals to Hippocrates were central to the creation and legitimation of a distinctive Paris medicine in the late eighteenth and early nineteenth centuries. For such reasons, La Berge suggests that Hippocrates served as an obligatory reference point for all physicians, even those who claimed to reject the ancients or tradition. She argues that, after the 1830s, explicit appeals to Hippocrates diminished because the identity of Paris medicine was secure and internal rivalries within Paris and between Paris and Montpellier had died down. Explicit references to Hippocrates played little part in the new rivalry between French clinical medicine and German medicine. As far as the French were concerned, Hippocratic medicine was Paris clinical medicine. The account concludes in the 1850s with the revival of interest in Hippocrates which accompanied the renewed interest in vitalism.

John Warner's account of the uses of Hippocrates in antebellum America shows how Hippocrates was deployed in a wider discourse about the state of American medicine and programmes for reform. In particular, Warner argues that, while most Americans depicted Hippocrates as a radical empiricist, this image was especially promoted by those who advocated French medicine. Warner links the interest in empiricism and observation to concerns about the medical marketplace as well as to attempts to unmask fraud and imposture within medicine. At the same time, he also explores a variety of alternative portrayals of the empirical Hippocrates. He shows how this Hippocrates was also invoked by opponents of French medicine, as well as by Southern physicians, attempting to create a distinctive identity for themselves as part of crusade for Southern nationalism.

The final four essays, in Part IV, explore various aspects of the revival of Hippocratism in the twentieth century, In particular, they focus on the ways in which Hippocrates was employed to express concerns about a crisis in modern medicine and society generated by the emergence of the laboratory, specialisation and mass medicine, as well as the growing role of the state and commerce in medicine. Susan Lederer suggests that American medical interest in Hippocrates must be seen in the context of the economic and social disruptions of the 1920s and 1930s, as well as of structural changes within the medical profession, such as the introduction of specialisation and group practice and the threat of collectivisation. In particular, Lederer focuses on dramatic and novelistic uses of the *Oath* to show how it provided a means for authors to discuss contentious issues such as abortion and medical competency and trust, though not always in ways with which the medical profession was comfortable.

If Lederer discusses the moral uses of the *Oath*, George Weisz examines the association of Hippocratism with holistic or synthetic medicine. Concentrating on interwar French medicine, Weisz argues that the majority of interwar works on Hippocrates associated him with critiques of orthodox medicine and with vitalism and various forms of alternative medicine especially homeopathy. He argues that non-orthodox physicians labelled their enterprise as 'Hippocratic' in an effort to enlist the support of a universally respected figure, and to enrich a variety of connected 'holistic' notions such as humanism, syncretism, vitalism and the healing power of nature, each capable of attracting different, but partially overlapping, degrees of assent. More generally, he also claims that it represented an appeal to the past which expressed a degree of discomfort with modern science and the world that it had brought into being.

David Cantor explores another aspect of medical responses to a perceived crisis in modern medicine among elite British clinicians. According to Cantor, British physicians feared that what they saw as an increasingly fragmented, mechanistic and specialised world was encouraging a narrow mental outlook, unable to see beyond the limits of its particular interests. Most worrying, they claimed, was that this narrow outlook was coming to dominate medical thinking as a result of the growing importance of the specialist, laboratory scientist and medical bureaucrat, all of whom (it was suggested) exhibited such an outlook, and confused the manmade category of disease with the reality of illness as expressed in the individual patient. In their view, the tyranny of disease labels, rather than the needs of the patient, dictated patient care. Cantor suggests that such arguments were often made by those elite clinicians who advocated broad, generalist and organic outlooks in medicine, and provided a means by which they sought to assert their authority over the 'narrow minds' they saw as below them. Such an organic and generalist view was often associated with Hippocrates who, these clinicians suggested, also asserted the primacy of experience and practice over the dictatorship of language.

Finally, Carsten Timmermann argues that Hippocratism emerged in Germany as part of a broader response to a crisis brought about by defeat in the First World War and the particular severity of the German economic crisis. However, in Germany Hippocratism took a different path to other countries. Right-wing commentators increasingly appropriated Hippocrates to legitimate an elitist medical ideology. In the hands of these physicians Hippocrates legitimated a new ethics that (unlike in Britain, France or America) focused on the collective rather than the individual: the *Volk* was an organism that had rights above the individual. In such ways, Hippocratic doctrines were quite reconcilable with eugenic ideas and ultimately with the programmes of human extermination and experimentation carried out by the Nazis. Timmermann thus questions essentialist readings of Hippocrates that suggest that Nazi doctors went against a timeless injunction expressed in the *Oath* against harming the individual. This controversial conclusion highlights many of the points of this collection of essays; that there is no one reading of Hippocrates; that he can be made to say more or less whatever a reader wants; and that portrayals of Hippocrates provide a valuable window on to the cultures and societies that produce them.

Acknowledgements

Many thanks to John Pickstone and Penny Gouk who read this paper, and to Helen King for her thoughtful commentary on Renaissance and early modern medicine. Of course, I am responsible for any errors and omissions.

Notes

1. The games are respectively: *Greyhawk* <http://vancouver.planeteer.com/~northgod/greyhawk.htm> accessed 15 September 1998; *EcoQuest. The Search for Cetus* <http://www.gamesdomain.co.uk/solution/EcoQuest1.txt> accessed 26 October 1999; *NetHack* <http://www.win.tue.nl/games/roguelike/nethack> accessed 26 October 1999; *RavenMUD* <http://www.geocities.com/~hasana2000/table.html> accessed 26 October 1999; *World of Darkness* <http://www.white-wolf.com/Home.html> accessed 15 April 1998; *Starwars: The Final Contingency* <http://www1.usa1.com/~davin/rpg/starwars/> accessed

20 November 1997; *Nanvaent* <http://www.nanvaent.org.uk/> accessed 9 April 1998; *Diplomacy* <http://www.netch.se/~ubbe/diplomacy/dip185.html> accessed 14 April 1998; *Stars of the Dark Well* <http://bbs.macnexus.org/~david_peterson/darkwell/darkwell.html> accessed 20 April 1998; *Star Trek* <http://www.holoworld.net/hwf/ships/hippocrates> accessed 27 November 1997; *Traveller* <http://www.interlog.com/~dmci104/GamingClub/Traveller/Hippocrates_Ambulance_TL11.html> accessed 16 June 1998; *Carrion Fields* <http://www.spellbook.net/cf/hell_dir.html> accessed 12 November 1997; *Blackstone Chronicles* <http://www.game-revolution.com/games/codes/pc/blackstone_chronicles_walk.htm> accessed 21 January 1999; *Third Rock MUSH* <http://members.xoom.com/3rdrock/index.html> accessed 11 June 1998; and *SpaceColonyH* <http://www.spacecolony.com/> accessed 9 April 1998.

The instructions on when a player should go mad are in 'The complete guide to sanity for fantasy role-playing games', 1996 <http://www.lysator.liu.se/~johol/netbooks/CompleteGuideTo/Sanity.txt> accessed 15 April 1998.
2. Erwin A. Ackerknecht, *A Short History of Medicine*, Baltimore: Johns Hopkins University Press, 1968, p. 74 and p. 106; G.A. Lindbloom, *Herman Boerhavve: The Man and His Work*, London: Methuen, 1968, pp. 55–56; Roselyne Rey, 'Anamorphoses d'Hippocrate au XVIIIème siècle', in Danielle Gourevitch (ed.), *Maladie et Maladies: Histoire et Conceptualisation. Mélanges en l'Honneur de Mirko Grmek*, Geneva: Droz, 1992, pp. 257–76.
3. So popular was the word 'Hippocrates' that innumerable web sites secretly incorporated his name in order to trick search engines into visiting: <http://www.enter.net/~butcher/engine.html> accessed 19 June 1998. For such reasons, one web site describes the term as one that makes life harder for search engines: <http://www.die.net/random/k/z/q/v/l/a/y/z/t/f/u/s/e/index.htm> accessed 12 November 1997. A Yahoo search on 16 April 1998 found 20 000 AltaVista web pages for the word 'hippocrates'.
4. See, for example, Poynter's discussion of Sydenham in F.N.L. Poynter, 'Sydenham's influence abroad', *Medical History*, 17, 1973, pp. 223–34 at p. 224.
5. Jacques Jouanna, *Hippocrates*, Baltimore and London: Johns Hopkins University Press, 1999, p. 364.
6. Leendert Jan Slikkerveer, *Plural Medical Systems in the Horn of Africa. The Legacy of 'Sheikh' Hippocrates*, London and New York: Kegan Paul International, 1990, esp. p. 279. George McClelland Foster, *Hippocrates' Latin American Legacy. Humoral Medicine in the New World*, Langhorne, PA.: Gordon and Breach, 1993. For a critical survey of this literature see Michael H. Logan, 'Anthropological research on the hot–cold theory of disease: Some methodological suggestions', *Medical Anthropology*, 1, 1977, pp. 87–112, esp. pp. 90–94.
7. For an excellent treatment of the reinvention of Hippocrates in the Renaissance see Nancy G. Siraisi, *The Clock and the Mirror. Girolamo Cardano and Renaissance Medicine*, Princeton NJ: Princeton University Press, 1997, Chapter 6.
8. Wesley D. Smith, *The Hippocratic Tradition*, Ithaca and London: Cornell University Press, 1979, p. 14.
9. Smith, *Hippocratic Tradition* (n. 8), p. 7.
10. Smith, *Hippocratic Tradition* (n. 8), p. 14.
11. The classic statement of such a view of tradition is Eric Hobsbawm and Terence Ranger (eds), *The Invention of Tradition*, Cambridge: Cambridge University Press, 1983.
12. See, for example, Christopher Stray, *Classics Transformed. Schools, Universities, and Society in England, 1830–1960*, Oxford: Clarendon Press, 1998. For the

importance of classical Greece to the Victorians, see Frank M. Turner, *The Greek Heritage in Victorian Britain*, New Haven and London: Yale University Press, 1981; Richard Jenkyns, *The Victorians and Ancient Greece*, Cambridge Mass: Harvard University Press, 1980; G.W. Clarke (ed.), *Rediscovering Hellenism. The Hellenic Inheritance and the English Imagination*, Cambridge: Cambridge University Press, 1989.

13. G.E.R. Lloyd, *Magic, Reason and Experience: Studies in the Origin and Development of Greek Science*, Cambridge: Cambridge University Press, 1979, p. 129.
14. Volker Langholf, *Medical Theories in Hippocrates. Early Texts and the 'Epidemics'*, Berlin: Walter de Gruyter, 1990, p. 193.
15. Ibid., p. 194.
16. Ibid., p. 190.
17. Ibid., p. 210.
18. Patricia Parsons and Arthur Parsons, *Hippocrates Now! Is Your Doctor Ethical?*, Toronto: University of Toronto Press, 1995; Roger J. Bulger (ed.), *Hippocrates Revisited. A Search for Meaning*, New York: Medcom, 1973.
19. *Round Springfield*, by Joshua Sternin and Jeffrey Ventimilia (teleplay) and Al Jean and Mike Reiss (story), directed by Steven Dean Moore, originally broadcast in North America on 30 April 1995, capsule revision G, 22 February1997. The script is at <http://www.snpp.com/episodes/2F32.html> accessed 24 April 1998.
20. Vivian Nutton, 'What's in an oath?', *Journal of the Royal College of Physicians of London*, **29**, 1995, pp. 518–24; Thomas Rütten, 'Receptions of the Hippocratic Oath in the Renaissance: the prohibition of abortion as a case study in reception', *Journal of the History of Medicine and Allied Sciences*, **51**, 1996, pp. 456–83; idem, *Hippokrates Im Gespräch. Anstellung des Instituts für Theorie und Geschichte der medizin und der Universitäts- und Landesbibliothek Münster (10.12.1993 bis 8.1.1994) analäßlich der Eröffnung der Zweigbibliothek Medizin*, Schriften der Universitäts- und Landesbibliothek Münster, Band 9 Münster, 1993.
21. Vivian Nutton, 'Hippocrates in the Renaissance', in *Sudhoffs Archiv Zeitschrift für Wissenschaftsgeschichte*, Beiheift 27, 1989, pp. 420–39.
22. Smith, *Hippocratic Tradition* (n. 8). Wesley D. Smith (ed. and trans.), *Hippocrates: Pseudepigraphic Writings*, Leiden and New York: Brill, 1990; Owsei Temkin, *Hippocrates in a World of Pagans and Christians*, Baltimore: Johns Hopkins University Press, 1991; Jody Rubin Pinault, *Hippocratic Lives and Legends*, Leiden, New York and London: E.J. Brill, 1992; Langholf, *Medical Theories* (n. 14), pp. 197–98.
23. Langholf, *Medical Theories* (n. 14), pp. 197–98.
24. Smith, *Hippocratic Tradition* (n. 8), *passim*.
25. Pearl Kibre, *Hippocrates Latinus. Repertorium of Hippocratic Writings in the Latin Middle Ages*, New York: Fordham University Press, 1985.
26. Michael R. McVaugh, and Nancy G. Siraisi, 'Renaissance Medical learning: Evolution of a Tradition', *Osiris*, **6**, 1990. Also, despite the title see Andrew Wear, R.K. French and I.M. Lonie (eds), *The Medical Renaissance of the Sixteenth Century*, Cambridge: Cambridge University Press, 1985.
27. Siraisi, *Clock and Mirror*, (n. 7), Chapter 6. Nancy G. Siraisi, 'Cardano, Hippocrates and Criticism of Galen', in *Girolamo Cardano: Philosoph, Naturforscher, Arzt*, Wolfenbütteler Abhandlungen zur Renaissanceforschung, Bd. 15, Wiesbaden: Harrassowitz, 1994, pp. 131–55.
28. For a catalogue of such publications see G. Maloney and R. Savoie, *Cinque Cent Ans de Bibliographie Hippocratique, 1483–1982*, St-Jerome-Chrysostome, Québec: Editions du Sphinx, 1982.

29. Nutton, 'Hippocrates in the Renaissance' (n. 33), p. 421. See also Vivian Nutton, 'John Caius and the Eton Galen: Medical philology in the Renaissance', *Medizinhistorisches Journal*, **20**, 1985, pp. 227–52, *passim*; idem, 'The legacy of Hippocrates: Greek medicine in the library of the Medical Society of London', *Transactions of the Medical Society of London*, **103**, 1986–87, pp. 21–30; idem, '"Prisci Dissectionum Professores": Greek texts and Renaissance anatomists', in A.C. Dionisotti, Anthony Grafton and Jill Kraye (eds), *The Uses of Greek and Latin. Historical Essays*, London: The Warburg Institute, University of London, 1988, pp. 111–26; idem, 'Greek science in the sixteenth-century', in J.V. Field and Frank A.J.L. James (eds), *Renaissance and Revolution. Humanists, Scholars, Craftsman and Natural Philosophers in Early Modern Europe*, Cambridge: Cambridge University Press, 1993, pp. 15–28. See also Helen King, 'Green sickness: Hippocrates, Galen and the origins of "The Disease of Virgins"', *International Journal of the Classical Tradition*, **2**, 1996, pp. 372–87 at p. 387. For the importance of Hippocrates to Renaissance understandings of the origins of Greek language see Anthony Grafton, *Joseph Scaliger: A Study in the History of Classical Scholarship. Volume 1. Critics and Exegesis*, Oxford: Clarendon Press, 1983, pp. 180–82.
30. On the complex place of Pliny in Renaissance medicine see R.K. French, 'Pliny and Renaissance medicine', in Roger French and Frank Greenaway, *Science in the Early Roman Empire: Pliny the Elder, his Sources and Influence*, London and Sydney, Croom Helm, 1986, pp. 252–81.
31. John Arrizabalaga, John Henderson and Roger French, *The Great Pox. The French Disease in Renaissance Europe*, New Haven and London: Yale University Press, 1997, p. 64. For a discussion of the attempts at a Hippocratic explanations of new diseases such as what came to be known as the French Disease in the late fifteenth century and the 'Green sickness' see p. 73. See also King, 'Green sickness' (n. 29), p. 387.
32. On the Hippocratic question see L. Edelstein, 'The genuine works of Hippocrates?', *Bulletin of the History of Medicine*, **7**, 1939, pp. 236–48; G.E.R. Lloyd, 'The Hippocratic question', in G.E.R. Lloyd, *Methods and Problems in Greek Science*, Cambridge: Cambridge University Press, 1991, pp. 194–223; Jouanna, *Hippocrates* (n. 5).
33. See also Smith, *Hippocratic Tradition* (n. 8), and Harold J. Cook, *The Decline of the Old Medical Regime in Stuart London*, Ithaca, NY: Cornell University Press, 1986, p. 185.
34. Thomas H. Broman, *The Transformation of German Academic Medicine, 1750–1820*, Cambridge: Cambridge University Press, 1996, pp. 140–41.
35. Michael A. Osborne, 'Resurrecting Hippocrates: Hygienic sciences and the French scientific expeditions to Egypt, Morea and Algeria', in David Arnold (ed.), *Warm Climates and Western Medicine*, Amsterdam: Rodopi, 1996, pp. 80–98 at p. 86.
36. Iain Lonie, 'Hippocrates the Iatromechanist', *Medical History*, **25**, 1981, pp. 113–50. Iain Lonie, 'The "Paris Hippocratics": Teaching and research in the second half of the sixteenth century' in Wear, French and Lonie, *Medical Renaissance* (n. 26), pp. 155–174.
37. Ludmilla Jordanova, 'Earth science and environmental medicine: the synthesis of the late Enlightenment', in Ludmilla Jordanova and Roy Porter (eds), *Images of the Earth. Essays in the History of the Environmental Sciences*, Chalfont St Giles: British Society for the History of Science, rev. edn 1997, pp. 127–51. Clarence J. Glacken, *Traces on the Rhodian Shore: Nature and Culture in Western Thought from Ancient Times to the End of the Eighteenth Century*, Berkeley, CA:

University of California Press, 1976.
38. See also Christopher Lawrence, 'Still incommunicable: clinical holists and medical knowledge in interwar Britain', in Christopher Lawrence and George Weisz, *Greater than the Parts. Holism in Biomedicine, 1920–1950*, New York and London: Oxford University Press, 1998, pp. 94–111.
39. However, some advocates of state and social medicine could focus on the individual patient. See Steve Sturdy, 'Hippocrates and State Medicine: George Newman outlines the founding policy of the Ministry of Health', in Lawrence and Weisz, *Greater than the Parts* (n. 38), pp. 112–34. Dorothy Porter, 'John Ryle: doctor of revolution?', in Dorothy and Roy Porter (eds), *Doctors, Politics and Society: Historical Essays*, Amsterdam and Atlanta: Rodopi, 1993, pp. 247–74.
40. J. Worth Estes, 'Samuel Thomson rewrites Hippocrates', in Peter Benes (ed.), *Medicine and Healing. The Dublin Seminar for New England Folklife. Annual Proceedings 1990*, Boston, MA: Boston University, 1990, pp. 113–32, at p. 120.
41. Plato, *Protagoras*, 311 b–c and *Phaedrus* 270 c–d; Aristotle, *Politics*, 7, 1326 a 15–16.
42. Temkin, *Pagans and Christians* (n. 22). Smith, *Hippocratic Tradition* (n. 8). Smith *Pseudepigraphic Writings* (n. 22). Pinault, *Lives and Legends* (n. 22).
43. Temkin, *Pagans and Christians* (n. 22), pp. 57–61.
44. Thomas Crow discusses some of these issues in his account of Girodet's painting *Hippocrates Refusing the Gifts of Artaxerxes* (1792). Crow shows how the meaning of this painting was shaped by Girodet's own relationships with figures of paternal authority, the importance of civic virtue and patriotism, and specific uses of Hippocratism in the political imagery of disease and health in revolutionary France. The painting was sufficiently well known to be referred to in passing by Victor Hugo, and Balzac referred to the Artaxerxes story almost casually, assuming that his readers would know the tale. See Thomas Crow, *Emulation: Making Artists for Revolutionary France*, New Haven and London: Yale University Press, 1995, pp. 140–44; Victor Hugo, *Les Misérables*, Vol I, Paris: Éditions Gallimard, 1995, p. 841. Honoré de Balzac, *Illusions Perdues*, Paris: Gallimard, 1972, p. 269.
45. On Farr see John M. Eyler, *Victorian Social Medicine. The Ideas and Methods of William Farr*, Baltimore and London: Johns Hopkins University Press, 1979.
46. William Farr, "Lecture on the history of hygiene", *Lancet*, 13 February 1836, pp. 773–80 at p. 779
47. J Rutherfurd Russell, *The History and Heroes of the Art of Medicine*, London: J. Murray, 1861, p. 25.
48. Ibid., pp. 25–26
49. Ibid., p. 26. The 'free' state in this example, however, was America, and Russell cites a modern parallel to the story of Hippocrates and Artaxerxes. In the modern example, an unnamed French geologist refused to return to France from America, his adopted country, although tempted by a personal and flattering invitation from Napoleon III.
50. Francis Adams, *The Genuine Works of Hippocrates Translated from the Greek with a Preliminary Discourse and Annotations*, Vol. 1, London: Sydenham Society, 1849, pp. 14–15.
51. J. Warburton Begbie, 'Hippocrates: his life and writings', *British Medical Journal*, 21 December 1872, pp. 674–77 at p. 676.
52. Adams, *Genuine Works* (n. 50), p. 15.
53. Begbie, 'Hippocrates' (n. 51), p. 676.
54. Wilder Penfield, *The Torch*, Boston: Little Brown, 1960.

Part I

Renaissance Constructions of Hippocratism

CHAPTER TWO

The Power of Paternity: The Father of Medicine Meets the Prince of Physicians

Helen King

Fathering medicine

Jonathan Sawday has recently argued that the Western medical tradition operates with 'twin fathers': Hippocrates, and Galen.[1] For Sawday, this reinforced paternity has been combined with a view of Eastern medicine that has devalued it by feminising it as a vessel passively carrying Western medicine through the centuries; only in the eleventh century was it able to give birth, when Constantine the African arrived in Italy with a cargo of books and proceeded to translate the lost texts of Galen from Arabic to Latin and thus restored Galenic medicine to the West.[2] The image of medical history in the western tradition therefore presents 'a doubly fathered masculine western knowledge of Greek medicine married to the passive, eastern tradition of transmission': Western medicine then proceeds by denying its 'fathers', in going beyond their medical ideas, while simultaneously claiming to recover them.

However, Sawday's cited source for the sixteenth-century recognition of the dual paternity of Western medicine – the Galenist, Thomas Gale, writing in 1586 – does not say exactly what Sawday wants to hear. Sawday states that the authority of knowledge is seen in terms of fatherhood: '... as Thomas Gale writes, it is the authority of the twin fathers, the "originall and foundacion", which each generation inherits from its predecessor'. But Gale does not go so far as to identify both Hippocrates and Galen as 'fathers' – in the passage cited by Sawday, Gale claims

> All these which I have spoken of, of what countrie so ever they were, they tooke their originall and foundacion, of our Father Hippocrates, and Galen, although they found out many thinges, appertaining to the arte of medicine ... all these men of what countrie so ever they were, they have drunk of the water that flowed out of their [Hippocrates's and Galen's] wells.[3]

Sawday may well have a valid point in his more general location of the 'father of medicine' theme within a view of science that represents it as a steady progress through the generations and modelled on biological paternity. But, despite his traditional role as one of the wells from which medicine has drunk, Galen is not usually given the title of 'father': for Gale, as for the dominant medical tradition from the late sixteenth century onwards, it is Hippocrates who is the father of medicine, while Galen is most commonly the Prince of physicians.

Variations on this theme occur. One of many references to Galen in William Harvey's *De Motu Cordis* labels him as '*vir divinus, pater medicorum*', 'a divine man, father of physicians'.[4] This tribute to Galen needs to be situated in the context of Harvey's carefully constructed rhetoric; these titles are not merely examples of what Peter Graham has called 'Harvey's gracious refusal to censure his mistaken colleagues',[5] but occur after a long passage in which Harvey uses extracts from Galen's *On the usefulness of parts* in support of the existence of the valves and of the pulmonary circuit. This section comes in chapter 7, at the end of the first half of *De Motu Cordis* and immediately before the central chapter 8 in which he claims hesitantly to move to the heart of his argument: 'so novel, and hitherto unmentioned ... I dread lest all men turn against me .... The die is cast.' One may therefore argue that Harvey praises Galen in a particularly effusive way in order to emphasise the commonly agreed certainties of chapter 7 before embarking on the heavily flagged novelty of chapter 8. However, Galen is not the father of physic, but the father of physicians. Many variations on the more common pattern of Galen as prince with Hippocrates as father come from seventeenth-century proponents of chemical medicine, such as Marchamont Nedham whose attack on those who think that citing a line of Hippocrates or Galen is sufficient justification for any medical action refers to Hippocrates as 'that ancient Prince of the Faculty' and to Galen as 'the *Usurper*'.[6]

Although in the preface to another of his works Gale refers to 'both the princes of phisicke Hippocrates and Galen',[7] when it comes to fatherhood it is Hippocrates alone who fills the role. In Gale's version of the history of medicine:

> Aesculapius dyd inlarge it and constitute it an Arte, but that noble man Hyppocrates dyd finish it, and make it perfect ... After all these, came that worthie manne, Galen, who was without any comparison, from the beginning of the worlde, unto this daye, except Hippocrates, not onely for his excellent learning, in so many famous Artes, which he was perfect in, but especially for this Arte of Medicine, which he was most excellently seene in, both in the Theorike, and Practike parte thereof ...[8]

Here Galen is clearly secondary to Hippocrates, an impression confirmed when Gale refers to '... Hippocrates, who was the Father and fountaine of all Medicine, as Galen himselfe doeth witnesse'.[9]

Medicine can only have one father, and that father is Hippocrates, a judgement conveniently supported by Galen's own endorsement of the

Hippocratic origins of all that is best in medicine. In this chapter, I will explore some of the implications of Hippocrates's fathering of medicine. As other contributors to this book demonstrate, one obvious advantage of installing Hippocrates as the father of medicine is that, due to the wide range of texts transmitted under his name, medicine can change radically while retaining the same father; change can disguise itself as continuity, as different texts from the Hippocratic *Corpus* are moved into the spotlight. Subsequent readers of the *Corpus* have managed to find a Hippocratic origin for a wide range of medical options – even branches of healing which consciously locate themselves as 'alternative' to orthodox medicine have been only too keen to 'discover' the principles of their own approach in the *Corpus*, so that it is possible to find homoeopathic, aromatherapist, chiropractic and osteopathic versions of Hippocrates, making him 'the "Father of Holistic Medicine"'.[10] After looking at the valuations of Hippocrates in the ancient and early modern periods, and in particular examining the sixteenth century, when the Hippocratic texts were first printed and began to be read by practising physicians who eventually discovered that their contents were not precisely what Galen had led them to expect, I will suggest here that it is the 'personality traits' of Hippocrates that are most valuable to those in the modern period who insist on his 'fatherhood'.

In the classical world, before the rise of the medical profession in its early modern sense, medicine remained unfathered. In ancient Greece, if medicine had any father at all, it was Asclepius or his own father, the god Apollo. According to the version most popular in antiquity, Asclepius' mother, Coronis, was killed by Apollo, because the god was jealous that she had left him for a mortal man. Her unborn child Asclepius was, however, spared, and sent by Apollo to be brought up by the wise centaur, Chiron. Asclepius learned from Chiron about the powers of herbs and also became a skilled surgeon. But he went too far; he did not just heal the sick but, in some versions of his myth, he also raised the dead to life. Angry at this challenge to the boundaries between mortal men and the immortal gods, Zeus killed him.[11] Hyginus' second-century AD summary of the origins of medicine claimed that

> Chiron son of Saturn first used herbs in the medical art of surgery; Apollo first practiced the art of treating eyes, and third, Asclepius, son of Apollo, began the art of clinical medicine.[12]

In classical Greek culture, medicine was seen as one of the *technai*,[13] the skills/crafts raising man from the level of the beasts and helping him to approach the immortality of the gods and, as such, it traced back its origins to the divine. However, Heinrich von Staden has recently argued that the Hippocratic *Oath*'s definition of a *technē* includes its creation of a sense of belonging to a collectivity extending over the generations;[14] here, the use of family models for medicine moves beyond its own paternity and becomes a part of the self-perception of the group of healers.

In another Greek story of the origin of medicine, however, it was Prometheus who was responsible for the *technê*, as part of his wider programme to help mankind against the will of the god Zeus. Prometheus' own father was Iapetos, one of the Titans, the gods who ruled before being defeated in battle by Zeus and his fellow Olympians. In some myths, Prometheus created mankind from clay; he was also the main culture-bringer of Greek myth, inaugurating many of the arts, crafts and sciences.

Apollo, Asclepius or Prometheus could each be seen as, in some sense, the father of medicine, but the Olympian Apollo, the Olympian-fathered Asclepius and the Titan-fathered Prometheus are all too distant from the entirely human concerns of medicine. It would be possible to argue that, if medicine is to have a father, he needs to be fully human. Hippocrates certainly began as a human being, although the genealogies created for him by writers such as the twelfth-century polymath Joannes Tzetzes traced the Hippocratic family tree back to Asclepius in 17 generations, and thus ultimately back to Apollo, while Christian interpreters found it easy to draw analogies between his medical work and that of Christ the Healer.[15] Moreover, the structural position of medicine in raising humanity from the level of the beasts and helping them towards the immortality of the gods meant that Hippocrates himself came to be seen as 'the divine Hippocrates'.

Tzetzes' genealogy is only one of several created for Hippocrates from perhaps the first century AD onwards.[16] The combination of a shortage of information about the historical Hippocrates and a culture concerned with origins and founders led to the fabrication of details, ranging from bare genealogies to full biographies complete with a physical description of Hippocrates and an annual ceremony at his tomb. The only testimony contemporary with Hippocrates comes from Plato: *Protagoras* 311b refers to Hippocrates of Cos, an Asclepiad, who charges a fee for teaching people medicine, and *Phaedrus* 270c–d claims that the understanding of the body found in Hippocrates the Asclepiad is based on knowledge of 'the whole'.[17] As Volker Langholf has pointed out, this does not make Plato a primary source for Hippocratic medicine; on the contrary, it makes him only the first of many to interpret 'the available information about Hippocrates's method on the basis of his own system of thought'.[18] While it is possible from Plato's references only to conclude that Hippocrates was sufficiently well known in the fourth century BC that the audience was expected to be familiar with him as a healer and instructor, the lack of information on the defining characteristics of 'Hippocratic medicine' has prevented neither ancient nor modern writers from trying to identify works in the Hippocratic *Corpus* as 'genuine' on the basis of their comments on 'the whole'.[19]

The Hippocratic *Corpus*, today seen as a disparate collection in terms of geographical origin, date of composition and theoretical position, existed as an entity from around 200 BC, when a group of heterogeneous early Greek medical texts was put together in the library at Alexandria and acquired the name 'Hippocrates', perhaps, as Wesley Smith suggests, simply because one of the texts in the pile happened to be a fake letter bearing his name.[20] The authority of Plato was enough to suggest that any medical text of any worth from the classical Greek world must be 'by Hippocrates', so the whole pile was classified as 'Hippocratic'. The subsequent discovery of blatant discrepancies in style or content between the texts of the *Corpus* could then be explained away by using the genealogies, with it being suggested that some works were directly 'by Hippocrates' and others edited by his sons. As both of his sons were supposed to have named their sons Hippocrates, this created further scope for a confused Alexandrian librarian to file works of an inferior quality under 'Hippocrates'.

Seneca, writing before Galen, called Hippocrates 'the greatest physician and the founder of medicine'.[21] For Galen, fighting to achieve superiority in the medical world of the Roman Empire of the second century AD, Hippocrates was not only the foremost of physicians, but also the precursor validating Galen's own medical position. As Wesley Smith convincingly demonstrated, when Galen announced which treatises attributed to Hippocrates were 'really' written by the great man, these conveniently turned out to be those which expressed views closest to those of Galen himself. The fifth-century BC past was reconstructed to fit Galen's second-century AD present, making those writers of the past most admired by his enemies into 'enemies of Hippocrates', while labelling the treatises that most resonated with his own ideas the 'genuine works of Hippocrates'.[22]

For the biography of Hippocrates, a further source is the fictional material transmitted in the Hippocratic *Pseudepigrapha*, including correspondence with the historical figures of the Persian king Artaxerxes and the philosopher Democritus, speeches and some fake decrees honouring Hippocrates. Published at the beginning of the sixteenth century, this material dates from perhaps 300 BC onwards, with the literary versions dating to the first century AD; its content may be traced back to stories created on Cos in order to claim authority for the Coan medical school.[23] In the *Pseudepigrapha*, Hippocrates even cures the famous plague which, according to the historian Thucydides, struck Athens in 431–30 BC. In the words of Wesley Smith, this whole enterprise should be seen as 'an etiological myth, an analytical scheme dressed up as a narrative of events'.[24]

But Hippocrates was not 'the father of medicine' in the *Pseudepigrapha*. He is 'the divine Hippocrates', because of his descent from Asclepius and thus from Zeus himself,[25] and he is 'father of health, saviour, soother of pain'.[26] But Asclepius, too, is described not only as 'the founder, Asklepios',[27] but also as 'father Asklepios',[28] while in another letter Hippocrates himself is supposed to have written 'Medicine and prophecy are very closely related, since of the two arts Apollo is the single father'.[29]

Who needs a father?

Hippocrates's own fictional claim that Apollo is the father of medicine is significant in the context of the wider discourse of fatherhood in science. What does it mean to be the father of medicine? Even a cursory glance at works on medicine and on its history will show that there are now considered to be many fathers within medicine. They can be fathers of just one operation or procedure, like Ephraim McDowell, 'father of ovariotomy' or Francis Henry Williams, 'father of cardiac fluoroscopy'. Here what is being claimed is simple priority of discovery; to be the father is to be the first.[30] In the case of women perceived as pioneers, it is possible to be the mother of one's speciality, as with Margaret McMillan, 'mother of child health'. Fatherhood can also be a more local claim, as in Nils Rosen, 'father of paediatrics in Sweden', or Dumitru Bagdasar, 'father of Romanian neurosurgery'. A new speciality needs its own parent.[31] But to father medicine – all of it, everywhere – is to enter a different league altogether.

Of course, in the fatherhood discourse of science, nobody ever describes himself as the father: fatherhood, as in Hippocrates's description of Apollo, is always imputed to earlier authorities. Jan Sapp's classic article on Gregor Mendel's role in the history of genetics traces a pattern by which 'founding fathers' are supposed to go through the stages of making a discovery 'ahead of their time', dying without recognition, and then being 'rediscovered' – preferably after a long period of neglect – in the context of a priority dispute, where the only solution to the problem of two scientists making apparently the same discovery is to project it back into the past and find an earlier, 'unrecognised' founding father.[32] Sapp argues in general that the accounts of history given by scientists should be understood as part of their process of persuasion, and in particular that Mendel is a valuable resource in this process because he published so little, making his experiments 'a flexible resource': 'The significance of Mendel's experiments lies in the diverse ways in which the commentators have constructed stories about them and used them in their knowledge making.' For the Hippocratic *Corpus*, one can instead argue that its value as a resource in constructing medicine is that there is so much of it, so that anyone looking for a foundation document for a medical approach will be sure to find something of use.

As Sawday was aware, the use of the image of fatherhood should be seen in terms of patriarchal values in a more general sense. Since the seventeenth century, knowledge has often been represented in terms of the male scientist imposing his will on a feminised nature.[33] Sapp suggests that the motif of the long neglect of the founding father gives us:

> ... the patriarchal image of how 'the founding fathers' penetrate Mother Nature to leave a child destined for greatness. However, the child is born 'premature' in an alien world. Underdeveloped and weak, it is left to die because no one is prepared or willing to take care of it.[34]

Brian Easlea's classic study of the rhetoric of masculinity in the nuclear arms race notes that the use of sexual and birth metaphors in the self-image of nuclear physicists could even extend to J. Robert Oppenheimer, 'father of the atomic bomb', being appointed Father of the Year by the National Baby Institution.[35] Easlea argues that we should see Francis Bacon's *The Masculine Birth of Time* (1603) as a key text in the search for a 'male' way of controlling a feminised nature by penetrating her 'secrets' or her 'recesses'.[36] Bacon argues that man can bind to his service 'Nature with all her children' and make her his slave; he must 'lay hold of her and capture her' in 'a chaste and lawful marriage between Mind and Nature, with the divine mercy as bride-woman'.[37] All the great names of the history of science are attacked for having fallen short of this goal of subduing nature in the service of man: Galen is 'the narrow-minded Galen, who deserted the path of experience and took to spinning idle theories of causation',[38] while Bacon's attack on Hippocrates deserves to be quoted in full:

> Now it is the turn of Hippocrates to appear, that product and puffer of ancient wisdom. Who would not laugh to see Galen and Paracelsus running to take shelter under his authority – under what the proverb calls the shadow of an ass? That fellow has the appearance of maintaining a steady gaze at experience. Too steady! His eyes never shift. They follow nothing. They are sunk in stupor. Then, still but half awake, he snatches up a few idols – not the monstrous idols of the great speculative thinkers, but a slim and elegant variety which haunts the surface of science. These he swallows, and swollen with this diet, half scientist and half sophist, protecting himself according to the fashion of his age by an oracular brevity, after long delay he brings out a few maxims, which Galen and Paracelsus take for oracles and quarrel with one another for the honour of interpreting. But in truth the oracle is dumb. He utters nothing but a few sophisms sheltered from correction by their curt ambiguity, or a few peasants' remedies made to sound imposing.[39]

Here Hippocrates is taken to represent an excess of experience, and Galen an excess of theory; Baconian science aims to take the middle way between the empirics who, 'like ants, gather and consume' and the rationalists who, 'like spiders, spin webs out of themselves', emulating instead the bee, who takes her material from nature, but transforms it by digestion and assimilation.[40] In particular here, Bacon attacks the 'few maxims' over which Galen and Paracelsus fight for the honour of interpreting; these are the Hippocratic *Aphorisms*, a text long held to be one of the 'most genuine' works of the Hippocratic *Corpus*, traditionally thought to have been composed by Hippocrates 'in his old age as a summary of his vast experience',[41] making it a distillation of the wisdom of a lifetime.

But it is not simply a question of why medicine has a father, but also why that father should be Hippocrates. Before the sixteenth century, Galen ruled: not as the father of medicine, but as the prince of physicians. Two aspects of this title could be emphasised. First, it focuses on the community of physicians rather than on the type of medicine they practise. It is perhaps in this sense that we should understand Harvey's Galen as 'father of physicians'. Second, Galen is not the prince in the sense of the next in line to the throne, but in the sense of the Roman aristocrat who is accepted by his peers as most fully embodying those qualities which they themselves share. *Princeps* is one of the most interesting of Latin titles for a ruler since, as Augustus found out in the first century BC when experimenting in order to find a position from which he could effectively rule Rome without alienating the senatorial class, the word conveys the sense of 'first among equals' rather than of control. As prince, the *princeps*, of physicians, Galen is not so far above the others that he has moved out of their reach. Augustus also accepted the title of 'Father of his Country', an ancient Roman honorary title carrying the sense of the *paterfamilias*, or head of household, firmly but fairly ruling over his family, slaves and possessions; here, fatherhood of the country brings every aspect of the life of Rome into Augustus' personal sphere of control.

Hippocrates's emergence as the father of medicine was a gradual and far from automatic process. Galen dominated Western medicine from the twelfth century until the sixteenth century, having synthesised those texts of Hippocrates which most resonated with his own theories to form a single 'grand theory' of humours, organs and *pepsis* that could explain anything in the body. In 1525 Marco Fabio Calvi's printed edition of the complete Hippocratic *Corpus* in Latin made the bulk of the Hippocratic *Corpus* available for the first time, creating the possibility of challenges to Galen's version of Hippocrates.[42] In the editions of both Calvi and Cornarius, the 'biography' attributed to Soranus appears before the texts themselves; this biography includes the Artaxerxes story in which Hippocrates refuses barbarian gold.

In 1526 the Aldine Greek edition was published, further raising the stakes in the competitive game of textual one-upmanship; now it was not just a question of comparing the Latin Galen with the Latin Hippocrates, but of mastering two ancient languages in order to prove one's points. Yet, as Vivian Nutton has shown, the Hippocratic publications at first made little stir in the Galenic universe; those who praised him rarely read him.[43]

An example not only of the positive evaluation of Hippocrates, but also of the tenacity of the Galenic model of the body, can be found in the field of gynaecology. Since Galen had not written any specifically gynaecological texts,[44] the particular Hippocratic contribution to this area of the two volumes on *Diseases of Women*, and the treatises *On Sterile Women* and *Nature of Woman*, was quickly recognised after they became available in full in 1525. By the 1580s it had become commonplace to praise Hippocrates for his gynaecological works; for example, the introduction to Jean Liébault's 1582 French version of his Latin treatise on gynaecology states that 'The divine Hippocrates, caring about the health and fertility of womankind, and stimulated by a charitable spirit to save her, wrote four separate books to help her'.[45]

Liébault then claims that few of Hippocrates's successors, ancient or modern, have been able to match his knowledge of gynaecology, because the subject is inherently shifting and unstable; the diseases of men are easier to treat because they remain constant.

This praise of Hippocratic gynaecology should not, however, blind us to what is going on behind the facade of enthusiasm. Before the second half of the sixteenth century, the newly available Hippocratic texts were simply read in Galenic terms;[46] the systematic Galenic model of the body, dominant since the twelfth century, guided the ways in which the new Hippocratic gynaecology was to be interpreted. So, when Liébault cites Hippocrates's 'livre des accidens des vierges' as saying that there are only two causes of diseases of virgins – namely, impeded menstruation and retention of seed – he is not reading the Hippocratic text *On the Diseases of Virgins*, which makes no mention of female seed; it was in fact Galen, in *De locis affectis*, who suggested that retained seed could be more dangerous than retained menses.[47] As I have discussed elsewhere, when in the 1550s Johannes Lange read the same Hippocratic text on menstrual retention in young girls, he also understood it within a Galenic model of the body, praising 'the divine Hippocrates' for what were Galenic views.[48]

For much of the sixteenth century, then, Hippocrates was named as supreme, but read through the eyes of Galen, who exalted him as a strategy to protect himself. In the prefatory material to the 1525 Calvi, Hippocrates is 'without dispute, of all physicians, the *princeps*', while the 1546 edition of Cornarius has 'Hippocrates and Galen, the *principes* of the best medical sect, namely the rational sect'.[49] There can be more than one *princeps*: but, *contra* Sawday, there is only one father.

Why Hippocrates?

In Hippocratic medicine, there are two main options for those looking for a theory of fatherhood. In the treatise *On Generation/Nature of the Child*, translated into Latin for the second time in the thirteenth century, both sexes contribute a 'seed' to the child, with its gender and other physical characteristics depending on the outcome of a battle for dominance between the father's seed and the mother's seed. However, this text consistently regards women's seed as weaker than men's seed.[50] In *Diseases of Women* female seed is not mentioned: women produce only menstrual blood, making these texts closer to the Aristotelian view that man is the carpenter, woman the wood, so that the male imposes form on the shapeless raw material of women's blood.[51] As I have already noted, Galen's woman produces both blood and seed: retention of female seed is seen as having far more serious consequences for health than retention of menstrual blood.

Over the course of the sixteenth century, Ian Maclean has argued, opinion shifted away from the Aristotelian version of female inadequacy towards what he calls 'a modified form of Galenism' in which woman was 'perfect of her kind'.[52] But one could argue that the return of the Hippocratic gynaecological texts to learned medicine shifted the image of fatherhood towards the view that the father plays a more significant part than the mother in forming the foetus. A suggestive parallel can be found in the preface to the first edition of Maurice de la Corde's commentary on the Hippocratic *Diseases of Women 1*.[53] The work of 'our divine Hippocrates' is singled out from the many other works available on how to provoke or restrain the menses, how to cope with a uterine prolapse, or how to calm down an inflammation of the womb, on the grounds not only that he alone has covered the diseases which affect woman throughout the whole course of her life, but also that he has arranged his findings in a particularly fitting manner. De la Corde seems to be arguing that Hippocrates alone has imposed form on the shapeless mass which is 'the diseases of women', a suggestion made even more attractive by the multiple meanings of the Greek title of the work on which de la Corde is commenting, *Gynaikeia*, which covers 'diseases of women', 'cures for women's diseases', and 'menstrual blood'. Hippocrates fathers medicine by shaping the human raw materials into coherent form.

But, as we have seen, Hippocrates is also the father of medicine because Galen needed to project his own views of medicine back into a conveniently distant past. The absence of any earlier surviving texts from ancient Greek medicine has subsequently helped maintain this situation. As Owsei Temkin put it: 'The fact that very little is known about Greek medicine before the Hippocratic writings has helped to put Hippocrates at the head of the tradition of Western medicine.'[54]

But there is more to Hippocrates's position than the authority of Galen or the absence of other contenders. The brilliance of hailing Hippocrates as the father of medicine lies also in the fact that it enabled medical writers from the late sixteenth century onwards to throw out the bathwater, while keeping the baby. As Galen had virtually insisted that Hippocrates was God, with Galen as his prophet, a return to Hippocrates could be represented as a move entirely consistent with Galenic medicine. This strategy is comparable to Vesalius' claim to have found over 200 errors in Galen, while engaged in precisely the same anatomy project that Galen had begun, so that, as Andrew Cunningham put it, 'Vesalius as vivisectionist was simply Galen restored to life'.[55] To abandon both Hippocrates and Galen, as Bacon recommended, was simply too dramatic; the medical profession needed a long and illustrious past to distinguish itself from other forms of healing.

The problem remained that Hippocrates is a name without a face. Later genealogists had done what they could to create a family for him: artists did their best to give him a face. But where Hippocrates scores as a potential father is in the variety of his offspring. There are so many texts in the 'Hippocratic *Corpus*', that disparate group of treatises going under his name, that virtually any form of medicine can claim to trace its roots back to Hippocrates. Every generation has been able to find a new Hippocrates: by resurrecting a previously neglected Hippocratic text, every medical newcomer can claim to be going back to the true fount of medicine.

But there is a further aspect of Hippocrates's fatherhood that should be considered. The fact that writers such as Thomas Gale could praise Hippocrates as 'divine' and hail him as father of medicine even when the Hippocratic *Corpus* was being understood in entirely Galenic terms demonstrates that the power of Hippocrates's fatherhood is not only based on the range of views expressed in the texts which bear his name. The contents of the Hippocratic *Corpus* can, paradoxically, become entirely irrelevant to the reputation of Hippocrates. Here I would suggest that to father medicine should be seen as giving it the traits of the father, an area where Hippocrates scores far more highly than Galen. Academic studies and popular histories are united: 'Galen was verbose, long-winded, doctrinaire', 'Galen as a man was conceited, dogmatic and abusive of those who disagreed with him'.[56] Galen was simply too pompous and too argumentative a character to be allowed to transmit his personal qualities to medicine.

What, then, are the superior moral qualities of Hippocrates – that name without a text and without a face? The ethical treatises such as *On Decorum*, taken with the *Oath* and the case histories of the *Epidemics*, can be used to give an impression of the personality of the man who did not, in fact, write any of them. In 1922 Charles Singer visualised Hippocrates as 'Learned, observant, humane ... orderly and calm ... grave, thoughtful and reticent, pure of mind and master of his passions'.[57] Not only medicine, but also its practitioners, need a father of this kind. The version of medical history put forward by E.J. Kempf in the *Medical Library and Historical Journal* of 1904 repeated the fictional biographical material from antiquity, and suggested that:

> Among the distinguished traits of Hippocrates were an exalted idea of medicine, its extent, its aim and its difficulties; a great regard for medical dignity, and a lively feeling of the duties and obligations of his profession; a deep aversion against those who in any way compromised it, either by quackery or immorality; and, in fine, his unceasing solicitude for the cure, or, failing in this, the relief of the sick ... Hippocrates was certainly entitled to his titles of 'The Great Physician' and 'The Father of Medicine'.[58]

Here Hippocrates even becomes a defender of his profession, a particularly extravagant claim when medicine in classical Greece functioned with no training system and no licensing, so that anyone claiming to be a doctor could attempt to treat the sick.[59]

Prominent among the supposed moral virtues of Hippocrates were his patriotism and his disdain for money, included in the fictions of the genealogies and biographies;[60] he refused to treat the Persian king Artaxerxes because he was the enemy of the Greeks, and preferred to treat the poor rather than taking up the position of court physician.[61] In one of the letters, Hippocrates replies to the Persian king:

> Send back to the King as quickly as possible that I have enough food, clothing, shelter and all substance sufficient for life, and I am unwilling to enjoy Persian opulence or to save Persians from disease, since they are enemies of the Greeks.[62]

The Hippocratic lack of concern for wealth is a comforting corrective to patients' criticism of medicine as an easy way to make money. The patriotism could, however, be questioned, on the grounds that a doctor should treat anyone needing his help, regardless of race or status.[63] But it has more commonly been positively valued. Thomas Crow has suggested, in his study of the interrelations between the personal and the political in Girodet's image of this scene, *Hippocrates Refusing the Gifts of Artaxerxes* (1792), that the choice of subject relates not only to Girodet's own relationships with figures of paternal authority, but also to the importance of civic virtue and patriotism, and to the specific uses of Hippocratism in the political imagery of disease and health in revolutionary France.[64]

The Hippocratic tradition does carry some doubts about the personality of Hippocrates – in particular, the rumour, mentioned in the biographies, that he burned the library at Cos before leaving. However, from whichever texts he is constructed, he comes across as a far more congenial person than Galen. He also lived at the best time; as Kempf put it, 'in the most brilliant period in the history of Greece – we might add, the most brilliant of all ages – in literature, philosophy, poetry and the fine arts',[65] making him a contemporary of many of the figures chosen as the ancestors of Western civilisation. Galen's origins were Greek, but he was unlucky enough to live under the Roman Empire and to serve the Roman emperors. In terms of his personality, his role for the medical profession, and the history of the greater glorification of classical Greek rather than Roman imperial culture, Hippocrates measures up to what is expected of the father of medicine.

Notes

1. Jonathan Sawday, *The Body Emblazoned: Dissection and the Human Body in Renaissance Culture*, London and New York: Routledge, 1995, p. 41.
2. Heinrich Schipperges, 'Die Assimilation der arabischen Medizin durch das lateinische Mittelalter', *Sudhoffs Archiv*, Beiheft 3, Wiesbaden: Franz Steiner, 1964; Monica H. Green, 'The *De Genecia* attributed to Constantine the African', *Speculum*, 62, 1987, pp. 299–323; idem, 'Constantinus Africanus and the conflict between religion and science' in G.R. Dunstan (ed.), *The Human Embryo:*

Aristotle and the Arabic and European Traditions, Exeter: University of Exeter Press, 1990, pp. 47–69.
3. Thomas Gale, Certaine Workes of Galens called Methodus Medendi, London: Thomas East, 1586, p. 6ᵛ cited in Sawday, The Body Emblazoned (n. 1), p. 40.
4. William Harvey, Exercitatio Anatomica de Motu Cordis et Sanguinis in Animalibus, Frankfurt: W. Fitzer, 1628, pp. 39–40.
5. P.W. Graham, 'Harvey's De motu cordis: the rhetoric of science and the science of rhetoric', Journal of the History of Medicine and Allied Sciences, 1978, pp. 469–76 at p. 473.
6. M.N. (Marchamont Nedham), Medela Medicinae. A Plea for the Free Profession, and a Renovation of the Art of Physick, London: Richard Lownds, 1665, p. 232, discussed by Cunningham, below.
7. Thomas Gale, Certaine Workes of Chirurgerie, London: Thomas East, 1586, author's preface.
8. Gale, Certaine Workes of Galens (n. 3), pp. 4ᵛ–5ʳ; not cited by Sawday. An edition of this work in the Wellcome Institute for the History of Medicine Library survives with the date 1566 or 1567; in this, the above sections appear on pp. 12–14.
9. Ibid., p5ʳ; in 1566–67 edition, p. 14.
10. Patricia Davis, Aromatherapy. An A–Z, Saffron Walden: C.W. Daniel, 1988, p. 158. Susan Moore, in A Guide to Chiropractic, London: Hamlyn, 1988, pp. 134–5, argues that 'Hippocrates was the first physician to identify a link between spinal problems and ill health', while Leon K. Chaitow, in Osteopathy. A Complete Health-care System, Wellingborough: Thorsons, 1982, p. 23, claims that 'Manipulative methods as part of medical treatment are known to date back to earliest times. Hippocrates wrote of their value.' Beth MacEoin, in Homoeopathy, Sevenoaks: Headway Lifeguides, Hodder and Stoughton, 1992, p. 8, makes homoeopathy 'a concept which had existed from the time of Hippocrates'. In some alternative health guides for a lay audience, the orthodox biomedical image of Hippocrates as the ideal doctor is both maintained and challenged with a claim that the medical profession ignored his 'observations on cure by "similars"' for a millennium, during which the folk medicine of ordinary people kept the principle alive; see Miranda Castro, The Complete Homeopathy Handbook: A Guide to Everyday Health Care, London: Macmillan, 1990, p. 3. On the development of a Hippocrates appropriate to the concerns of the nursing profession, see Helen King, Hippocrates' Woman: Reading the Female Body in Ancient Greece, London and New York: Routledge, 1998, ch. 8.
11. The variants on the myth of Asclepius' birth are given in full in Emma J. Edelstein and Ludwig Edelstein, Asclepius: Collection and Interpretation of the Testimonies, Baltimore and London: Johns Hopkins University Press, 1945 (reprinted 1998), I, pp. 1–59 and discussed in detail in II, pp. 1–64.
12. Hyginus, Fabula 274, trans. Mary Grant, The Myths of Hyginus, Lawrence: University of Kansas Press, 1960.
13. Gian A. Ferrari and Mario Vegetti, in 'Science, technology and medicine in the classical tradition' in Pietro Corsi and Paul Weindling (eds), Information Sources in the History of Science and Medicine, London and Boston: Butterworth Scientific, 1983, pp. 197–220, have characterised a technê as a 'practical activity that required intellectual competence as well as manual dexterity, was based on scientific knowledge, produced results that it was possible to verify, and was governed by well-defined rules that could be transmitted by teaching' (p. 202).
14. Heinrich von Staden, '"In a pure and holy way": personal and professional

conduct in the Hippocratic Oath?,' *Journal of the History of Medicine and Allied Sciences*, **51**, 1996, pp. 404–37 at pp. 412, 416.
15. Tzetzes, *Chiliades*, 7.944–958, cited in Edelstein and Edelstein, *Asclepius*, (n. 11), I, pp. 102–3; on Christian interpretations of Hippocrates, see Owsei Temkin, *Hippocrates in a World of Pagans and Christians*, Baltimore: Johns Hopkins University Press, 1991.
16. Jody Rubin Pinault, *Hippocratic Lives and Legends*, Leiden and New York: Brill, 1992, gives translations of all the ancient genealogies.
17. Jaap Mansfeld, 'Plato and the method of Hippocrates,' *Greek, Roman and Byzantine Studies*, **21**, 1980, pp. 341–62.
18. Volker Langholf, *Medical Theories in Hippocrates: Early Texts and the 'Epidemics'*, Berlin and New York: de Gruyter, 1990, p. 197.
19. Wesley D. Smith, *The Hippocratic Tradition*, Ithaca, NY: Cornell University Press, 1979; cf. Robert Joly, 'Hippocrates and the school of Cos' in Michael Ruse (ed.), *Nature Animated: papers of the Third International Conference on the History and Philosophy of Science, Montreal, Canada 1980*, Vol. 2, Dordrecht: Reidel, 1983, pp. 29–47; Jaap Mansfeld, 'The historical Hippocrates and the origins of scientific medicine' in Ruse (ed.), *Nature Animated*, pp. 49–76. Ludwig Edelstein, 'The genuine works of Hippocrates', *Bulletin of the History of Medicine*, **7**, 1939, pp. 236–48, reprinted in Owsei and C.L. Temkin (eds), *Ancient Medicine: Selected Papers of Ludwig Edelstein*, Baltimore, MD: Johns Hopkins University Press, 1967, pp. 133–44 conveniently summarises earlier scholars' claims for the authenticity of the works in the *Corpus*.
20. Wesley D. Smith (ed. and trans.), *Hippocrates: Pseudepigraphic Writings*, Leiden and New York: Brill, 1990, pp. 6–8.
21. Seneca, *Epistulae*, 95.20.
22. Smith, *Hippocratic Tradition* (n. 19), p. 121.
23. Ibid., pp. 215–21.
24. Ibid., p. 30.
25. *Epistula* 2; Smith, *Pseudepigraphic Writings* (n. 20), p. 49.
26. *Patêr hygeias*, *Epistula* 2; Smith, *Pseudepigraphic Writings*, p. 51. 'Saviour' is a common title for Asclepius.
27. *Epistula* 20; Smith, *Pseudepigraphic Writings*, p. 97.
28. *Epistula* 10.2; Smith, *Pseudepigraphic Writings*, p. 59.
29. *Epistula* 15; Smith, *Pseudepigraphic Writings*, p. 71.
30. Robert K. Merton, 'Priorities in scientific discovery,' *American Sociological Review*, **22**, 1957, pp. 635–59, reprinted in Robert K. Merton, *The Sociology of Science: Theoretical and Empirical Investigations*, Chicago and London: University of Chicago Press, 1973. For the range of claims to father a speciality, I am using the catalogue of the Wellcome Institute for the History of Medicine.
31. Merton, 'Priorities' (n. 30), p. 299 cites some extreme examples of the need for new specialities to claim their own parents.
32. Jan Sapp, 'The nine lives of Gregor Mendel' in Homer E. Le Grand (ed.), *Experimental Inquiries: Historical, Philosophical and Social Studies of Experimentation in Science*, Dordrecht: Reidel, 1990, pp. 137–66; available on <http:www.netspace.org/MendelWeb>.
33. Ludmilla Jordanova, *Sexual Visions: Images of Gender in Science and Medicine between the Eighteenth and Twentieth Centuries*, London: Harvester Wheatsheaf, 1989.
34. Jan Sapp, *Where the Truth Lies: Franz Moewus and the Origins of Molecular Biology*, Cambridge: Cambridge University Press, 1990, pp. 28–29.

35. Brian Easlea, *Fathering the Unthinkable: Masculinity, Scientists and the Nuclear Arms Race*, London: Pluto Press, 1983, p. 115.
36. Ibid., pp. 25–6.
37. Francis Bacon, *The Masculine Birth of Time, or Three Books on the Interpretation of Nature*, in Benjamin Farrington, *The Philosophy of Francis Bacon*, Liverpool: Liverpool University Press, 1964, p. 62 at pp. 130–31.
38. Ibid., p. 64.
39. Ibid., pp. 67–68.
40. Ibid., p. 131.
41. W.H.S. Jones, 'Introduction,' *Hippocrates*, Vol. IV (Loeb edition), London: Heinemann, 1931, p. xxxiv; cf. Francis Adams, *The Genuine Works of Hippocrates*, 2 vols, London: Sydenham Society, 1849, pp. 50–54; also Burton Chance, 'On Hippocrates and the Aphorisms', *Annals of Medical History*, 2, 1930, pp. 31–46.
42. Marco Fabio Calvi, *Hippocratis Coi medicorum omnium longe principis, Octoginta volumina*, Rome: Franciscus Minitius, p. 1525.
43. Vivian Nutton, 'Hippocrates in the Renaissance' in Gerhaad Baader and Rolf Winau (eds), *Die Hippokratischen Epidemien: Theorie–Praxis–Tradition*, Verhandlung des Ve Colloque international hippocratique, Berlin, 10–15 September 1984, *Sudhoffs Archiv*, Beiheft 27, Stuttgart: Franz Steiner, 1989, pp. 420–39 at p. 426.
44. Israel Spach, *Nomenclator scriptorum medicorum. Hoc est, Elenchus eorem, qui artem medicam suis scriptis illustrarunt*, Frankfurt, 1591, p. 130 includes 'Galeni liber spurius' in his listing of works on the diseases of women known at that time. In the Arabic tradition, a pseudo-Galenic work *On the Secrets of Women* existed, dating from before the ninth century, but this does not appear to have been known in the West. See Martin Levey and Safwat S. Souryal, 'Galen's *On the Secrets of Women* and *On the Secrets of Men*,' *Janus*, 55, 1968, pp. 208–19.
45. Jean Liébault, *Trois Livres appartenant aux infirmitez et maladies des femmes, pris du Latin de M. Jean Liebaut, Docteur Médecin à Paris, et faicts François*, Paris: Jacques de Puys, 1582. This work is listed in the catalogues of the British Library and the Wellcome Institute for the History of Medicine as having been compiled from Giovanni Marinello, *Le medicine partenenti alle infermità delle donne*, Venice: Francesco de Franceschi Senese, 1563. However, as Iain Lonie pointed out, the originality of Liébault's work is defended in Bayle's *Dictionary*; see 'The "Paris Hippocratics": teaching and research in Paris in the second half of the sixteenth century' in Andrew Wear, Roger K. French and Iain M. Lonie (eds), *The Medical Renaissance of the Sixteenth Century*, Cambridge: Cambridge University Press, pp. 155–74 at p. 321 n. 23.
46. Nutton, 'Hippocrates in the Renaissance' (n. 43), pp. 422, 426.
47. Jean Liébault, *Thrésor des remèdes secrets pour les maladies des femmes*, Paris: Robert Jacques de Puys, 1597, p. 8 (first edition 1585). [Hippocrates], *On the Diseases of Virgins* (Littré 8.466–71); Galen, *De locis affectis* 6.5 (Kühn 8.420, 424 and 432–3).
48. Johannes Lange, *Medicinalium epistolarum miscellanea*, Basel: J. Oporinus, 1554; *Ep.* 1.21. See King, *Hippocrates' Woman* (n. 10), ch. 10.
49. Janus Cornarius, *Hippocratis Coi medicorum omnium longe principis, opera quae ad nos extant omnia*, Basel: Froben, 1546, Epistola Nuncupatoria.
50. Iain M. Lonie, *The Hippocratic Treatises 'On Generation', 'On the Nature of the Child', 'Diseases IV'*, Berlin and New York: De Gruyter, 1981; King, *Hippocrates' Woman* (n. 10), pp. 8–9.

51. King, *Hippocrates' Woman* (n. 10), pp. 10–11.
52. Ian Maclean, *The Renaissance Notion of Woman: a Study in the Fortunes of Scholasticism and Medical Science in European Intellectual Life*, Cambridge and New York: Cambridge University Press, 1980, p. 44. On the Renaissance medical debate about the removal of excess female seed, see Winfried Schleiner, *Medical Ethics in the Renaissance*, Washington DC: Georgetown University Press, 1995, chapter 5.
53. Maurice de la Corde, *Hippocratis Coi, Medicorum Principis, liber prior de morbis mulierum*, Paris: Dionysius Duvallius, 1585.
54. Temkin, *Hippocrates* (n. 15), p. 41.
55. Andrew Cunningham, *The Anatomical Renaissance: The Resurrection of the Anatomical Projects of the Ancients*, Aldershot, England: Scolar Press; Brookfield, VT, USA: Ashfield Publishing Co., 1997, p. 115.
56. Nutton, 'Hippocrates in the Renaissance' (n. 43), p. 435; F.N.L. Poynter and K.D. Keele, *A Short History of Medicine*, London: Scientific Book Club, p. 21.
57. *Greek Biology and Greek Medicine*, Clarendon Press, Oxford.
58. E.J. Kempf, 'From Hippocrates to Galen', *Medical Library and Historical Journal*, **2**, 1904, 282–307, pp. 286–87 and p. 291. Kempf includes a list of eight works 'certainly written by Hippocrates'.
59. See, for example, Geoffrey Lloyd, *Magic, Reason and Experience: Studies in the Origin and Development of Greek Science*, Cambridge: Cambridge University Press, 1979 and *Science, Folklore and Ideology: Studies in the Life Sciences in Ancient Greece*, Cambridge: Cambridge University Press, 1983.
60. See Pinault, *Hippocratic Lives* (n. 16), pp. 70–94; Temkin, *Hippocrates* (n. 15), p. 56; Johannis Ravisius Textor, *Officina*, Venice, 1588, p. 191^v.
61. *Epistula* 11; Smith, *Pseudepigraphic Writings* (n. 30), p. 61; Temkin, *Hippocrates* (n. 15), pp. 47–48.
62. *Epistula* 5; Smith, *Pseudepigraphic Writings*, p. 53.
63. Temkin, *Hippocrates* (n. 15), pp. 59–60.
64. Thomas Crow, *Emulation: Making Artists for Revolutionary France*, New Haven and London: Yale University Press, 1995, pp. 140–44. Crow underestimates the sources available in this period containing the story of Hippocrates and Artaxerxes.
65. Kempf, 'Hippocrates to Galen', p. 286.

CHAPTER THREE

Hippocrates and the Construction of 'Progress' in Sixteenth- and Seventeenth-century Medicine

Thomas Rütten

It might seem paradoxical to link Hippocratism with early modern ideas of progress, since the term 'progress' is generally taken to imply an outlook that is future-oriented.[1] Thus, it would seem highly unlikely that Hippocrates would have ever caught the attention of those we regard today as early modern 'progressives'. Surely it would be more appropriate to associate him with reactionaries, those opposed to or openly obstructing progress. It might also seem paradoxical to link sixteenth- and early seventeenth-century medicine with 'progress' because historians have denied the era between Petrarch and Descartes any claim to the idea of progress.[2] Although this verdict has been challenged,[3] it is true that the idea of progress has received relatively little attention from Renaissance scholars.[4]

The two putative paradoxes in the title of this paper call for a preliminary clarification which can be obtained through a definition. The concept of progress assumed here is not identical with a process that is unequivocally linear, historically continuous and cumulative. It does not aim, as Nisbet puts it, at 'those works external to subjective consciousness which are, of course, the fundamental data of any theory of historical progress'.[5] It is not 'progress' as propagated in modern scientific medicine, where new techno-scientific developments combine to raise an indefinite number of possibilities.[6] By using the term 'progress' in quotation marks, I would like to indicate that I do not use the word as a universal historical–philosophical general term, but adhere to a different understanding of this concept, such as is offered, for example, by Alistair Crombie:

> The concept of progress expresses an attitude to man's place in time and history, to the relation of his past to his future, that is both descriptive and prescriptive. It involves insights both into the progress of knowledge, and also into the sources and progress or regress of happiness, power or moral virtue. The concept implies a desirable direction, hence the possibility of deviation, and value judgements about what ought and ought not to have been, and to be, done in man's dealings with nature, with himself and his fellow creatures, or with God. In other words, the concept

of progress is at once profane and sacred, at once epistemological, cosmological and religious, in that it implies beliefs about knowledge, about what exists, and about man's origins, expectations and responsibilities within whatever is accepted as the scheme of knowledge and existence.[7]

Applied to medicine this definition boils down to a simple formula: 'Progress is making medicine better.'[8] And since 'progress implies a goal, or at any rate a direction, and a goal or direction implies a value judgement',[9] it could be argued that anything that was formulated, in terms of goals within medicine, including the means recommended or propagated to achieve them, relates to a concept of progress. The term 'progressive', therefore, should be applied to any idea that was perceived as, or proclaimed to hold out the promise of, something new or discontinuous. From this perspective, 'progress' is undoubtedly a relational term, defined, often for polemical or ideological reasons, not only by those who advocate what they term progress, but also by those who oppose new endeavours or pronounce them doomed to failure.

In order to define a role for Hippocrates and Hippocratic medicine within our considerations of progress, let us first turn to those representatives of Renaissance and early modern medicine who are most readily associated with ideas of progress. This, I hope, will address some of the problems posed by the juxtaposition of the three key elements of my title – Hippocrates, progress, and sixteenth- and seventeenth-century medicine.

Paracelsus, Vesalius and Harvey: the warrantors of 'progress' and their supposed anti-Hippocratism

Medical historiography of the late nineteenth and early twentieth centuries regarded three figures in particular as 'progressive': Paracelsus (1493/94–1541), Andreas Vesalius (1514–1564) and William Harvey (1578–1657).[10] The dominant medico-historical narrative portrayed these three as the founding fathers of the key disciplines of contemporary medicine – chemistry, anatomy and physiology. They are seen as emblematic of a shift in medicine that occurred between 1530 and 1630 – a century that supposedly saw the decline of dogmatic medicine rooted in the canonical concepts of humoral pathology and blind faith in authority. What emerged instead were the beginnings of a modern medicine based on pathological, physiological–anatomical, experimental and inductive science, and the idea of a linear, constant and cumulative advance, devaluing tradition. Accordingly, Paracelsus, Vesalius and Harvey were revered for opposing those authorities perceived to be standing in the way of progress in the modern sense – notably Aristotle, Galen and Hippocrates. From this perspective, defenders of Hippocrates must indeed appear reactionary, traditionalist or, at best, obstructive to 'progress'. As a result, sixteenth- and seventeenth-century Hippocratism is all too often reduced to a chronicle of prejudice against the human intellect.[11]

However, a closer reading of the writings of the triumvirate mentioned above reveals that their relationship to Hippocrates was not as strained as some accounts suggest. Upon a first reading, Paracelsus seems to have been the most inclined to criticise Hippocrates: 'Who does not know that most doctors in this age, to the patients' detriment, have lapsed most disgracefully since they stuck to the words of Hippocrates, Galen, Avicenna and others too slavishly?'[12] he asked his medical colleagues at Basel in 1527. On the basis of this supposedly anti-Hippocratic dictum, even recent commentators are inclined to regard Paracelsus as a 'revolutionary, unorthodox, oppositional-critical' spirit, a 'sceptic against any printed and taught knowledge'.[13] As a matter of fact, however, Paracelsus was taking up an issue which had already been under discussion in the late Middle Ages.[14] Moreover, as some scholars have pointed out, this polemic is not representative of Paracelsus' general attitude towards Hippocrates. In fact, he tends to exempt Hippocrates from the criticism he directs against other figures of authority and accords him a special status in his *oeuvre*. For Paracelsus, it is obvious that 'even in Hippocrates's times, people have erred',[15] but he nevertheless believed that, with the help of Apollo, Machaon, Podaleirios and Hippocrates, medicine had set off on the right path.[16] 'Which fallen person', argues Paracelsus, 'cries: help Juvenal, help? – None; but: help Hippocrates, help; as it is he whom God has ordered to do so, who lives in Nature and is a master of the light of Nature'.[17] And, in his 'Greeting to the Hippocratic doctors' in the *Labyrinthus*, Paracelsus expresses his veneration for Hippocrates in the form of a rhetorical question: 'When has medicine ever stood higher than where Hippocrates was?'.[18] In addition, probably around 1528, he wrote commentaries on a few passages in the Hippocratic *Aphorisms*.[19] The choice of genre alone indicates that his relationship to Hippocrates was far from being straightforwardly antagonistic.[20] Paracelsus' starting point, according to J.-P. Pittion, W. Smith, O. Temkin and others, was to dissociate Hippocratic from Galenic medicine.[21] Indeed, as Walter Pagel asserts, Hippocrates was among the few whom Paracelsus refrained from mocking.[22]

If Paracelsus cannot be seen as entirely antipathetic to Hippocrates, neither can Vesalius. His biographer Charles O'Malley refers to him as a devout follower of the revival of Hippocratic medicine – at least in 1536.[23] At that time, Vesalius had just spent three years studying at the University of Paris, one of the early sixteenth-century strongholds of the Hippocratics.[24] He had become well versed not only in the Hippocratic texts taught as part of the curriculum[25] (*De victu in morbis acutis*, *Aphorisms*, *Prognostic*, *De victu*) but in others as well. His next stop was Padua, where Hippocratic medicine was also held in high esteem.[26] It is therefore hardly surprising that, in his writings, Vesalius repeatedly refers to Hippocratic texts[27] or to the author himself as his personal authority.[28] Vesalius' invocation of Hippocrates 'divinus'[29] in the preface to his *Fabrica* may simply be a *captatio benevolentiae* directed towards the dedicatee, especially considering the popularity of this epithet in the medical literature of his time. But this does not explain his emphatic praise of a professor of Hippocratic medicine in Bologna.[30] Vesalius' *oeurve* suggests only a few, almost imperceptible alterations to the Hippocratic teachings[31] and, throughout his works, there is a notable absence of fundamental critique of Hippocrates or any polemic against him. This is true not only of the 28 year-old author of the *Fabrica*, but also of the older Vesalius, who refers to Hippocrates in a consilium sent to his pupil Pieter van Foreest, known as the 'Dutch Hippocrates',[32] some time in the 1550s.

Likewise, Harvey, far from criticising Hippocrates, holds him in high esteem. In his lectures on anatomy in 1618 he even calls him 'amazing'.[33] Moreover, in both his lectures and his major work *De motu cordis*, he repeatedly refers to Hippocrates's *De corde*,[34] part of the *Corpus Hippocraticum*, in favourable terms. In fact, his entire work is interspersed with commendations to the Hippocratic texts.[35] In his *Exercitationes de Generatione Animalium* (1651) alone, Harvey mentions a Hippocratic account of an aborted foetus on three separate occasions in order to confirm and authorise his own experience.[36] An extensive reference to Hippocrates reads as follows:

> I think that in the first month there is little of the foetus extant in the womb; at least, I never found anything. But at the end of that month, I have quite frequently seen a conception cast out like the one that Hippocrates mentions as having been dropped by a woman flute player, of the size of a pheasant's or pigeon's egg. It was oval in shape, just like an egg with the shell pulled off, but the thicker membrane, called the chorion, that surrounded it was plastered on the outside as it were with a white mucous substance, especially at the blunt end, but inside it was slimy and filled with clear, sticky water and nothing else at all.[37]

This passage clearly refers to the Hippocratic treatise *De natura pueri*:

> As a matter of fact I myself have seen an embryo which was aborted after remaining in the womb for six days. It is upon its nature, as I observed it then, that I base the rest of my inferences. It was in the following way that I came to see a six day old embryo. A kinswoman of mine owned a very valuable singer, who used to go with men. It was important that this girl should not become pregnant and thereby lose her value. Now this girl had heard the sort of thing women say to each other – that when a woman is going to conceive, the seed remains inside her and does not fall out. She digested this information, and kept a watch. One day she noticed that the seed had not come out again. She told her mistress, and the story came to me. When I heard it, I told her to jump up and down, touching her buttocks with her heels at each leap. After she had done this no more than seven times, there was a noise, the seed fell out on the ground, and the girl looked at it in great surprise. It looked like this: it was as though someone had removed the shell from a raw egg, so that the fluid inside showed through

the inner membrane – a reasonably good description of its appearance. It was round, and red; and within the membrane could be seen thick white fibres, surrounded by a thick red serum; while on the outer surface of the membrane was a small projection: it looked to me like an umbilicus, and I considered that it was through this that the embryo first breathed in and out. From it, the membrane stretched all around the seed. Such then was the six day embryo that I saw, and a little further on I intend to describe another observation which will give a clear insight into the subject. It will also serve as evidence for the truth of my whole argument – so far as is humanly possible in such a matter. So much then for this subject.[38]

The parallels between the structure and content of the two accounts are obvious, as are the small alterations which Harvey undertakes: the end of the first month instead of six days, a woman flute player instead of a singer, an oval pheasant's or pigeon's egg instead of a round one, and so on. What is particularly interesting about Harvey's borrowing is the fact that he stresses Hippocrates's observational skills as a means of legitimising his own experimental mode of research.

If Paracelsus, Vesalius and Harvey thus by no means opposed Hippocrates and the writings attributed to him, we will also need to adopt a more cautious attitude towards the assumption that 'progress' in early modern medicine was only achieved by breaking with the Hippocratic tradition. On the contrary, it could be argued that Hippocrates remained quite present to the 'moderns', in the sense of Christian Meier's term '*Könnensbewußtsein*',[39] a neologism which roughly translates as 'ability awareness'. In other words, the division between conservative or reactionary parties on the one hand, and their progressive or revolutionary counterparts on the other, does not coincide with the dichotomy set up between Hippocratism and anti-Hippocratism.

Indeed quite the opposite seems to have been the case: Hippocrates found entry into any number of imaginable concepts of progress. He provided a role model for medical biographies, a source for often highly divergent cosmological and anthropological concepts, a rich store of experiential testimony in need of interpretation and systematisation and an almost inexhaustible well of wisdom. The scarcity of biographical data, his fame (more often than not elevated into realms of mythical vagueness), his compressed style of writing, and his heterogeneous and unstructured *oeuvre* left ample room for creating a Hippocrates who fitted the label 'patron of progress' only too well. For early modern commentators, the fact that Hippocrates had died almost 2000 years before was of little consequence in the construction of his persona as a 'progressive'. Furthermore, the role he was accorded was twofold: he was considered both the origin of medical progress and its ultimate goal.

Hippocrates as the origin of medical 'progress'

A cyclical concept of history, theories of degeneration, the idea of revelation transposed on to medicine and a pattern of thinking focused on *'Personalautorität'* and seniority could lead to the seemingly paradoxical situation in which the future goal of progress was perceived to beckon from the golden Hippocratic age. The imagery and iconography of the late Middle Ages are quite telling in this context: Hippocrates was, for example, portrayed as the spring of medical art leading on to a hot Galenic summer which was followed by the autumn of Persian Arabic medicine until winter descended in the Latin Middle Ages.[40] Such imagery seems to imply that the dawn of the medical Renaissance also heralded the return of spring. Or, to draw on an artisan metaphor, Hippocrates, or rather Hippocratism, was, according to Henri de Mondeville or Guy de Chauliac, like a house which had to be continuously maintained, renovated and refurbished, but which still remained basically unchanged in form, dimensions and substantial solidity.[41]

If late medieval writers looked to the past to bring about 'progress', so too did Renaissance and early modern humanist scholars. Their research aimed to reconstruct the former glorious days of ancient medicine in the hope of thus distinguishing their own endeavours from those of the scholastic or Arabic world of medicine.[42] In true humanist fashion,[43] they took up the slogan '*Redite ad fontes*' ('back to the sources') as the battle-cry for a moral and programmatic revival of medicine. To interpret this *'redite'* as regression, however, would be to misunderstand the ideological and programmatic connotations of this call to arms. To reconstruct texts, to decipher their contents by using humanist philology and to historicise the result was considered to be an extremely promising and progressively fruitful endeavour of medicine between 1480 and 1550.[44] In a sense, the philological approach became the primary scientific focus of a medicine which was eager for 'progress' and which sought – due to the language barrier that classical Greek represented to physicians – the support of humanists who were not physicians. Although this line of inquiry could only develop with considerable delay[45] and eventually turned out to be of little use as a primary branch of medical research, at the time, it nevertheless held out the promise of a much needed and widely called for moral revival and increased efficacy.

For medicine, Hippocrates provided the focal point for this effort to recover a wiser past as an essential step towards a more prosperous future. Humanists associated him above everyone else with the Golden Age of ancient medicine. Hippocrates was the father of medicine,[46] and while his standing and personal authority were generally reinforced by a mindset given to deference towards seniority,[47] his contemporaneity with Plato, who testifies to Hippocrates's existence and was himself crucial to the humanistic movement,[48] could only add to his credentials. Furthermore, Hippocrates was thought to have been a key figure in peripatetic philosophy⁴⁹ and humanists accorded him authority because all ancient schools of medicine, including – *ex negativo* – the Methodists and, of course, Galen,⁵⁰ had invoked his name. The Christianisation of his figure during late ancient times and the Middle Ages eventually also qualified him for appropriation by Christian humanism.⁵¹

The tendency to view Hippocrates as the origin of medical progress was also strengthened by cyclical understandings of history and by theories of degeneration. For humanists, Hippocrates, his works and his time represented the first peak (in the theory of historical recurrence)⁵² or sometimes even the only peak (in the theory of permanent degeneration) in the history of medicine. Furthermore, by applying theological imagery to medicine, Hippocrates was thought to have acquired his medical knowledge by means of a revelation that was directly comparable to divine revelation. Similarly, the figure of Hippocrates was constructed in analogy to the *Christus medicus* and he was stylised as an initiate of the Creator's will as manifest in unadulterated nature. Medical tradition was thus constructed analogously to the theological tradition which was marked by a hierarchical succession with God at the top, followed by the apostles who were in turn followed by the patristic elders of the Church.⁵³ Against this backdrop, 'Hippocrates closes the series of author–discoverers', whereas 'Galen begins that of the author–commentators';⁵⁴ Hippocratic writings acquired the character of gospel for physicians and were occasionally considered to be infallible canonical texts; the *Oath* became analogous to the Decalogue. In keeping with this analogy, the *Corpus Galencium* corresponded, for the field of medicine, to the exegetic work of the elders of the church and, from the mid-sixteenth century, became the target of 'medical anti-clericalism'.

An example might help to clarify this tendency to view Hippocrates as the origin of all medical 'progress'. The open enmity with which Vesalius' teacher, Jacques Dubois (Jacobus Sylvius, 1478–1555), greeted the publication of the *Fabrica* in Paris is well known.⁵⁵ Sylvius' charges against Vesalius included ignorance, ingratitude, arrogance and a lack of belief and piety.⁵⁶ Furthermore, he called his student a monster, a breath of the plague on to Europe and many other insulting names. Vesalius, the *calumniator* ('the distorter of the law') and *vesanus* ('madman') is presented as a dissident, while Sylvius flatters his own readers by addressing them as *pius* ('holy') and *candidus* ('pure'). Much like a prosecuting attorney or an Inquisitor, Sylvius demanded that the emperor punish Vesalius but that his students be granted amnesty provided that they returned to the guidance of their teachers (*praeceptorum suorum vexilla*) who thus far had taught them *liberalissime* ('most liberally'), *humanissime* ('most humanely') and *integerrime* ('with the utmost integrity, most justly'). Although the crucial bone of contention in this dispute was Vesalius' criticism of Galen, Sylvius felt compelled, as the title of his defamatory pamphlet indicates, to deliver an apologia of Hippocrates, whom he called *divus* and *divinus* ('divine').⁵⁷

The reason for bringing Hippocrates into this dispute in the first place was very simple. As a Catholic physician and professor, Sylvius insisted on recovering tradition as a prerequisite to ensuring quality in medicine. He aimed at unity of teaching, unity of science and unity of belief, to underscore his authority, an authority that finds its grounds in his self-proclaimed role as 'vicar' of Hippocrates and disciple of Galen. Sylvius thus tried Vesalius on behalf of Hippocrates, who is presented as the highest and quasi-divine authority of medicine. Having taken the Hippocratic *Oath*, Sylvius argued in his programmatic preface, Vesalius had pledged fidelity to Hippocrates and all his followers.

For him, the 'teacher' referred to in the *Oath*'s covenant of instruction stands, *pars pro toto*, for all successive links in the chain of medical knowledge and tradition. Among these revered teachers, Galen deserved the rank of an Augustine or Hieronymus, which is why any fundamental critique of Galen was tantamount to a breach of the *Oath*. Furthermore, under the precept of purity and holiness, Vesalius had sworn before the gods and goddesses to keep his life and his art uncorrupted. As I have mentioned above, 'pure and holy' are precisely the attributes which Sylvius, alluding to the wording of the *Oath*, ascribed to the readers of his book. Sylvius naturally linked this vow of purity to Catholic doctrine which, in terms of anatomy, was Galenic. Criticising Galen, thus amounted to doubting Church doctrine and sinning against genuine faith. In light of this charge, Vesalius could not even be protected by the fact that, in his work, he continuously referred to God as *opifex* ('maker'), *creator* ('creator'), *rerum conditor* ('founder of all that is'), *rerum Parens* ('begetter of all that is'), *fabricator membrorum et naturae* ('fabricator of the members and of nature').[58]

From a contemporary point of view, the theology underpinning Sylvius' argument[59] was by no means regressive. Considering Sylvius' past-oriented concept of 'progress', it is hardly surprising that he believed Vesalius' criticism of Galen to have missed its target completely. Sylvius attributed findings that differed from Galen's to editorial error or to the degeneration of human nature since Galen's day. However, it was not simply that Vesalius pointed out errors in Galen's writings that upset Sylvius so much; what Sylvius took issue with was the fact that Vesalius tried to promote medical 'progress' in opposition to medical tradition and that he sought to achieve it not by *permutatio* (transformation), but by *reformatio* (in the sense of renewal). For Sylvius the Catholic, salvation was anchored in Christ; for Sylvius the physician, the 'progressive' future of medicine stood and fell with following Hippocrates and Galen. His life's work was dedicated to, and focused on, a Second Coming of the Hippocratic–Galenic era. Regardless of history's subsequent verdict, his was a valid concept of 'progress' too, and one that was commonly held in the first half of the sixteenth century.

Hippocrates as the ultimate goal of medical 'progress'

If past-oriented concepts of 'progress' looked to Hippocrates, so too did future-oriented ones. From this perspective, Hippocrates was a forerunner who had set medicine on a certain course – a course which had to be followed through into the future; Hippocrates became the ultimate yardstick of technological, moral or social advance and a timeless figure predestined to serve as a contemporary companion to any physician. Again, a common metaphor might help in understanding this future-oriented Hippocratism: Hippocrates was regarded as the 'good farmer who first sowed this art'.[60] This, of course, implied that he had not yet harvested all the fruits that he had planted.[61] After all, his First Aphorism suggested a concept of 'progress' that was only taken seriously and set in motion in the sixteenth and seventeenth centuries. And the contrast between the brevity of life and the longevity of art, as pronounced in this aphorism, could only result in a concept of continuous advance in knowledge and experience.[62] This interpretation can be further supported by other Hippocratic writings.[63]

Hippocrates's reputation in Renaissance and early modern thought was further enhanced by his admission of fallibility,[64] which not only earned him the epithet 'φιλαλήϑης' ('the lover of truth'), but by which he also indirectly invited his successors to correct his mistakes, challenge him and even surpass him. He thus committed them to uphold truth rather than his authority. Sixteenth- and seventeenth-century writers therefore did not perceive the fact that their search for truth in the book of nature (Galileo, Bacon, Descartes) and in time (Bacon) contradicted Hippocratic teachings. The theories of the development of cultures and the concept of 'progress', tentatively outlined in the *Corpus Hippocraticum*, made Hippocratism appealing even to those progressive elements that were future-oriented rather than past-oriented. Hippocrates came to play an important role not only in the *Re*naissance and *re*construction of the ancient world, but also in the *Re*formation and Scientific *Re*volution. Or, to put it another way, wherever the prefix *re-* in its broadest sense took centre-stage, Hippocrates was sure to be waiting in the wings. The shaping of those parts of the medical profession that adhered to the concept of a past-oriented *imitatio* ('*imitation*') was thus as closely linked to his name as the emerging self-image of early modern physicians who relied on the more future-oriented concepts of *aemulatio* ('emulation' – that is, appropriation/ assimilation) and *superatio* ('surpassing the past').

Ultimately, Hippocrates and his writings served not only as both origin and ultimate goal for highly divergent concepts of 'progress', but also as the benchmark against which any kind of 'progress' could be measured. Whatever had been achieved at a given point in time was only put into proper perspective when compared with the Hippocratic legacy. This held true not only for Hippocratic philology, but also for methods of empirical or experimental verification or falsification of Hippocratic doctrine or the integration of

Hippocratic writings into contemporary natural philosophy, moral philosophy, anthropology and theology.

Thus, whereas for some Renaissance and early modern physicians the goal of medical 'progress' lay in a past to be recovered, other devotees of medical 'progress' began, as of the mid-sixteenth century, to direct their efforts and value judgements towards a goal located in the future. Humanists felt increasingly confident that they had come closer to the humanist ideal of perfection than their ancient forerunners. Theirs was an age in which new plants, new instruments, new continents – in other words, new worlds, even on the map of the human body – were being discovered, and they not only perceived the history of the world as having two peak points – one in ancient times, the other in their present day – but they also gradually emancipated themselves from ancient role models. The horizon of medical 'progress' was gradually beginning to expand, if not infinitely, then at least unpredictably, beyond the lost, but recoverable, range of expectations of Hippocratic medicine.

And yet this new vision of 'progress' did not necessarily entail a complete abandonment of Hippocrates. The physician from Cos still offered so much inspiration and guidance, and his writings harboured a wealth of further suggestions and ideas, without being explicit (unlike Galen) or systematic about the as yet unrealised potential of the medicine projected in them. Early modern readers approached the *Corpus Hippocraticum* with the full horizon of their own medical, natural-philosophical and anthropological expectations and thus exposed it to a process of assimilation and modernisation. In this sense, the *re*naissance of Hippocrates proclaimed by the humanists is more appropriately described as a *neo*-naissance,[65] albeit under altered historical conditions. The 'new Hippocrates' suddenly became a contemporary, providing medicine with Hippocratic impulses and giving it orientation and goals for the future.[66]

As the appellation suggests, the 'new Hippocrates'[67] was not the same as he used to be. Contemporary biographical drafts and representations of Hippocrates reveal the shaping hand of the respective biographer.[68] The newly created Hippocrates can therefore be seen to be familiar with all those contemporary medical accomplishments and phenomena which, in fact, had been completely unknown in ancient times. As had already occasionally been the case in the medieval period,[69] Hippocrates could now be credited with some of the 'progress' that had been achieved since his day, such as differentiations in the concept of the four humours and temperaments,[70] advancement in the status of medical astrology,[71] the introduction of new nosological entities,[72] the reintroduction of therapeutic procedures,[73] and new developments in surgical techniques,[74] to name but a few of the anachronisms contained in early modern versions of Hippocrates. Embellishments and attributions such as these, along with countless others, render Hippocrates prone to any number of rejuvenations that ultimately dehistoricise him and introduce permanent stylisations that typify an ideal. As a timeless ideal, Hippocrates is thus always just ahead of reality and epitomizes whatever the current 'progressive' trend proclaims as its goal: be it the power of eloquence or virtue, scholarliness or experience, the one proper method or comprehensive knowledge, genuine faith or true morality, Hippocrates can be seen to stand for any or all of these. In other words, the entire metahistorical dimension of 'progressive' thinking could find embodiment in the person of Hippocrates.

Towards a reconsideration of Paracelsus', Vesalius', and Harvey's attitude towards Hippocrates

On the basis of such a dehistoricisation, even the anti-traditionalist Paracelsus, could advocate adherence to the Hippocratic *Oath*. In the context of his critique of his peers, Paracelsus, for whom a physician's virtue was one of the four pillars of medicine,[75] wrote:

> That which the peasant likes, which you [doctor] know well, that's why you do it, implies that a doctor shall be dressed well, shall wear his gown with buttons, his red hooded cloak and a lot of red (why red? because the peasant likes it) and his hair nicely combed and a red baret on top, rings on the fingers, turquoise, emerald, sapphire, or glass at least; so will the sick have a faith in you. and the stones have such a splendid nature that they inflame the heart of the sick with love towards you; Oh you my love, Oh you my doctor! is this physick? is this iusiurandum Hippocratis? is this surgical? is this art?[76]

With words such as these, Paracelsus draws attention to the gap between the demands on, and the reality of, the art of his day. In his opinion, medicine was to be based on *philosophia*, *astronomia*, *alchimia* and *virtus* (or *proprietas*).[77] The Hippocratic *Oath* was part of the latter concept, which has since occasionally been classified as the most distinctly 'progressive' element in Paracelsian thought.[78]

As far as Vesalius is concerned, his *Fabrica* contains, among other things, a passionate call for every kind of dissection, thereby paradoxically energising the critical forces that had been mounting against the dissection of human corpses and against vivisection in particular, ever since the days of Herophilus and Erasistratus of Ceos. Those sixteenth- and seventeenth-century physicians who, in the name of medical 'progress', then championed such autoptic practices had to spend a great deal of time and energy trying to convince colleagues, authorities and the public of the validity of their work. Hippocrates or his writings could not, *prima facie*, offer much help in this future-oriented enterprise, since the 'anatomical knowledge in the Corpus Hippocraticum [is] extremely deficient, with exception of reasonably accurate descriptions of the skeletal structure of the limbs'[79] contained in the books on orthopaedic surgery.

Nevertheless, Hippocrates was frequently called on to legitimise and validate the moral and scientific purpose of human dissection, zootomy and vivisection; the debate that had flared up, particularly in the wake of the publication of the *Fabrica*, invoked Hippocrates as an important reference point and high authority, thereby accelerating the rate at which autoptic procedures would finally be accepted. Physicians such as Marcus Aurelius Severinus, Werner Rolfinck, Johannes Timme, Jacques Mentel, Johann Conrad Barchusen and Christian Gottfried Gruner further fuelled the debate by relating an anecdote from the Hippocratic letters, which, although primarily not concerned with anatomy, could be used as a vehicle for promoting dissection. In this anecdote, Hippocrates meets Democritus, who is dissecting animals for research purposes, and eventually convinces the physician of Cos of the usefulness of this endeavour. Ultimately, Hippocrates, who had himself never dissected anything and whose writings, as mentioned above, displayed an extremely modest knowledge of anatomy, became the standard-bearer of the practice of dissection, and the 'modern' proponents of dissection, animal experiments and vivisection enthusiastically gathered under his banner during the sixteenth, seventeenth and eighteenth centuries.[80]

Harvey, the last of the three warrantors of 'progress', took the principle of personal authority and seniority to its logical end and came to the conclusion that the objective authority of nature was the highest authority of all.[81] Nevertheless, his approach did not completely replace Hippocrates's authority. Rather, Harvey relegated Hippocrates to second place in the hierarchy of authority. In a letter on *De calculo renum et vesicae* ('On the kidney- and bladder-stone'), dated 20 April 1638, Harvey congratulated Johann Beverwijk (1594–1647), a colleague and relative of Vesalius practicing in Dordrecht, on having treated Hippocrates's and Galen's views with 'such reverence' 'that (if the knowledge and opinions of the ancient princes of medicine are not to be refuted so much as candidly explained) you judge them acceptable in a better sense.'[82]

Conclusion

This paper suggests that Renaissance and early modern Hippocratism demonstrate that the category 'progress' was not necessarily linked to an abandonment of traditions and their founders. 'Progress' was not automatically accompanied by an exclusive orientation towards the future or by a crisis of authority. In other words, the promise of the idea of 'progress' was not necessarily eschatological. A view of progress as linear and cumulative might encourage an image of early modern Hippocratism as a history of obstructionism in Renaissance medicine that could only be interrupted by such key figures of new medicine as Vesalius, Paracelsus and Harvey. A closer examination, however, reveals that the Hippocratism of the sixteenth and early seventeenth centuries should be considered as an integral part of contemporary medical concepts of 'progress', as well as the midwife of *nova scientia*.

Acknowledgements

I am deeply indebted to Leonie von Reppert-Bismarck, Alexa Alfer and Carsten Timmermann for their invaluable help with the translation. I am also most grateful to the Institute for Advanced Study in Princeton for making it possible to complete this article under excellent working conditions. My thanks also to David Cantor for his initiative and patience, and to Heinrich von Staden, Stephen Jaeger and Susan G. Lewis for reading the entire manuscript and their helpful suggestions.

Notes

1. On the history of this term, see Morris Ginsberg, 'Progress in the Modern Era', in Philip P. Wiener, *Dictionary of the History of Ideas*, 4 vols, New York: Charles Scribner's Sons 1973–74, Vol. 3, pp. 633–50; Reinhart Koselleck, 'Fortschritt', in Otto Brunner, Werner Conze and Reinhart Koselleck, *Geschichtliche Grundbegriffe. Historisches Lexikon zur politisch-sozialen Sprache in Deutschland*, Vols 1–8/2, Stuttgart: Klett-Cotta, 1972–97, Vol. 2, 1975, pp. 351–423; Joachim Ritter in collaboration with Günther Bier, 'Fortschritt', in Joachim Ritter and Karlfried Gründer (eds) in collaboration with Günther Bien, *Historisches Wörterbuch der Philosophie*, 9 vols, Basel: Schwabe, 1971–95, Vol. 2, 1972, pp. 1032–60.
2. Robert Nisbet, *History of the Idea of Progress*, London: Heinemann, 1980, pp. 104 and 118. For further secondary literature on the idea of progress from Antiquity to the Enlightenment, see Alistair Cameron Crombie, *Styles of Scientific Thinking in the European Tradition. The History of Argument and Explanation Especially in the Mathematical and Biomedical Sciences and Arts*, 3 vols, London: Duckworth, 1994, Vol. 3, p. 1776, n. 8.
3. See Hans Robert Jauß, 'Ursprung und Bedeutung der Fortschrittsidee in der "Querelle des Anciens et des Modernes"', in Helmut Kuhn and Franz Wiedmann (eds), *Die Philosophie und die Frage nach dem Fortschritt*, Munich: Anton Pustet, 1964, pp. 51–72, esp. p. 52.
4. See, for example, G. Sarton, 'The quest for truth: scientific progress during the Renaissance', in Wallace K. Ferguson *et al.* (eds), *The Renaissance: Six Essays*, reprint, New York: Harper & Row, 1962, pp. 55–76; Paolo Rossi, *I filosofi e le macchine (1400–1700)*, 2nd edn, Milan: Feltrinelli, 1971. The idea of progress has received much more attention in different fields. Compare E. R. Dodds, 'Progress in Classical Antiquity', in Philip P. Wiener, *Dictionary of the History of Ideas*, 4 vols, New York: Charles Scribner's Sons, 1973–74, Vol. 3, pp. 623–33; Wolfram Kinzig, *Novitas Christiana. Die Idee des Fortschritts in der Alten Kirche bis Eusebius*, Forschungen zur Kirchen- und Dogmengeschichte, Vol. 58,

Göttingen: Vandenhoeck & Ruprecht, 1994; Chiara Crisciani, 'History, novelty, and progress in scholastic medicine,' in *Osiris*, **6**, 1990, pp. 118–39.
5. Nisbet, *History* (n. 2), p. 104.
6. With its promissory character and orientation towards the future, this modern notion of progress represents the secular form of the Christian promise of salvation and reveals itself as being indifferent to history, reflecting the medieval Christian relationship to secular history. The same historical indifference holds true for today's concept of progress, where the past is always considered to be obsolete and surpassed or, at best, represented by the curious or antique.
7. Alistair C. Crombie, 'Some attitudes to scientific progress: ancient, medieval and early modern', *History of Science*, **13**, 1975, pp. 213–30, at p. 213.
8. Andrew Wear, Roger K. French, Iain M. Lonie (eds), 'Introduction', *The Medical Renaissance of the Sixteenth Century*, Cambridge and London: Cambridge University Press, 1985, p. xi.
9. Dodds, 'Progress' (n. 4), p. 624.
10. On this outdated picture of the three luminaries, see, for Paracelsus, Karl Sudhoff, *Paracelsus. Ein deutsches Lebensbild aus den Tagen der Renaissance*, Meyers Kleine Handbücher 1, Leipzig: Bibliographisches Institut AG, 1936, pp. 11 and 156; for Vesalius, Ernest Sigerist, *Große Ärzte. Eine Geschichte der Heilkunde in Lebensbildern*, Munich: J. F. Lehmanns, 1954, pp. 98–107 at pp. 104–5; idem, 'Commemorating Andreas Vesalius', *Bulletin of the History of Medicine*, **14**, 1943, pp. 541–46 at p. 542; for Harvey, Fielding H. Garrison, *An Introduction to the History of Medicine*, 4th edn, Philadelphia and London: W. B. Saunders, 1929, p. 246; Charles Joseph Singer and E. Ashworth Underwood, *A Short History of Medicine*, 2nd edn, Oxford: Clarendon Press, 1962, pp. 120 and 122.
11. Although the last few years have seen numerous attempts to demystify Paracelsus', Vesalius' and Harvey's role as forerunners of modern medicine, their supposed enmity towards Hippocrates and Hippocratic teachings has not been sufficiently refuted. For a demystification of Paracelsus, see Franz Rueb, *Mythos Paracelsus. Werk und Leben von Philippus Aureolus Theophrastus Bombastus von Hohenheim*, Berlin and Munich: Quintessenz, 1995, especially p. 320, where Paracelsus is demystified while Vesalius and Harvey remain the forerunners of modern medicine. For a demystification of Vesalius, see Juan José Barcia Goyanes, *El mito de Vesalio*, València: Real Academia de Medicina de la Comunidad Valenciana. Universitat de València, 1994. For a demystification of Harvey, see Walter Pagel, *William Harvey's Biological Ideas*, Basel: S. Karger AG, 1967; idem, *New Light on William Harvey*, Basel: S. Karger AG, 1976, esp. p. 1; Thomas Fuchs, *Die Mechanisierung des Herzens. Harvey und Descartes – der vitale und der mechanische Aspekt des Kreislaufs*, Frankfurt am Main: Suhrkamp, 1992; and Roger French, *William Harvey's Natural Philosophy*, Cambridge: Cambridge University Press, 1994. A clear characterization of Vesalius as a humanist adhering to Hippocrates is given by Richard Toellner, ' "Renata dissectionis ars". Vesals Stellung zu Galen in ihren wissenschaftsgeschichtlichen Voraussetzungen und Folgen' in August Buck, *Die Rezeption der Antike. Zum Problem der Kontinuität zwischen Mittelalter und Renaissance. Vorträge gehalten anläßlich des ersten Kongresses des Wolfenbütteler Arbeitskreises für Renaissanceforschung in der Herzog August Bibliothek Wolfenbüttel vom 2. bis 5. September 1978*, Hamburg: Hauswedell, 1981, pp. 85–95 at p. 88.
12. Compare Sudhoff, *Paracelsus* (n. 10), pp. 28–29.
13. Stefan Rhein, 'Melanchthon und Paracelsus', in Joachim Telle, *Parerga Paracelsica. Paracelsus in Vergangenheit und Gegenwart*, Heidelberger Studien

zur Naturkunde der frühen Neuzeit, 3, Stuttgart: Franz Steiner, 1991, pp. 57–73 at p. 59 attempts to illustrate the differences between Melanchthon and Paracelsus by pointing out, among other things, their diverging concept of Hippocrates. But this is one of the rare instances in which their mutual regard for Hippocrates allows them to agree. See also Robert Seidel, 'Caspar Dornau und der Paracelsismus in Basel. Schulhumanismus und Medizin im frühen 17. Jahrhundert', in Telle, *Parerga Paracelsica* (this note), pp. 249–63 at p. 249, who is also uncritical in his mentioning of Paracelsus' dismissal of the 'schulmedizinische(n) Hauptautoritäten' Hippocrates, Galen, and Avicenna.

14. See the recent article by Antoni Jonecko (with the collaboration of Gundolf Keil), 'Studien zum Dichterarzt Nikolaus von Polen. Eine Skizze des mittelalterlichen Arztes und Dichters unter besonderer Akzentuierung seiner "Antipocras"–Streitschrift, seiner "Experiment", der "Chirurgie" sowie seiner Verbindungen nach Schlesien', *Würzburger Medizinhistorische Mitteilungen*, 11, 1993, pp. 205–25.
15. Theophrast von Hohenheim gen. Paracelsus, *Sämtliche Werke*, I. Abteilung: *Medizinische naturwissenschaftliche und philosophische Schriften*, ed. Karl Sudhoff, 12 vols, Munich, Berlin: R. Oldenbourg, 1922–31, Vol. IV (1931), p. 494.
16. Ibid., XI (1928), p. 125.
17. Ibid., VIII (1924), p. 321.
18. Ibid., XII (1929), p. 476.
19. *Aphorisms*, I, II.1–5, III.76–84.
20. Udo Benzenhöfer and Michaela Triebs, 'Zu Theophrast von Hohenheims Auslegungen der "Aphorismen" des Hippokrates', in Telle, *Parerga Paracelsica* (n. 13), pp. 27–37 at p. 27. See also Lucien Braun, 'Paracelsus und sein Hippokrates-Kommentar', in Sepp Domandl, *Paracelsus im Blickfeld heutiger wissenschaftsgeschichtlicher Betrachtung (Ein Rundgespräch)*, Salzburger Beiträge zur Paracelsusforschung, 12, Wien: Verband der wissenschaftlichen Gesellschaften Österreichs, 1974, pp. 1–13 at p. 4.
21. J.-P. Pittion, 'Scepticism and Medicine in the Renaissance', in Richard H. Popkin and Charles B. Schmitt, *Scepticism from the Renaissance to the Enlightenment*, Wolfenbütteler Forschungen, 35, Wiesbaden: Otto Harrassowitz, 1987, pp. 103–32 at p. 104.
22. Walter Pagel, *Paracelsus. An Introduction to the Philosophical Medicine in the Era of the Renaissance*, 2nd rev. edn, Basel, Munich: S. Karger AG, 1982, p. 218.
23. Charles Donald O'Malley, *Andreas Vesalius of Brussels. 1514–1564*, Berkeley and Los Angeles: University of California Press, 1964, p. 71.
24. For Hippocratism and its exponents Houllier, Duret, Baillou and others see Ian Malcolm Lonie, 'The "Paris Hippocratics": teaching and research in Paris in the second half of the sixteenth century', in Wear et al., *Medical Renaissance* (n. 8), pp. 155–74. Vesalius studied under both Fernel (c. 1497–1558) and the Galenists, Jacques Dubois (1478–1555) and Günther of Andernach (1505–1574).
25. It might be noted that the counterseal of the medical faculty, engraved in 1274, bore the legend 'Secret. gloriosissim. Ypocratis'. See O' Malley, *Andreas Vesalius* (n. 23), p. 425, note 23.
26. Giuseppe Ongaro, 'La medicina nello studio di Padova e nel Veneto', in *Storia della Cultura Veneta dal Primo Quattrocento al concilio di Trento*, Vol. 3, Vicenza: Neri Pozza Editore, 1981, pp. 75–134. See also Nancy Siraisi, *The Clock*

and the Mirror. Girolamo Cardano and Renaissance Medicine, Princeton, NJ: Princeton University Press, 1997, especially the chapter entitled 'The New Hippocrates', pp. 119–45.
27. In the Fabrica, for example, he explicitly refers to De Articulis and to the Aphorisms. See Andreas Vesal, De Humani Corporis Fabrica Libri Septem, Basel: Oporinus, 1543, ff. 58, 66, and 538.
28. In the Fabrica, when discussing the different shapes of the skull, he agrees with Hippocrates that injuries of the temple muscles result in spasms, fever and delirium and are very dangerous. This is also the case with regard to the right ventricle: Vesal, Fabrica (n. 27), ff. 19, 33, and 602.
29. Ibid., f. 2.
30. Ibid., f. 78.
31. See the rejection of the cotyledons as described by Hippocrates, Aphorisms V, 45 (IV. 548 L.) and Galen, De uteri dissectione 10, 8–11 (II. 904–6 K.; 54 Nickel, Corpus Medicorum Graecorum (hereafter CMG) V, 2, 1) in Vesal's Fabrica (n. 27), ff. 539–40 which, however, in itself has an ancient tradition.
32. See O'Malley, Andreas Vesalius (n. 23), p. 395. For the most recent volume on Pieter van Foreest, see Hendrik Leonard Houtzager (ed.), Pieter van Foreest: Een Hollands medicus in de zestiende eeuw. Bundeling van de voordrachten gehouden op het symposium ter gelegenheid van het 25-jarig bestaan van de Pieter van Foreeststichting (Delft, 18. Nov. 1989), Serie-uitgaave van de Stichting Historia Medicinae, 3, Amsterdam and Atlanta: Rodopi, 1989.
33. Charles Donald O'Malley, Frederick Noel Lawrence and Kenneth Fitzpatrick Russell, William Harvey. Lectures on the Whole of Anatomy. An Annotated Translation of Prelectiones Anatomiae Universalis, Berkeley and Los Angeles: University of California Press, 1961, p. 181. For the dating of these lecture notes and the first mentioning of the circulation of the blood, see the introduction of the translators at pp. 6–11.
34. 'Finally, it was not without justice that Hippocrates in his book, De Corde, styled the heart a muscle, for it has an identical action and office, namely, to contract and to move something, in this case the blood contained within it.' Quoted from William Harvey. The Circulation of the Blood and Other Writings, trans. Kenneth James Franklin, New York: Everyman's Library, 1977, p. 107.
35. He thus mentions Epidemics VI, Aphorisms, On Joints, Prognostic, Heart, and Wounds in the Head in the lectures on anatomy, noted above (n. 33).
36. Gweneth Whitteridge, Disputations Touching the Generation of Animals by William Harvey, Oxford: Blackwell, 1981, pp. 287, 335, and 357.
37. Ibid., p. 287.
38. Hippocrates, Nature of the Child, ch. 13. Quoted from Iain Malcolm Lonie, The Hippocratic Treatises 'On Generation', 'On the Nature of the Child', 'Diseases IV'. A Commentary, Ars Medica II, 7, Berlin and New York: W. de Gruyter, 1981, p. 7. For Lonie's comment on this passage see pp. 158–68. See also French, William Harvey (n. 11), p. 323.
39. Christian Meier, 'Ein antikes Äquivalent des Fortschrittsgedankens: das "Könnens-Bewußtsein" des 5. Jahrhunderts v. Chr.', Historische Zeitschrift, 226, 1978, pp. 265–316. Enlarged and revised in idem, Die Entstehung des Politischen bei den Griechen, Frankfurt-am-Main: Suhrkamp, 1980, pp. 435–99 at pp. 469–84.
40. London, British Library, Add. 15697 (1443–1444), Astrological Misc. (in German) f. 30–50^v: (illustrating monthly horoscopes) Hippocrates (February); Galen (March); Avicenna (May); Constantinus Africanus (November). See Loren

MacKinney, *Medical Illustrations in Medieval Manuscripts*, Berkeley and Los Angeles: University of California Press, 1965, p. 134.

41. See Crisciani 'History' (n. 4), p. 139.
42. As far as the reconstruction of ancient worlds is concerned, it is typical that the first humanist to publish the entire *Corpus Hippocraticum* in Latin also belonged to the coterie surrounding Pope Leo X, who himself was interested in the artistic reconstruction of Ancient Rome. (Calvo himself created a transcription (= Vat. gr. 278) of Hippocratic writings; this manuscript then served as the basis for the translation written between 1510 and 1515 and printed in 1525 in Rome.) See *Archäologie der Antike. Aus den Beständen der Herzog August Bibliothek. 1500–1700. Ausstellung im Zeughaus der Herzog August Bibliothek Wolfenbüttel vom 16.7.–2.10.1994*, (Exhibition Catalogue Margaret Daly Davis), Exhibition Catalogues of the Herzog August Library, 71, Wiesbaden: Harrassowitz, 1994, pp. 39–42 (with further references). On Calvo's work on Hippocrates, see *Hippocratis (...) octoginta volumina, quibus maxima ex parte, annorum circiter duo milia Latina caruit lingua, Graeci vero, Arabes, & Prisci nostri medici, plurimis tamen utilibus praetermissis, scripta sua illustrarunt, nunc tandem per M. Fabium Calvum Latinitate donata ac nunc primum in lucem aedita*, Romae: Ex Aedibus Francisci Minitii Calvi, 1525; A. Campana, 'Manente Leontini fiorentino, medico e traduttore di medici greci', *La Rinascita*, **20**, 1941, pp. 499–515; for Calvo's biography, see Aguzzi-Barbagli, D., s.v. 'Marco Fabio Calvo', in P.G. Bietenholz and T.B. Deutscher (eds), *Contemporaries of Erasmus. A Biographical Register of the Renaissance and Reformation*, 3 vols, Toronto and Buffalo: University of Toronto Press, 1985–87, Vol. 1, pp. 246–47; Gualdo, R., s.v. 'Fabio Calvo, Marco', in *Dizionario biografico degli italiani*, Vol. 43, Rome: Istituto della Enciclopedia Italiana, 1993, pp. 723–27.
43. 'Humanist' is used here in the approximate sense of Roberto Weiss: 'the scholar who studied the writings of ancient authors ... searched for manuscripts of lost or rare classical texts, collected the works of classical writers, and attempted to learn Greek and write like the ancient authors of Rome.' Quoted in Richard J. Durling, 'Linacre and Medical Humanism', in Francis Maddison, Margaret Pelling and Charles Webster, *Essays on the Life and Work of Thomas Linacre c. 1460–1524*, Oxford: Clarendon Press, 1977, pp. 76–106 at p. 76. But compare also Paul Oskar Kristeller, 'Humanism', in Charles B. Schmitt (ed.), *The Cambridge History of Renaissance Philosophy*, Cambridge: Cambridge University Press, 1988, pp. 113–37.
44. See Durling, *Linacre* (n. 43), p. 77: 'Galenism at this period [i.e. c. 1480–c. 1520] was considered synonymous with progress.' In trailing behind this Galenism, Hippocratism naturally also received considerable momentum in the form of Galenic Hippocratism before the two schools drifted further apart during the sixteenth century. See also Ann Blair and Anthony Grafton, 'Reassessing Humanism and Science', *Journal of the History of Ideas*, **53**, 1992, pp. 535–40 at pp. 537 and 539.
45. Vivian Nutton, 'Hellenism postponed: some aspects of Renaissance medicine, 1490–1530', *Sudhoffs Archiv*, **81**, 1997, pp. 158–170 at p. 163. See also idem, 'Greek science in the sixteenth-century Renaissance', in J.V. Field, Frank A.J.L. James, *Renaissance and Revolution: Humanists, Scholars, Craftsmen and Natural Philosophers in Early Modern Europe*, Cambridge: Cambridge University Press, 1993, pp. 15–28 at pp. 16–24. The first edition of the Hippocratic writings was published in 1526 by Francesco Asolano in Venice. However, certain individual texts had already appeared in first editions, such as the

Hippocratic *Letters* in 1499, or the Hippocratic *Oath* in 1508 (1509, n. st.). For the *editio princeps* of the letters see Thomas Rütten, 'Zur Anverwandlungsgeschichte eines Textes aus dem Corpus Hippocraticum in der Renaissance', *Journal of the Classical Tradition* **1** (2), 1995, pp. 75–91 at p. 85; on the *editio princeps* of the oath, see Jean Irigoin, 'La véritable (?) édition princeps du *Serment* d'Hippocrate', *Revue des Études Grecques*, **112**, 1999, pp. 715–18. It is typical that the first texts to appear were intended to appeal to a broad audience including non-physicians. This means that humanistic Hippocratism breaks new ground in a manner that is comparable to the effect of humanistic Galenism. See Nutton, *Greek Science* (this note), p. 22, n. 31.

46. The fifteenth- to seventeenth-century propagation of Hippocrates as a Πρῶτος εὑρετής ('first discoverer') is largely to be credited to Celsus and Pliny. Celsus refers to him as 'primus ex omnibus memoria dignus' and 'vetustissimus auctor' (*De medicina*, Prooem. 8 and 66), and Pliny similarly wrote 'princeps medicinae' (HN 7, 123), 'princeps medicorum' (HN 7, 171) and 'primus medendi' (HN 26, 2). Both authors were well received by humanists and physicians as early as the fifteenth century; the *editio princeps* of *De medicina* appeared in 1478 in Florence and of *Historia naturalis* presumably in 1469. On Celsus' legacy, see Leighton D. Reynolds, *Texts and Transmission. A Survey of the Latin Classics*, Oxford: Clarendon Press, 1983, pp. 46–47; Danielle Jacquart, 'Du Moyen Age à la Renaissance: Pietro d'Abano et Berengario da Carpi lecteurs de la Préface de Celse', in Guy Sabbah and Philippe Mudry, *La médecine de Celse. Aspects historiques, scientifiques et littéraires*, (Mémoires XIII), Saint-Étienne: Publications de l'Université de Saint-Étienne, 1994, pp. 343–358 at p. 353; on Pliny's legacy, see Daniela Mugnai Carrara, *La biblioteca di Nicolò Leoniceno. Tra Aristotle e Galeno: cultura e libri di un medico umanista*, Florenz: Olschki 1991, p. 159.

47. Richard Toellner, 'Zum Begriff der Autorität in der Medizin der Renaissance', in Rudolf Schmitz and Gundolf Keil, *Humanismus und Medizin*, Deutsche Forschungsgemeinschaft: Mitteilungen der Kommission für Humanismusforschung, Vol. 11, Weinheim: Acta Humaniora, 1984, pp. 159–80. On securing medical knowledge in accordance with the theologically mandated principle of tradition or authority during the Middle Ages, see Gundolf Keil, 'Ipokras. Personalautoritative Legitimation in der mittelalterlichen Medizin', in Peter Wunderli, *Herkunft und Ursprung. Historische und mythische Formen der Legitimation* (files of the Gerda Henkel Kolloquium, organised by the Research Institute for the Middle Ages and Renaissance at the Heinrich-Heine-Universität. Düsseldorf, 13–15 October 1991), Sigmaringen: Jan Thorbeke, 1994, pp. 157–77.

48. See J. Hankins, *Plato in the Italian Renaissance*, 2 vols, Leiden: Brill, 1991.

49. Cardano, Champier and Melanchthon, to mention only a few, saw Aristotleism in such filiations.

50. The extent to which Galen's works are oriented towards Hippocrates was recently documented: Anargyros Anastassiou and Dieter Irmer, *Testimonien zum Corpus Hippocraticum. Part II: Galen. Vol. 1: Hippokrateszitate in den Kommentaren und im Glossar*, Göttingen: Vandenhoeck und Ruprecht, 1997. To this end, every form of Galenism brought with it some Hippocratism, albeit a Galenic Hippocratism.

51. Patristic literature mentions Hippocrates's living conditions and individual writings of his as well as therapeutic procedures (see 'Hippocratic straitjacket') that have nearly become proverbial. Furthermore, Hippocrates is esteemed as a medical authority, experienced therapist and founder of the school of the four

elements and *contraria–contrariis* principle (principle of opposites), although he is occasionally criticised for proposing the brain theory in the context of teachings about the soul as well as for his medical practices. See Tertullian *De anima*, 15, 3 (ed. Waszink, pp. 60–61); Clemens Alexandrinus *Stromata*, 2, 126, 4 (GCS Clement of Alexandria 2, p. 181]; idem, *Stromata*, 6, 22, 1 (GCS Clement of Alexandria 2, p. 439); Cyprianus *Epistolae*, 69, 13 (CC Ser. Lat. IIIC, p. 490); Methodius, *De resurrectione*, 1, 9, 14 (GCS Method., p. 233); Ambrosius, *De Noe*, 92 (CSEL 32, 1, p. 478); Gregory of Nazianzus, *De oratore*, 7, 10 (BKV 59, p. 218); Hieronymus, *Epistolae*, 52, 15 (CSEL, 54, p. 438–39); Nemesius of Emesa, *De natura hominis*, 4 (146 Matthaei); Augustine, *De civitate dei*, 5, 2 (CC Ser. Lat. 47, pp. 129–30]; Theodoretus, *Graecarum affectionum curatio*, 5, 22 (Raeder, p. 128).
52. See G.W. Trompf, *The Idea of Historical Recurrence in Western Thought: From Antiquity to the Reformation*, Berkeley and Los Angeles: University of California Press, 1979.
53. On the *Christus medicus*, see Ignatius, *Ad Ephesos*, 7, 2 (= *Die apostolischen Väter. Eingeleitet, herausgegeben, übertragen und erläutert von Joseph A. Fischer*, Darmstadt: Wissenschaftliche Buchgesellschaft 1956, new edn 1981, pp. 142–61 at p. 147); Ambrosius in PL 16, col. 307; Augustine in PL 37, col. 1708, 38, cols 495, 789 and 1270; Petrus Chrysologus in PL 52, col. 339; Maximus Taurinensis in PL 57, col. 502; Hieronymus Stridonensis in PL 95, col. 1430; Walafridus Strabo in PL 114, 258. As redeemer and saviour, Christ is not only declared a physician in a metaphorical sense, however; rather, he is also made the physician of the soul (Ambrosius, Augustine as relayed by Philo of Alexandria) and, as the incarnate Son of God, is comparable to Hippocrates, incarnate nature (see Flashar in *Hermes*, **90**, 1962, p. 415), whose domain is the body.
54. Crisciani, 'History' (n. 4), p. 125.
55. On Sylvius, see Gerhard Baader, 'Jacques Dubois as a practitioner', in Wear et al., *Medical Renaissance* (n. 8), pp. 146–54.
56. Meaning, in accordance with Cicero, *De natura deorum*, 1, 116 lack of *iustitia adversum deos* ('doing the gods justice').
57. These quotes were found in the following edition: Iacobus Sylvius, *Vaesani cvivsdam calvmniarvm in Hippocratis Galenique rem anatomicam depulsio* (1551), in Renatus Henerus, *Adversus Iacobi Sylvii depvlsionvm anatomicarvm calvmnias, pro Andrea Vesalio apologia (...)*, Venice, 1555, pp. 71–135, at pp. 73 and 133 *et seq*. On the dispute between Vesalius and Sylvius, see also O'Malley, *Andreas Vesalius* (n. 23), pp. 246–51.
58. See also Jackie Pigeaud, *L'Art et le Vivant*, Paris: Gallimard 1995, pp. 155–61.
59. See French, *William Harvey*, (n. 11), pp. 31–50.
60. Crisciani 'History' (n. 4), p. 138–39 with references to Nicolò Bertucci (d. 1347), Matteolo da Perugia (d. before 1473) and the introduction to the 1515 Latin Pavia edition of Galen's works prepared by Rusticus Placentinus.
61. Compare Falcucci's image of medicine as a tree 'in which there are at once flowers and fruits, some green and some ripe'. See Criciani, 'History' (n. 4), p. 131.
62. Ibid., p. 127 *et seq*.
63. See Hippocrates, *On Ancient Medicine*, 2, 12, 14 (1.570 sqq. L.): 'Many splendid medical discoveries have been made over the years, and the rest will be discovered if a competent man, familiar with past findings, takes them as basis for his inquiries.' Similarly Hippocrates, *On Joints*, 1 (6.2 sqq. L.): 'To make new discoveries of a useful kind, or to perfect what is still only half worked out, is the

ambition and the task of intelligence.' Quoted from Eric Robertson Dodds, *The Ancient Concept of Progress and other Essays on Greek Literature and Belief*, Oxford: Clarendon Press, 1985, pp. 11–12. But even non-medical literature ascribes concepts of progress to medicine; a good example is the famous choral music Πολλὰ τὰ δεινά in Sophocles' Antigone (vv. 363 *et seq.*).

64. See Hippocrates, *Epidemics* 5, 27. It is recorded in Apollonius of Citium, *Commentary on the Joints of Hippocrates*, 92, 26–94, 1; Celsus, *On Medicine*, 8.4.3–4; Quintilianus, *Institutio Oratoria*, 3.6.64; Plutarch, *Moralia* 82d; Julian, *Letters*, 59 d; *Subfiguratio empirica* 69, 17sq.

65. See Rütten, 'Zur Anverwandlungsgeschichte' (n. 45), p. 81, n. 29, who quotes the Foreword of Rinuccio d'Arezzo's Latin translation of the seventeenth Hippocratic letter. In this programmatic text from the early 1440s, we find the phrase: '*ab imis sepulcralibus excitatum*' ('conjured up from sepulchral depths'). In his 1518 preface to Peter Burckhard's 'Parva Tabula', Melanchthon also expresses the wish that Hippocrates might '*reviviscere*' ('come to life again'). See Petrus Burckhard and Philipp Melanchthon, *Parva [...] tabula per [...] Petrum Burckhard Ingolstatensem [...] quibusdam familiaribus scholiis et aucta et illustrata*, Witenbergae: In Officina Joannis Grunenbergii, 1519.

66. When 28-year-old Janus Cornarius (1500–1558) longs to be able to '*consenescere*' with Hippocrates – that is, grow old with him – then this wish implies that Hippocrates is also young, perhaps even eternally young. See *In divi Hippocratis laudem praefatio ante eiusdem prognostica per Janum Cornarium Zuiccauien. habita*, Basileae, 1529 (Dedication to Bonifacius Amerbach). In a way, reaching such a biblical age, Hippocrates crossed over the boundary of transience, and perhaps indeed succeeded in defying death itself; he underwent a transfiguration into an unaging god. This led Cornarius to ask Amerbach in the cited dedication whether Hippocrates was not more of a deity than a human. Here the Hellenistic epithet θεῖος becomes a complete predicate of divinisation. For references see Thomas Rütten, *Hippokrates im Gespräch. Ausstellung des Instituts für Theorie und Geschichte der Medizin und der Universitäts- und Landesbibliothek Münster (10.12.1993–8.1.1994) anläßlich der Eröffnung der Zweigbibliothek Medizin*, Schriften der Universitäts- und Landesbibliothek Münster, Münster: Selbstverlag der Universitäts- und Landesbibliothek, 1993, p. 26. For Cornarius, see most recently, Brigitte Mondrain, 'Éditer et traduire les médecins grecs au XVIe siècle. L'exemple de Janus Cornarius', in Danielle Jacquart, *Les voies de la science grecque. Études sur la transmission des textes de l'Antiquité au dix-neuvième siècle*, Hautes Études Médiévales et Modernes, 78, Genève: Librairie Droz SA, 1997, pp. 391–417; Marie-Laure Monfort, 'L'apport de Janus Cornarius (ca. 1500–1558) à l' édition et à la traduction de la collection hippocratique', Thèse de doctorat, Paris, 1998. Marie-Laure Monfort very kindly sent me a copy of her dissertation which is yet unpublished.

67. As such, the title of the chapter about Cardano's relationship to Hippocrates in Siraisi, *The Clock* (n. 26), pp. 119–45, is particularly fitting.

68. The recorded fragments from Isidor de Sevilla (c. 570–636; especially *orig.* 4), from the *Speculum maius* by Vincent de Beauvais (c. 1184/94–1264), from the *Vita omnium philosophorum et poetarum* by Walter Burleigh (c. 1275–c. 1346; ed. Knust, 1886, pp. 180–86), and from the Hippocratic *Pseudoepigrapha* were resynthesized into 'biographies' in the hands of such humanists as Symphorien Champier, Pierre Verney, Otto Brunfels, Philip Melanchthon and Konrad Gesner. The result is a Hippocrates who exhibits the qualities of a Renaissance physician in an avid age of discovery, a man who has encyclopaedic knowledge, is

cosmopolitan, well versed in rhetoric, philosophically trained and a duly appointed court physician – in a word, a man who displays contemporary characteristics. Franciscus Asulanus' dedication of the *editio princeps* of the Hippocratic works demonstrates the concentration of such a rendering of Hippocrates into the present day. See Beriah Botfield, *Praefationes et epistolae editionibus principibus auctorum veterum praepositae*, Cantabrigiae: e Prelo Academico, 1861, pp. 365–66 at p. 366.

69. In this fashion, in the fourteenth century alcohol distillation was attributed to Hippocrates. See Gundolf Keil, 'Der deutsche Branntweintraktat im Mittelalter. Texte und Quellenuntersuchungen', *Centaurus*, 7, 1960–61, pp. 53–100.

70. Thomas Rütten, 'Die Entdeckung eines pseudohippokratischen Briefromans als Melancholieschrift', in Juan Antonio López Férez, *Tratados Hipocráticos. Estudios acerca de su contenido, forma e influencia*, Actas del VIIe Colloque International Hippocratique, Madrid, 24–29 September de 1990, Madrid, 1992, pp. 437–52 at pp. 445–52; idem, *Demokrit – lachender Philosoph und sanguinischer Melancholiker. Eine pseudohippokratische Geschichte*, Mnemosyne, Bibliotheca Classica Batava, Collegerunt A.D. Leeman, H.W. Pleket and C.J. Ruijgh. Supplementum T. 118, Leiden, New York, Kopenhagen, Köln: E.J. Brill, 1992, pp. 168–87.

71. See, for example, Cardano's astrological interpretations of *Airs, Waters, Places*: Siraisi, *The Clock* (n. 26), pp. 128–31.

72. This is demonstrated by the example of chlorosis found in Helen King, 'Green sickness: Hippocrates, Galen and the origins of the "disease of virgins"', *Journal of the Classical Tradition*, 2 (3), 1996, pp. 372–87. A revised version of this article appeared very recently: eadem, *Hippocrates' Woman. Reading the Female Body in Ancient Greece*, London, New York: Routledge, 1998, pp. 188–204.

73. For example, letting blood from a vein near the afflicted organ while invoking Hippocrates. See Leonhart Fuchs, *Errata recentiorum medicorum*, Hagenau: Johann Setzer, 1530, f. 46^v. Siehe Eberhard Stübler, *Leonhart Fuchs. Leben und Werk*, Münchener Beiträge zur Geschichte und Literatur der Naturwissenschaften und Medizin, Fasc. 13/14, München: Verlag der Münchner Drucke, 1928, p. 193.

74. For example, in the case of cutting the bladder stone according to the new technique propagated by Mariano di Santo (1488–1565) in his *Libellus aureus de lapide a vesica per incisionem extrahendo* published 1522. Of course, Mariano di Santo did not ascribe this new technique to Hippocrates. On the contrary, his preface tries to reconcile Hippocrates's proscription against cutting the stone as outlined in his *Oath* with his own surgical practice. In this context, Hippocrates is not mentioned as an opponent to surgical interventions, but as a forerunner of those who managed to solve the technical problems inherent in cutting the bladder stone. The author implies that Hippocrates prohibits cutting the bladder stone out of a concern for quality rather than with a categorical interdiction. Since Hippocrates could not perform the operation to his satisfaction he preferred to refrain from operating on the bladder, but nevertheless stimulated his successors to develop an acceptable and efficient method of operation. Mariano claims that his teacher Giovanni de Romanis and he himself brought to a good end what Hippocrates had begun. Thus, Hippocrates is considered to be part of the team, so to speak, and can be partially credited with the 'progressive' achievements that eventually resulted in the Marian operation with the *grand appareil* or *apparatus major*.

75. Wolfgang U. Eckart, 'Medizin und Ethik', in Robert Jütte, *Paracelsus heute – im Lichte der Natur*, Heidelberg, Karl F. Haug, 1994, pp. 111–23 at pp. 115–16.
76. Paracelsus (n. 15), VIII (1924), p. 153.
77. Paracelsus developed his theory of the four pillars in his 1529–30 book, *Paragranum*.
78. See Eckart, 'Medizin und Ethik' (n. 75), p. 121:

> Das fortschrittliche Element in der Deontologie des Paracelsus drückt sich als ärztliche Pflicht zur Liebe der Arzneikunst aus. Diese Arzneikunst kann nur die erneuerte Arzneikunst sein, eine Arzneikunst, die gereinigt ist von den Irrlehren der antiken Autoritäten. Dieser Teil der paracelsischen Pflichtenlehre verfügt über keine älteren Traditionen und weist in die Zukunft.

Here it seems that a conclusion was reached too quickly, for Hippocrates was not only, as is shown above, in the centre of Paracelsus' deontology; he was also the predecessor of the Paracelsian 'Love of Art of Medicine'. See Hippocrates, *Precepts* 6 (ed. Heiberg, CMG I, 1, p. 32): 'For if love of men is present, love of the art is also present.' Translated from Owsei Temkin, *Hippocrates in a World of Pagans and Christians*, Baltimore and London: The Johns Hopkins University Press, 1991, p. 30.

79. Georg Harig and Jutta Kollesch, 'Galen und Hippokrates', in *La Collection hippocratique et son rôle dans l'histoire de la médecine. Colloque de Strasbourg (23–27 oct. 1972) organisé par le Centre de Recherches sur la Grèce Antique, avec le concours des Facultés de Philosophie et des Langues Classiques*, Leiden: Brill, 1975, pp. 257–74 at p. 260.
80. Compare Andreas-Holger Maehle, *Kritik und Verteidigung des Tierversuchs. Die Anfänge der Diskussion im 17. und 18. Jahrhundert*, Stuttgart: Steiner, 1992, pp. 56–59; Thomas Rütten, 'Zootomieren im hippokratischen Briefroman. Motivgeschichtliche Untersuchungen zur Verhältnisbestimmung von Medizin und Philosophie', in Renate Wittern and Pierre Pellegrin, *Hippokratische Medizin und antike Philosophie. Verhandlungen des VIII. Internationalen Hippokrates-Kolloquiums in Kloster Banz/Staffelstein vom 23. bis 28. September 1993*, Hildesheim, Zürich, New York: Georg Olms AG, 1996, pp. 561–82 at pp. 567–72.
81. See, for example, Harvey's response to Riolan's accusation in 1649 quoted in Toellner, 'Zum Begriff' (n. 47), pp. 163–64.
82. Geoffrey Keynes, *The Life of William Harvey*, Oxford: Clarendon Press, 1978, p. 272.

CHAPTER FOUR

The Chemical Hippocrates: Paracelsian and Hippocratic Theory in Petrus Severinus' Medical Philosophy

Jole Shackelford

The name Hippocrates, being associated with the literary remains of a flourishing school of Hellenic medicine to which Western scientific medicine traces its roots, is surely the most famous in the history of medicine. It designates a rational approach to diagnosis and healing and – perhaps most important today – it signifies the moral integrity of a profession that has a unique ethical status in the Judeo-Christian world. But in the past, Hippocrates – the supposed author of the Hippocratic treatises – was looked to as a source of medical theory as well as method, and this theory was to serve many masters. In this paper I will specifically address how Hippocrates was enlisted to support Paracelsian medicine, as Petrus Severinus expounded it in his 1571 treatise, the *Idea medicinæ*.[1] By so doing, I will reveal that the reading and reevaluation of Hippocratic texts was implicated in the formation of Paracelsian chemical philosophy during the 1560s.

The story of how Hippocratic medicine was shaped in antiquity by the great Greco-Roman physician and writer, Galen of Pergamon, and assimilated to a Christianising Roman Empire, has been told by Wesley Smith and Owsei Temkin.[2] Galen emerged from the European Middle Ages as the leading medical authority in the West; his tomes were supplemented by the work of Arabic physicians and commentators who extended his rational system of humoral pathology to embrace more complex pathologies and new herbal compounds. Hippocrates, inasmuch as he was known in the late Middle Ages, was largely Galen's Hippocrates. Then, as Renaissance humanists pored over and standardised the Galenic corpus in the fifteenth and sixteenth centuries, academic physicians sought to learn about ancient medicine and began to study the Hippocratic treatises anew. This attracted renewed attention to the antiquity of the art and detracted from the near monopoly that Galen's books had come to exert on academic medicine with the result that Hippocrates's authority was reborn in early modern Europe. Thus, physicians like Thomas Sydenham, the 'English Hippocrates', drew on the authority of the Hippocratic tradition, with its emphasis on making prognoses based on accumulated case histories, in order to promote the role of observation and empirical experience in medicine, in contradiction to an elaborate practice based on a Galenic theoretical apparatus, with its qualities and humours. But Hippocrates's name was also involved in the long-running debate between traditional humoral medicine and the chemical medicine of the Paracelsians and Helmontians, so that, in Sydenham's day, a 'chemical Hippocrates' – to borrow the title of Otto Tachenius' book – existed alongside Hippocrates the clinical observer and model physician and Hippocrates the forerunner of Galenic disease theory.[3] Indeed, as Temkin and Smith have observed, Paracelsus was largely responsible for causing medical scholars to suspect the validity of Galen's version of Hippocrates and to use other sources as well to begin reconstructing the historical writer or writers to whom we now attribute the Hippocratic writing.[4] But how Hippocrates, who had been construed to support Galen's qualities and humours, became a champion of chemical medicine has not been adequately explained.

Vivian Nutton located the resurgence of interest in Hippocratic medicine early in the second half of the sixteenth century, which Iain Lonie connected specifically with study of the *Epidemics*.[5] Nutton's chronology supposes that a Hippocratic revival was underway before Paracelsian ideas became widely known, beginning in the 1570s.[6] The Paracelsian interpretation of Hippocrates, in his view, was not a cause, but a strong stimulus to an already existing process that he called the 'emancipation of Hippocrates' from Galen's version.[7] Wesley Smith, however, perceived Paracelsus as a decisive figure in this story, but then skipped a century, to the world of Jan Baptist van Helmont, to whom he gives credit for finding support for a chemical reading of Hippocrates in *Ancient Medicine*.[8]

There is no doubt that van Helmont's work was very influential in seventeenth-century Europe, especially so in England, where Helmontian medical theory informed a whole generation of chemical physicians and experimental philosophers, from Walter Charleton to Robert Boyle.[9] Presumably, Hippocrates's reputation among the English chemical physicians was also partly shaped by van Helmont's vision of Hippocrates as a chemist. However, I believe that the great work of extracting a chemical Hippocrates, or separating him from the corrupt base matter of Galenism and exalting him as an important *priscus medicus*, had already begun in the second half of the sixteenth century, as scholars began to assess and assimilate Paracelsus' ideas. This view fits with Nutton's chronology and generally supports his analysis, but it may well be that discussion of Paracelsus' ideas was implicated in the renewal of Hippocratism earlier than Nutton's account allows.

Here, I will focus on the use of Hippocrates as a source of ideas and authority by one of the earliest writers to go beyond transcribing and publishing Paracelsus' tracts to actually assimilating the master's ideas – a Danish medical student named Petrus Severinus. In so doing I am following in the footsteps of Walter Pagel, who viewed Severinus as a founder of a Paracelsian neo-Hippocratism, which was nourished and sustained by Roderigo Castro and J.B. van Helmont.[10] As I will demonstrate, the basic framework for van Helmont's reading of Hippocrates was already in place in Severinus' 1571 treatise, the *Idea medicinæ*. Severinus' book was widely read and undoubtedly contributed to van Helmont's understanding of chemical philosophy, as it did to other medical writers of the early seventeenth century.[11]

Severinus' views were probably shaped while he was a student in France, Germany, Switzerland, and Italy in the 1560s, where he studied Paracelsian and Hippocratic treatises and discussed their meanings. This suggests that either Severinus was a lonely pioneer in the task of assimilating Paracelsian doctrines to Hippocratic readings, or – as I suspect – there was already an established intellectual dialogue about Hippocratism and Paracelsianism. His contemporary sources must await further study; for now, it is enough to establish how Severinus brought Hippocratic theory into agreement with Paracelsian doctrine – and why.

Severinus, Paracelsus and Hippocrates

Petrus Severinus was among the first generation of Paracelsians, those who went beyond gathering, editing, translating and publishing Paracelsus' manuscripts and began to synthesise the master's utterances into a coherent chemical philosophy. This process necessarily entailed a confrontation between Paracelsian ideas – which were Platonic, sometimes gnostic and couched in the language of miners, lay preachers and alchemists – and the scholastic Galenism and Aristotelianism that Severinus and his contemporaries had learned in the universities. The collision between the divergent philosophies and methods of the chemists and the Galenists resulted in a violent disagreement over medical education, practice and control of the profession that lasted for a century and a half.[12] But in Severinus' day it must have seemed as though bringing together the old and new medicines would produce a reformed method of diagnosis and healing, judging by the titles of the early treatises: for example, *De concordia Hippocraticorum et Paracelsistarum* (1569) and *De medicina veteri et nova tum cognoscendi tum facienda* (1571).[13] As suggested by its title,[14] the *Idea medicinæ* itself was ostensibly such a synthetic effort, drawing the best elements from Paracelsian, Hippocratic and Galenic medicine to create a framework, an ideal, for a new medical theory. However, it is quickly evident from reading Severinus' book that he was an ardent Paracelsian and very critical of received medicine. Although elements of Galenic and Aristotelian theory can be readily identified by the reader, they are not salient in Severinus' rhetoric, which repeatedly emphasises the chemical nature of the world and the basis of true medicine in a biological metaphysics that is unambiguously

Paracelsian and Neoplatonist. Yet Severinus did not see himself as a pioneer or innovator, but rather as a restorer of medicine, much as his countryman and friend, Tycho Brahe, saw himself as a restorer of astronomy, and Marsilio Ficino, 100 years previously, saw himself as restoring the true ancient theology.[15] For Severinus, Paracelsus was not so much an innovator as a wise physician who had perceived that medicine had drifted from its ancient moorings – its twin basis in the observation of nature and in divine revelation. And this is where Hippocrates comes in.

Severinus opens the first chapter of the *Idea medicinæ* with praise for the healing abilities of the earliest recorded physicians Asclepius, Podalyrius and Machaon – the legendary healers of Homeric Greece.[16] The fact that medicine was a very old human activity gave it a twofold authority. On the one hand, medical knowledge was handed down from very ancient divinely inspired sources, in an unbroken line of *prisci philosophi* that parallels the lineage of the *prisci theologi* revered by Platonist religious philosophers such as Marsilio Ficino.[17] In fact, the two lines were presumed to derive from the same very early sages and they represent a religio-philosophical view that can justifiably be called Hermetic, since, in the sixteenth century, this term was generally applied to alchemists, students of ancient theology (including the actual Hermetic treatises) and Paracelsian physicians.[18] On the other hand, the antiquity of medicine also implied an accumulation of knowledge, which gave practitioners a credibility that was based on generations of experience. This is not a Hermetic quality, but an empirical one, inasmuch as it is independent of any particular hypothesis about the origins of health and disease. This aspect of medical history, the discovery of causes by means of careful and collective observations, was also important to Severinus, as is evident from his words:

> There was great industry and concord among men in those times. Everyone openly brought his observations into the public eye. For indeed, they judged that the brevity of life was not at all sufficient for the perfection of the art, for coming forth with a collection of so many observations. On that account, these students, who were instructed in the observations, rules, and methods of their teachers, then added their own, confirmed the truth of the former, illuminated the darkness, and enlarged the narrow scope of natural philosophy.[19]

Severinus placed this eloquent statement of scientific method in the dedication to his book, where it would stand out as an ideal. We see in it a spirit of cooperation among researchers that better resembles the collective science of Francis Bacon's *New Atlantis* than what we normally think of as the closed world of the Paracelsian adept.

Severinus understood that Hippocrates did not invent medicine; the fact that he disputed competing methods, especially those based on particular 'hypotheses', as he called them, tells us that a plurality of opinions existed before him. However, Hippocrates was the first among the known ancient physicians to openly declare the principles of his medicine and leave his observations to posterity. Hippocrates rejected the 'hypotheses' of his contemporaries and established a method that was based on observation, case studies, and experience.[20]

Severinus must have supposed that a pluralistic, cooperative and empirical medical inquiry existed between Hippocrates's time and that of Galen, for he credits the latter with the desire to bring order to medicine by forcing it to become a 'geometrical' science that is derived from basic axioms, with the result that medicine was set on the wrong track.[21] In the process, Galen misread Hippocrates and used his name to lend weight to his own system, which was syllogistic (derived) rather than empirical in nature.[22] Galen's followers, including the Arabic physicians who inherited the Galenic system, also abused Hippocrates's name: 'they placed Hippocrates's name on their ignorance' and forced his words to submit to 'strange and violent interpretations'. Furthermore, they even used his authority as a weapon against the empirics, to whom Severinus credited the actual discovery of medicines.[23] So successful was this stratagem that in Severinus' opinion, the university-educated Galenist physicians had become nothing but 'heaters and bathers', seeking merely to affect the patient's superficial qualities; they were not healers.[24]

Fortunately, wrote Severinus, a chain of 'greater physicians and philosophers' brought the principles of true healing down through the ages. However, because they shunned fame and buried their wisdom in 'commentaries full of obscurities and riddles', these men 'remain unknown to the common people and to popular society'.[25] Thus, although public medicine – that is, university medicine – followed Galen's false lead, unnamed occult philosophers preserved and cultivated a true Hippocratic medicine which they left behind as an 'immortal seed' that will endure for all time. The inadequacy of Galenic medicine became more apparent as new diseases appeared. Because these maladies defied Galenic explanations, some physicians explained the new diseases in terms of occult properties and Hippocratic 'powers' which they reintroduced into medicine.[26] But it was Paracelsus who followed in the footsteps of the unnamed adepts and used their precepts to completely reshape medicine.[27]

Severinus' praise of Hippocrates as a proponent of empirical medicine fits well with what historians have told us about the renewed interest in Hippocratism around the mid-sixteenth century – namely, that study of those Hippocratic treatises that preserved case histories and an objective empiricism, which did not depend on a particular medical theory, helped reorient medicine. In a sense, this new advocacy of observation is in keeping with a more general trend, during the first half of the century, toward attention to natural fact, which was exemplified at the time by the anatomical work of Vesalius and Paracelsus' challenge to scholastic philosophy, which may be related. This change in attitude towards the methods of investigation ultimately helped lay the foundations for a natural philosophy that was based on experiment, which flourished in the seventeenth century. This particular approach to neo-Hippocratism –that is, as an epistemological renewal – has received scholars' attention because of its connection with clinical observation, which is considered an essential element of medical progress. The idea, I suppose, is that a public avowal of a scientific inquiry that is tied to no particular hypotheses freed early modern philosophers from the yoke of medieval scholasticism. This view of Hippocrates as providing justification for a methodological reform is supported by the *Epidemics* and *Coan Prognostications* and, as an ideal, found expression in Sydenham's empirical medicine, for which he was dubbed the 'English Hippocrates'.[28]

Severinus was also a proponent of observation and hands-on experience, to which the most oft-quoted passage from the *Idea medicinæ* bears witness:

> Go, my sons, sell your fields, your houses, your clothes, and your rings. Burn your books, buy shoes, come to the mountains, investigate the valleys, the wildernesses, the shores of the sea, and the deep hollows of the earth. Observe the distinctions among the animals, the differences of the plants, the orders of the minerals, and the properties of all things and the ways they come into existence. Carefully learn the astronomy and terrestrial philosophy of the peasants, and do not be ashamed. Finally, purchase coals, build furnaces, be vigilant and tend to your preparations without weariness. For thus will you come to an understanding of bodies and their properties, and not otherwise.[29]

This is Paracelsian rhetoric at its finest, and it also agrees with Severinus' reading of Hippocrates as an empirical observer, except of course for the part about building furnaces and tending them untiringly, which belongs to a later age.[30] However, Severinus also found in the Hippocratic treatises an ontological basis for Paracelsian medicine, and this, I believe, marks a departure from the interest Hippocrates generated among the Parisian physicians, which was more methodologically oriented and tied to study of case histories, chiefly in the *Epidemics* and the *Coan Prognostics*.[31] However, to understand better how Severinus read Hippocrates, we must first understand the fundamentals of Severinus' chemical philosophy.

A metaphysics for health, disease and cure

Severinus' genius was to organise Paracelsian ideas into a coherent natural–philosophical system; to place a mainly chemical theory of medical pathology and pharmacology into the context of a general metaphysics of existence and change. As an organised theoretical system, Paracelsian doctrine and methods could hope to compete with the prevailing scholastic medicine. Moreover, Severinus' system was better suited to a Christian physician than was the pagan materialism of Galen – at least, in his opinion. Without a basis in natural philosophy, Paracelsus' methods were doomed to the empirical fringes of elite medicine; with such an integration between ancient wisdom and new therapy, chemical medicine became a doctrine to be reckoned with at the highest levels of academic discourse. Severinus' *Idea medicinæ* was a key element of this effort to establish Paracelsian theory in the world of learning, and he can therefore be considered one of the founders of chemical philosophy.[32]

At the very centre of Severinus' philosophical system lies what I call his *semina* theory. Severinus believed that the visible world of bodies – corporeal existence – was an unfolding or manifestation of a divinely created and ordained ideal world. This supposition owed much to the Christian Neoplatonism of St Augustine, which was handed down through the Middle Ages in the Hexaemeral literature, where Augustine's *rationes seminales* (seminal reasons) enjoyed longevity as an explanation for creation.[33] Indeed, for Severinus and his kind, Moses was one of the early sources of natural philosophy, and a good philosophical system needed to accommodate or explain his account of the creation of the world in Genesis.[34]

According to Severinus, all bodies grow or develop from seeds (*semina*), which contain within them their predestined life and all the information necessary for their development. This is an ongoing process, allowing for the possibility of the future germination of long-dormant seeds, which would give rise to apparently new species.[35] Although Severinus did not draw specific parallels between his *semina* and Augustine's *rationes seminales*, he sometimes calls them that, and the resemblance is obvious to us, just as it was readily apparent to Severinus' critic, Thomas Erastus, soon after the *Idea medicinæ* was published.[36]

The ontological status that Severinus gives to *semina* is somewhat equivocal. That is, it is not unambiguously stated whether they are form or matter or some hylomorphic combination. Although at the beginning of the world they were dimensionless centres around which bodies would be constructed, they took on various stages of corporeal development, and even the most undeveloped of them might already have become subtly corporeal soon after their initial implantation in a dimensionless material substrate. The *Idea medicinæ* is not clear on this point, since Severinus did not relate a specific cosmogony, but *semina* are without doubt formal in essence, with their material nature supervening – or, more correctly, emanating – as a husk or vestment. Severinus indicates this somewhat ambiguous status by repeatedly referring to *semina* as the chains that bind the visible to the invisible, bodies to non-bodies.[37]

All seeds have cycles of development. The metaphor is clearly biological and surely owes its elaboration in Severinus' hands to traditions in natural history stretching back to Pliny and Theophrastus and before. *Semina* lie dormant until the time for their swelling and sprouting, which is predestined in them by the Creator.[38] At this point, the spiritual efficient agent, the alchemist or *archeus* within the seed, begins to draw in matter from the elemental *matrix* or womb in which the seed is located and sets about unfolding the divine plan by constructing the rudiments of a body. In general terms, Severinus' vision is an extension of Nicholas of Cusa's theory, in which reality is an unfolding or *explicatio* of potential that is enfolded in the seed, but interpreted in a biological sense.[39] When a form is unfolded it becomes increasingly more specific and concrete, and the range of its possible development is successively restricted until reification is complete. So it is with Severinus' *semina*: they unfold according to limitations placed on them by their predestinations, the elemental substrate, and various other factors until they achieve an individual body. And then at the appointed time, the body decays, enfolding and returning to its seminal potential, which is a state of darkness and chaos.

Severinus envisioned the actual developmental process as 'mechanical' and repeatedly refers to bodies as developing in a 'mechanical liturgy' (*lithurgia mechanica*) that is carried out by 'mechanical spirits' (*spiritus mechanici*) according to the 'mechanical knowledge' (*scientia mechanica*) or blueprint within the *semina*.[40] The generative process is therefore analogous to the way in which a technician or mechanic assembles an object from material resources and plans. However, although I would not rule out an intellectual filament connecting the *Idea medicinæ* to the construction of 'mechanical philosophy' in the following century, Severinus' doctrine is clearly *not* mechanical in the later Cartesian sense, inasmuch as, for Severinus, all 'mechanical' causation is fundamentally spiritual and powered by a non-material vitality.[41]

Seminal development or progression depends on the material and spiritual resources available to the *archeus*. Matter is dimensionless, passive and elemental; like Paracelsus, Severinus denied the Aristotelian elements an active role in generation – they are but containers for the seed. Spiritual resources are identified with the Paracelsian principles – namely salt, sulphur and mercury. But, at a more fundamental level, a vital substance is required that is variously called mummia, balsam, vital sulphur, radical moisture, quintessence, vital heat, among other names. This balsam is associated with the basic activity of seminal development.

The generative process, the mechanical liturgy of seminal explication, may be altered by a supervening form or impression that is brought by a hostile tincture. Such impressions affect the seed's growth plan or *scientia* and result in what Severinus calls a transplantation (*transplantatio*). Thus, he says, wheat is always potentially darnel (a weed), since no matter how carefully the farmer selects his seed, some darnel will appear in the sown field as a result of a natural transplantation, by which some of the wheat becomes darnel.[42]

Transplantation can be regarded as a deviation or aberration in the normal process of generation and is, in that sense, pathological. Indeed, Severinus defines some kinds of diseases as arising from transplantations that occur when a hostile tincture supervenes. This pathological process accounts for the existence of diseases in the world as entities rather than as physiological failures or privations of function that are induced by humoral imbalances, as in the Galenic view. Seminal pathogens, the seeds of diseases (*semina morborum*), arose after the fall of Adam, when morbific tinctures were introduced to some of the previously innocuous and harmonious *semina* that were sown into the cosmos at creation. All diseases, then, owe their origin to the divine curse.[43] This, however, does not explain how healthy individuals become sick or get well again.

Diseases have various causes, and I am considering here only those that are seminal in nature. Severinus himself recognised that diseases arising from external injuries were not seminal, although seminal diseases might supervene in the case of a wound, which is one reason why Paracelsian physicians must also be surgeons.[44] However, the *Idea medicinæ* is concerned only with internal disease. Some of these – hereditary or congenital diseases – arise from the sudden development of dormant seminal pathogens that have been a part of the individual from the beginning. Their growth might be triggered by environmental factors or they may merely have reached their predestined times for sprouting. In any case, their growth might itself be subjected to a transplantation – in other words, altered – which provides theoretical justification for the Paracelsian belief that epilepsy and other 'incurable' diseases could be successfully treated.[45]

More commonly, according to Severinus, diseases arise from the sprouting of seeds taken into our bodies in our food, drink and air. These may settle into various 'anatomies' (organs or tissues), sprout and begin to set down roots. As they grow, they send out supervening impressions and attempt to transplant the normal developmental processes of the body, resulting in dysfunction and symptoms. However – and Severinus is very clear on this – it is not the dysfunctions or the symptoms that are the disease, and a true cure will not merely restore function or ameliorate symptoms; to do that is to treat the effect and not remove the cause.

The success or failure of a disease can depend on several factors, including the number of morbific seeds present, how long they are present, the availability of a fertile field (an appropriate organ or tissue) in which to root, the resistance offered by the host, and whether the pathological plan is itself altered by a supervening tincture and transplanted. Therefore, the physician aims to cure the disease by fortifying the patient's natural vitality or innate balsam, by expelling the harmful seeds or eradicating them if they are already rooted, and by introducing drugs with tinctures that can transplant the pathogen's development by imposing its therapeutic impressions on the seeds of the disease. Like a horticultural transplantation, *transplantatio*, whether curative or pathogenic, is most successful when it occurs at an early stage of development.[46]

None of this sounds particularly chemical, but rather like an extended biological metaphor drawn from classical natural history and from many generations of agricultural practice and empirical medicine. But it is chemical philosophy, because the defining characteristics of seminal activity are chemical. Diseases and drugs have chemical properties or signatures that are observable in the laboratory and *in vivo*, and these provide a more certain indication of the inner, spiritual activity of things than do the 'empty qualities' of the Galenists – hot, cold, wet, and dry – and the associated humours – blood, black bile, yellow bile and phlegm. One does not observe bile in the test tube, but rather nitrosulphurous, aluminous or vitriolic salts. Furthermore, diseases affect not only humans, but all animals, vegetables and minerals, all of which reveal chemical signatures in the laboratory.

The chemical properties of diseases that are growing in the body produce symptoms that indicate their presence, and therefore the diseases themselves might well be classified chemically. More importantly, one chooses the proper remedy for a disease by finding a drug with the proper chemical characteristics to transplant the disease or expel it. Chemical drugs are especially well suited for these purposes, particularly if the disease is well rooted.[47] It must be remembered that Severinus, and quite likely most physicians whom we could call Paracelsian, did not insist on chemical remedies for all occasions. Chemical therapy existed as a supplement, or corrective, to an eclectic practice that grew organically from generations of practical medical experience.

Theory, however, was a different matter. Severinus' doctrine was quite incompatible with Galenic medicine on at least two fundamental points. First, it was not materialistic, like Galenic and Aristotelian theory in Severinus' opinion. Second, it wholly rejected humoral pathology and the qualitative physics on which Galenic physiology depended. Thus, when Galenists sought to 'compromise' with chemical medicine, it usually entailed adapting the chemical drugs to humoral pathology and throwing the Paracelsian theory out of the window.[48] Not surprisingly, Paracelsian attempts to compromise entailed coopting traditional methods, explaining them chemically, and throwing out Galenic theory – or at least the parts that depended on the four humours and four qualities.[49] Galen himself had elaborated and refined humoral pathology from its earlier basis in the Hippocratic treatises. So, how, then, did Severinus manage to recruit Hippocrates in support of a Paracelsian theory that rejected the medical importance of the humours?

Severinus' reading of Hippocrates

We might begin by establishing that Severinus was acquainted with Hippocratic medicine and its relationship to Galenism. He mentions 18 titles that are considered part of the Hippocratic *Corpus* today, and quotes – in Greek – from nine of them. Often these quotations are a few words or a short phrase, but substantial passages are reproduced in some cases, notably from *Regimen I*, which he referred to as *On Diet* (*De Diæta*).[50] I have compared several of the quotations from *Ancient Medicine* and *Regimen* to modern standard versions and found that they correspond quite well, especially when the major variants are taken into account.[51] This suggests to me that Severinus had access to a stable manuscript tradition or to printed texts at some time prior to finishing the *Idea medicinæ* in 1570.[52]

We do not know how well Severinus knew Greek. Melanchthonian humanism reached Denmark early in the second half of the sixteenth century, bringing with it an emphasis on letters. Ribe Latin School, where he was schooled, lay on the main overland trade route from Jutland to Germany and was probably influenced by developments at Wittenberg as early as any school in Denmark, which leaves open the possibility that he may have been introduced to the fundamentals of Greek as a primary student. He may also have learned Greek as an undergraduate at the University of Copenhagen, where he distinguished himself quite early in classical literature and rhetoric (pedagogy). The fact that he accompanied his longer Greek quotations in the *Idea medicinæ* with Latin paraphrases indicates that he did not expect his readers to command the language and suggests that he possessed sufficient reading competence in Greek to enable him to read the Hippocratic treatises in the original. In any case, his inclusion of these quotations attested to his abilities as a scholar and lent authority to his interpretation of Hippocrates.[53]

Severinus seems to have had a special affinity with two Hippocratic treatises in particular, *Ancient Medicine*, and *Regimen I*. After discussing Hippocrates's rejection of the qualities in *Ancient Medicine*, he referred to his own 'paraphrase on that same book of Hippocrates', implying that he had made a special study of that tract during his years as a student.[54] Since sixteenth-century scholars did not think that Galen mentioned this treatise, we can expect that it figured prominently in humanist attempts to distinguish the true Hippocrates from Galen's version.[55] But Severinus quoted more extensively and more often from *Regimen I* than from other sources, indicating its salient importance for his interpretation of Hippocrates. Although Galen knew of *Regimen I*, he considered it not to be consistent with other Hippocratic texts.[56] Severinus, however, argued that the books of *Regimen* should be accepted as legitimate since they were not listed among the pseudonymous tracts by Galen, 'and because they have the manner of speech usual to Hippocrates and contain doctrines by that same author'.[57]

Severinus did not quote Galen as he did Hippocrates, but that does not mean that he was unfamiliar with Galen's medicine. In fact, Severinus cited few authorities, and quoted only the most ancient sources – chiefly Hippocrates, with a couple of passages from Orpheus and the Scriptures here and there. He studied medicine for years, both in Denmark and abroad, and although we do not know precisely where he studied or what, it is inconceivable that he was not conversant with university medicine, which to a large measure was Galenic. In the *Idea medicinæ* he pointed to the obvious success of Galenic method and observed that it was therefore difficult for anyone to contradict it. Furthermore, it was widely known that many of Galen's ideas were drawn from Hippocratic sources, which were generally revered. However, Severinus also understood that Galen had interpreted Hippocrates, giving weight to the widely known *Aphorisms* and other texts that agreed with his own ideas, while disputing and suppressing ideas that supported the precepts of other sects.[58] Or perhaps Galen simply misunderstood Hippocrates.

On the one hand, Hippocrates had clearly written that man was composed of blood, phlegm and the two biles. Furthermore, he had applied the qualities hot, cold, wet and dry to these humours, saying that generation requires a balance of these, and that an imbalance, deficiency or surfeit causes disease.[59] In Book I of *Diseases*, as also at the very beginning of *Affections*, Hippocrates stated that diseases derive from bile and phlegm that are provoked by excessively hot, cold, wet or dry foods.[60] And in Book I of *Regimen*, Hippocrates 'is satisfied with fewer elements', explaining generation in terms of only fire and water, which are hot and wet, and therefore both moved things and nourished them.[61] However, in *Ancient Medicine*, Hippocrates wrote that all actions come from inner forces and not hot, cold, wet and dry, which in themselves have no power to cure diseases.[62] Clearly, Hippocrates had failed to express himself univocally, and Galen had opted to emphasise Hippocrates's statements in support of humoral pathology and the efficacy of the four primary Aristotelian qualities rather than his speculations about invisible forces. For his part, Severinus aimed to reinterpret these texts and set forth 'the true and genuine opinion of Hippocrates, agreeing with ancient philosophy and worthy of so great a philosopher'.[63] He expected that this would arouse opposition: 'I know that some who attempt to place the Galenic Hippocrates on an exalted throne will strenuously repudiate an interpretation of this kind to the extent that they can'.[64] However, in his own defence, Severinus claimed the freedom to interpret Hippocrates anew: if Hippocrates can be compared to Galen, he wrote, why cannot Galen be compared to Hippocrates?[65] In other words, why should we privilege Galen's reading of Hippocrates when we can read him for ourselves?

Severinus believed that Hippocrates was speaking loosely when he wrote about the role of the humours and the four elements in generation and corruption in causing and curing disease. In *The Nature of Man*, for example, where Hippocrates laid out the foundations for a humoral pathology, he admitted that he had not investigated the nature of the elements as deeply as medicine and the study of human nature demand.[66] Severinus concluded that when Hippocrates had indiscriminately applied the term 'element' to the humours, he was 'relying on the freedom and example of the philosophers' rather than speaking concisely, for 'it is absurd to confuse the notions of things and to assess the simple natures of the elements from the things that are compounded and heavily clothed'.⁶⁷ Implicit here is the idea that thick and obviously complex mixtures, such as the humours, cannot possibly be elementary. Hippocrates would never have called the humours 'elements' nor would he have attributed the four primary qualities to them had he foreseen the abuse of these ideas by posterity.⁶⁸

Severinus must have believed that Galen depended too heavily on this account in *The Nature of Man*, the genuineness of which he brings into doubt by adding 'or whoever is proclaimed to be the author'.⁶⁹ This is demonstrated by his announcement that he is presenting another interpretation of Hippocrates, one 'agreeing with the whole Hippocratic doctrine' and depending principally on the tracts *Ancient Medicine, Regimen I, The Nature of the Child* and *Diseases*, 'so that we can more easily observe the rashness of those who, with remarkable subtlety, have deduced the absolute definitions and properties of the elements' from *The Nature of Man*.⁷⁰

On the assumption that Hippocrates was being practical rather than philosophically profound when he associated healing with the addition or removal of visible substances, Severinus presented various passages in which Hippocrates indicated the real agents of disease and cure – spiritual forces or virtues (*dynameis*). Hippocrates identified these powers with characteristic flavours – namely, sharp, sour, biting, salty, bitter, sweet and so on – which Severinus associated with the chemical characteristics or signatures of substances.⁷¹ For example, when Hippocrates referred to the south winds as βαρήκοοι, νωθροί, καρυβαρηκοί, διαλυτικοί, it was not because they are hot and wet, but because they are endowed with the properties of opium, hemlock and other powerful drugs. And when he called the north wind ἦν δὲ βόρτιον ἰ βῆθες φάρυγγεο, κοιλίαι σκληραί, δύο κρέας φρικώδεες ὀδύναι πλευρέων στηθέων, it was not because of its cold and dry qualities, but because of its acetic quality, much like the properties of bar-berry and acacia.⁷² Hotness, dryness, wetness and coldness are not causes, but merely outward characteristics or 'shadows and companions of the powers, properties, and tinctures' that lie within, which expressed themselves as flavours, odours and other strong signatures.⁷³

In Hippocrates's ideas on the generation and growth of organisms, Severinus found support for his belief that an inner efficient acts on the elemental matter: 'Hippocrates described this divine administration of generation in a learned and deep explanation in his treatise *On Diet* [*Regimen I*]. There he also set forth the general nature of all generation and seeds'.⁷⁴ Severinus associated his own doctrine of seminal development with Hippocrates's statements of the role of the soul in directing the proper aliments to the proper places, a process that Severinus envisioned as chemical, involving separations and resolutions:

> He called these vital principles, radical tinctures, and mechanical spirits in which knowledge, life, and power thrive ψυχην, elsewhere θερμὸν, as in his book *Fleshes*, and here [*On Diet*] often πῦρ.⁷⁵

This soul, or heat, is the vital principle of the organic body, which 'flows' from it: by its virtue 'the elements and principles are mixed, increased, and changed from spiritual into corporeal'.[76] Thus Severinus interpreted what Hippocrates had termed 'aliment' (nutriment) to be elemental matter that is endowed with the tinctures and vital principles from which the rudiments of the body are formed. This agrees with Hippocrates's figurative use of fire and water as principles of action and nutrition, respectively, which correspond to the Paracelsian vital spiritual agent and passive material matrix or elemental womb. Severinus strengthened this connection by noting that Hippocrates and Aristotle both viewed seminal matter as merely a container for the actual seed, which is a spirit that thickens into husks and shells.[77]

In *The Nature of Man* Hippocrates said that diseases arise from food and air. Diseases that come with the air explain those cases where many people fall victim to the same disease at the same time, whereas diseases coming with food are responsible for individual or idiopathic conditions. He affirmed this in *Breaths*, where he stated that general diseases arise from air or spirits, and that individual diseases depend on diet. Yet, in *Diseases* and *Affections*, he wrote that diseases are caused by phlegm or bile that has been provoked by foods that are too hot, cold, wet or dry.[78] Severinus interpreted this to mean that Hippocrates thought of bile and phlegm not as causes but as 'wombs' for internal seeds, which Severinus associated with the spiritual *dynameis* or *semina*. For, in *Ancient Medicine*, Hippocrates divided the causation of diseases into two classes, ἀπὸ δυνάμεων and ἀπὸ σχημάτων, the former being associated with the exaltation of the humours. Therefore, bile causes disease not because it is hot and dry, but because it contains *dynameis* which cause disease when they are separated and exalted. Whilst it is true that this process is accelerated or retarded by hot, cold, wet and dry foods, and by other kinds of regimen, these are merely accidental factors.[79] Severinus found confirmation of this view in Book IV of *Diseases*, where Hippocrates explained that the elements were not mere qualities of the humours, but properties of all kinds, and in *The Nature of Man*, where he said that each humour naturally dominates the body at certain times of the year, and that different properties dwell within them – namely, the sweet, sour, bitter, sharp, and so on, the exaltation of which he claimed in *Ancient Medicine* causes diseases.[80]

By legitimising and privileging *Ancient Medicine*, Severinus elevated Hippocrates's statements about the inner forces or virtues, the *dynameis* within things, giving them priority over what he had written elsewhere concerning the empty and impotent superficial qualities of Galenic medicine. The former he associated with the Paracelsian *chærionia*, a potency, and the latter with *relollaceum*, another of Paracelsus' peculiar terms, meaning without developmental power or potential.[81]

Severinus credited Hippocrates with the recognition that dynamic forces and vital heat were implicated in generation and therefore also with diseases and their curing, and moreover that things vary in the degree of vitality they exhibit.[82] Yet he was unsure whether Hippocrates had fully understood the true nature of the vital substance, although clearly he had 'expounded its properties and characteristics', which are readily apparent in nature.[83] Later philosophers refined the concept:

> Theophrastus the Greek, the student of Aristotelian philosophy, touched on this matter in his book *On the Causes of Plants*, and he called it τὸ ἔμβιον τῆς φύσεως, the vital principle in nature, by whose virtue all things live and grow: the rest are dead. But Theophrastus Paracelsus, the pride of Germany, adorned this fruitful treasury of nature with many names: he named it Balsam, Mummy, Mercury, also Quintessence, Arcanum, Elixir, perfected matter, Manna, etc.[84]

Severinus asserted that the need for this multiplicity of names for one substance would become evident when he had 'brought the purposes of each ... back to the anvil' to hammer out their significance.[85]

Once Severinus had equated Hippocrates's innate heat with the Paracelsian vital balsam, it was an easy step to associate this quintessential power with the *scientia mechanica* or knowledge that governs the separation and exaltation of elemental matter, which he believed Hippocrates had expressed as 'the nature of man' when he was explaining how aliment is utilised by the body.[86] This nature or seminal virtue accounted for how bodies know to acquire what they need from foods, so that when a man eats bread it is used to make human tissue, but when a dog eats that same bread, it acquires nutriment suitable for generating dog tissue. Likewise, the knowledge resident in our bodies knows to separate and exalt matter suitable for the different kinds of tissues that are required in us.[87] Thus, Severinus found justification for his Paracelsian vision of mechanical spirits using innate knowledge to fashion bodies from raw materials in the ancient idea that the wholes contain the parts, and the parts the wholes.[88]

Specifically, Hippocrates had stated, in *On the Places in Man*, that each part of the body contains the whole – that even the smallest part contains all the parts. Severinus interpreted this to mean that each part of the body possesses the mechanical knowledge of the whole body and thus has the potency to become any part or all the parts.[89] This reading is further supported by Hippocrates's statement that the human soul is the principle of the body and contains within it the necessary equipment for the whole body. Since this knowledge exists throughout the body, it is obviously present in human semen.[90] Aristotle agreed that semen must carry the human form within it, but both he and Galen had, according to Severinus, put forth incorrect accounts of generation. Aristotle had claimed that the heart was fashioned first and then it nourished the growth of the other parts. Galen claimed that the three principal organs successively generated the three principal systems of the body. However, Severinus regarded both as 'falling short of Hippocrates and the truth', because they did not understand the mechanical process and the power of the innate knowledge. Hippocrates had said, in *On Diet*, that the parts of the embryo form simultaneously, even if they do not all become visible at the same time.[91] Severinus used Hippocrates's embryology, which maintained that the individual seed contains all the knowledge necessary to form a complete organism, to strengthen his general claim that all bodies grow from invisible *semina*. Each seed is a centre at which separations and exaltations are carried out, which he supports with quotations from *Regimen I*. Severinus refers the curious reader to Paracelsus' *Philosophy to the Athenians* for a fuller account of these processes.[92]

Hippocrates also wrote, in *Regimen I*, that nothing ever perishes, but that everything is just mixed and separated, an idea that readily lends itself to chemical interpretation. Also, he spoke of generation as a proceeding from the world of darkness, *Orcus*, to the world of light, *Jove*, or from potency to actuality.[93] According to *Regimen I*, generation and corruption are an alternation between *Orcus* and *Jove*, and this holds true for all things, even the sun and the moon, which gives Severinus an opportunity to suggest that even the celestial bodies are not immune to change.[94] This basic concept, that beings never die but undergo cyclical changes between a state of pure spirit – a potential body – and a fully realised corporeal individual, underlies the whole of Severinus' doctrine. He frequently referred to the state of potency as *Orcus*, which he also equated with Orpheus' 'Night' (non-existence) and with Paracelsus' terms '*Iliadus*' and '*Iliaster*', all of which are the same as 'natural seminal reasons'.[95] This is not to say that a *particular* individual is reborn again and again, but rather that its essential being, which is connected with its species, remains in the 'root' of the individual – namely in the *ratio seminalis*. Severinus supported this assertion with an appeal to 'horror vacui', which would prevent an entire species from becoming extinct, and with a quotation from *The Nature of Man*.[96]

Severinus explained the generation of bodies from *semina* in agricultural terms: the individual seed requires a period of dormancy, during which it ferments, if it is to sprout and be fruitful. He interpreted Hippocrates's account of how a single seed can produce a man, in *The Nature of the Child*, as supporting this theory.[97] The fermentation, or spiritual activity, within the dormant seed resembles what Hippocrates regarded as the 'skillful dispensation of generation' that is carried out in the stillness of night by craftsmen who work in silence.[98] For Severinus, this process applied to diseases as well: when the *semina morborum* sprout, they cause symptoms to become manifest, as, Severinus claimed, Hippocrates had implied in *Aphorisms*, where he discussed weariness, loss of appetite and so on, as signs of illness.[99]

Specific Paracelsian doctrines

In the course of laying out the fundamentals of his medical philosophy, Severinus found support for particular ideas and doctrines that scholars today closely associate with Paracelsus and Paracelsian medicine, and these are worth noting here, inasmuch as they shed light on how Severinus implicated Hippocratic medicine as a basis for chemical medicine. One such concept that serves as a hallmark of Paracelsian medicine is the therapeutic preference for treating a disease with a remedy that has similar characteristics (*similia similibus*), rather than trying to restore a patient's qualitative and humoral balance by means of a contrary medication (*contraria contrariis*). These methods are not diametrically opposed, because *similia* refers to a similarity between manifest characteristics of drug and disease, thereby indicating a similarity in their spiritual essences, whereas the Galenic indication presumes that the actual qualities of the drug will alter the qualities of the patient. The former view is based on a semiological view, in which the chemical characteristics are taken as signs of the underlying spiritual powers, which are the true agents of disease and cure, and the latter assumes no such occult virtues but instead presupposes a simple arithmetic of matter and form: if a problem is caused by an excess, the solution is to subtract, but if it is caused by a deficiency, the solution is to add. The latter view led the Galenists to establish an elaborate system of identifying *materia medica* by qualitative compositions and degrees. Thus, whether to cure by similars or by contraries becomes a kind of code for two distinct ontologies, rather than merely denoting competing therapeutic choices. That is, a Paracelsian and Galenist might choose the same drug in a given situation, but ascribe that choice to different methods, the one identifying it as having signatures similar to those of the disease essence, the other classifying it as having qualities that are contrary to those that define the disease. The eclecticism of Paracelsian physicians, like Severinus, who used Galenic and Paracelsian methods and presumably explained Galenic cures in terms of chemical philosophy, suggests that, in many cases, the differences were theoretical and ideological rather than practical.[100]

For Severinus, however, the choices and meanings were not so clear, and true healing could be viewed in terms of both *similia similibus* and *contraria contrariis*, both of which he considered to be expounded by Hippocrates. Severinus claimed that his approach maintains the 'Oracle' of Hippocrates, since he aimed to cure both by removing the pathological impurities that contain the *semina morborum*, which might be construed as removing an excess, and by restoring the body's innate forces and vital balsam, which is to correct a deficiency. However, he was adamant that this is not to be explained by augmenting or diminishing hotness or any other of the 'dead qualities', in which there is no Hippocratic *dynameis* or Paracelsian *chærionia*.[101]

Hippocrates had indeed advocated curing with contraries, as when he said in

Breaths that hunger is a disease and that food is the cure. Severinus interpreted this to mean that, inasmuch as remedies are aliments and restore deficiencies in the inner balsam by means of their spiritual tinctures, they are contraries.[102] But here Paracelsian and Hippocratic doctrine are in agreement. Hippocrates identified an aliment as that which nourishes; but a substance that has been separated, digested, matured and changed into 'spiritual vapours' provides nourishment for the vital spirits, for we are what we eat, and inasmuch as we are spiritual, we are nourished by spirits.[103] Therefore, Paracelsus' claim that similars cure similars does not conflict with Hippocrates, since it was established earlier that nutriment or aliment is the same as that which is nourished:

> For this reason, when Paracelsus says that similars are cured by similars, he does not rave, he does not speak foolishly, but thinks correctly and speaks philosophically: he does not oppose Hippocrates [who said] ... that contraries are the remedies for contraries.[104]

But Paracelsus did oppose Galen who applied the theory of *contraria contrariis* to 'mere qualities' which were 'condemned by Hippocrates in his book *Ancient Medicine*'![105] Severinus, in effect, understood that the real issue was not how one interpreted *similia* and *contraria*, but rather whether or not the primary qualities were considered reliable indicators for the true natures of diseases and drugs.

Another characteristic idea of Paracelsian philosophy is that active agents are 'astral' in some sense – an idea that is embodied in Paracelsus' concept of *astrum* and an astral body that exists with or within the elemental body.[106] Severinus interpreted Paracelsus to mean that there are 'stars' everywhere in the cosmos, including in man. The defining characteristic of 'stars' in Severinus' philosophy is that they exhibit cyclical behaviour. Therefore, the 'stars' within man also have revolutions that govern his cyclical nature and the 'stars' within diseases account for their particular timings. Indeed, the physician might attempt to alter the course of a disease by imposing a tincture on it and transplanting its timing.

Severinus claimed, in the *Idea medicinæ*, that 'Hippocrates has adduced these resolutions of the stars in human physiology before us', and pointed to a quotation from *Dreams* (*Regimen IV*) that identifies the circuit of the fixed stars with man's extremities, the circuit of the sun with the middle, and that of the moon with the abdomen. By middle, Hippocrates meant the heart, brain and blood, where there are purer, more stable motions that imitate the nature of the sun. The cycles of the synovia (fluids in the joints), muscles, ligaments, bones and so on have slower development, imitating the stars. Abdominal cycles are faster, more like the moon.[107] Hippocrates affirmed this theory in *On Diet* (*Regimen I*), where he said that the nature of fire has a threefold circuit in the generation of man, which Severinus quoted.[108] It is clear from this account that

Severinus identified the correspondences between stars and various parts of the human body – a widely known Hermetic idea that Robert Fludd exhibited with a famous illustration showing a human body superimposed on a Ptolemaic cosmos – as a legitimately Hippocratic concept.[109] Severinus adapted this idea to his Paracelsian theory: astral diseases are characterised by long periods of inactivity, but the *semina* in the stomach and intestines, which have taken on thicker, more corporeal vestments, have shorter periods and faster cycles, like the moon, as Hippocrates said.[110] Hippocrates had adduced these correspondences to explain the correlation of the onset and remission of certain diseases with the seasons.[111] Severinus illuminated this by quoting from *Humors* to defend the idea that if one has observed the correlation between weather and the celestial risings and settings and diseases, one can predict it.[112] In *Epidemics* Hippocrates had associated the timings of diseases with the 'intemperate resolutions of the stars'. Severinus explained this as occurring from 'celestial impressions' or 'fruits' which cause diseases not by heating, moistening, cooling or drying, but by introducing chemical properties that cause diseases.[113]

The cycles exhibited by all things are also connected with the *semina* in Severinus' philosophy, and in fact *semina* and *astra* are often spoken of similarly. He noted that there are certain appointed times of growth and decay for all things, which Hippocrates had called τὴν πεπρωμένην μοίρην, and Paracelsus referred to as their predestined or appointed times.[114] Severinus in fact claimed that Paracelsus had got the idea that *semina* contain divine 'predestinations', by which the laws of development are implanted in the very essence of nature, from Hippocrates and Orpheus who had said that the development of all seeds is propelled by divine necessity, as if they are 'furnished with the laws of the fates'.[115] Thus Severinus found support for his idea that *semina* are the loci for divine predestination – a basically Augustinian idea – in the ancient authority of Hippocrates and Orpheus.[116]

Unlike the peripatetics, who followed Aristotle in dividing the world into two distinct realms – the sublunary containing the four terrestrial elements and the superlunary filled with a fifth element – Severinus permitted quintessence to exist everywhere, as the vital balsam or *astra* in things. He lumped the four terrestrial elemental zones into two homocentric spheres – an inner sphere consisting of earth and water and an outer one containing air and fire, encompassing also the celestial bodies. Severinus claimed that humans are nourished by both regions, inasmuch as we take in spirits with the air we breathe, as well as earth and water in our corporeal foods. In support, Severinus cited *Breaths*, where Hippocrates pointed out that inhaling spirit is necessary for life.[117]

Part of Severinus' objection to the Galenic theory of disease as a qualitative imbalance involved his belief that names should bear a relationship to the things they denote – that they should capture something of the essences of the things themselves. The fact that he wrote a tract on this subject as a student suggests that consideration of realism and nominalism helped persuade him that a chemical nomenclature was suitable to describe the inner, active virtues of things.[118] He supports this idea in the *Idea medicinæ* by referring to Hippocrates's *Nutriment* (*De alimento*), which states that something cannot be called an aliment unless it nourishes – that is, that words must relate to actions.[119] Severinus generalised Hippocrates's definition of certain diseases as ἀπὸ δυνάμεων to mean that diseases should be named according to the chemical properties they exhibit,[120] thereby, locating precedents for a chemical nomenclature as well as the underlying chemical operation of nature in Hippocratic treatises. By assigning weight to passages that seemed to agree with his understanding of Paracelsian medicine, Severinus was able to fashion a *chemical* Hippocrates who had grasped the true nature of causes before Galen obscured them.

Conclusion

From the evidence presented above it is clear that Severinus quoted Hippocratic treatises to clarify and support the medical philosophy that he put forth in the *Idea medicinæ*, which was largely based on Paracelsus' theories. This use of Hippocrates's name served an intentional, rhetorical purpose. That he expected Hippocrates's authority to help mute criticism of his ideas by those who were antagonistic to Paracelsus is clear from Chapter VIII, where he expounded his doctrine of generation:

> These theories are Paracelsian, they are not inconsistent with Christian religion, and they are close to the decrees of the Platonists. But if they have been supported by the authority of Hippocrates, who can accuse them of novelty?[121]

However, Severinus also believed that there was a genuine 'consensus of Hippocrates and the ancient philosophers' with Paracelsus' ideas as he had expressed them in the *Idea medicinæ*.[122] I believe that it was Severinus' underlying commitment to shaping a new medicine that could address the new diseases of early modern Europe, incorporate the chemically prepared 'Paracelsian' drugs that had proven themselves effective in the hands of empirical practitioners, and better conform to the religious and philosophical reforms of the Age of Reformation, that motivated him and like-minded contemporaries to oppose what he called the 12 centuries of medical tradition. In other words, for a small group of medical writers and practitioners, Paracelsus and Hippocrates were part of a reformation of medical theory and practice that Pagel has labelled 'a Paracelsian neo-Hippocratism'.

Severinus' place within this movement is plain: he made a solid link between

Hippocratic *dynameis* and the seminal forces that manifest themselves as chemical properties. Furthermore, it is likely that those who later interpreted Hippocrates as a chemical philosopher were influenced by the *Idea medicinæ* and accepted Severinus' legitimation and prioritisation of the views expressed in *Ancient Medicine* and *Regimen* and other tracts that mentioned the *dynameis* as active principles. The English Paracelsian, Thomas Moffet, must be numbered among these. The title of his *Nosomantica Hippocratea* (Frankfurt, 1584) itself reveals his reverence for Hippocratic medicine. Moffet had met Severinus in Denmark and was sufficiently impressed by him and his philosophy to dedicate his *De iure et præstantia chymicorum medicamentorum*, a Latin defence of Paracelsus and iatrochemistry, to the Dane and to request his help in refuting the claims of the anti-Paracelsians.[123] Nevertheless, this does not prove that Moffet was first persuaded by the new Hippocratism by reading the *Idea medicinæ*. He was educated in southern Germany and Switzerland, where interest in Hippocratism was established early, and he may have been affected by the same intellectual forces and lines of inquiry that caused Severinus to closely study the Hippocratic treatises.[124] One of the medical professors at Basel who supported Moffet's PhD, Theodor Zwinger, was himself interested in both Hippocratic and Paracelsian medicine and corresponded with Severinus about his ideas.[125] Further examination of this milieu may reveal a discussion about Hippocrates in and around the universities and among learned humanist physicians in northern Italy, France, and particularly the German–Swiss area, during the 1550s and 1560s that provides a context for the emergence of Severinus' ideas. The analysis of the *Idea medicinæ* presented here establishes that a reinterpretation of Hippocrates in terms amenable to Paracelsian chemical philosophy was already well underway by the late 1560s – perhaps further study will discover that attempts to understand and assimilate Paracelsus' ideas were more intimately connected with the process of distinguishing the 'true' Hippocrates from Galen's Hippocrates than has been hitherto suggested.

Finally, I would speculate that the process that led to a new, chemical understanding of Hippocrates was not just motivated by the desire of humanists to reform medicine, but was embedded in the great moral and religious conversations that occupied the European intelligentsia in the wake of Luther's Reformation. Owsei Temkin, in his thoughtful analysis of Hippocratic medicine and its relationship to pagan and Christian mentalities, has emphasised that the Hippocratic writings are built around a world-view that invests nature with divine powers and relegates the physician to the role of a minister who assists the natural processes. I suspect that this feature of Hippocratic thought was attractive to the Paracelsians and other proponents of Renaissance naturalism. This would explain their desire to create philosophical and medical systems that were agreeable to the Mosaic account of creation, which began with the divine infusion of ideas into matter and the predestination of the natural world.[126] Thus, the Paracelsians' search for an integrated theology and chemical philosophy led them to reread and interpret the old philosophers and to re-create Hippocrates as a chemical physician.

Notes:

1. Petrus Severinus, *Idea medicinæ philosophicæ fundamenta continens totius doctrinæ Paracelsicæ, Hippocraticæ et Galenicæ*, Basel: Henric Petri, 1571.
2. Wesley D. Smith, *The Hippocratic Tradition*, Ithaca, NY: Cornell University Press, 1979; also Owsei Temkin, *Hippocrates in a World of Pagans and Christians*, Baltimore: Johns Hopkins University Press, 1991.
3. Otto Tachenius, *Hippocrates Chymicus*, Venice, 1669.
4. Owsei Temkin, *Galenism: The Rise and Decline of a Medical Philosophy*, Ithaca, NY: Cornell University Press, 1973; also Smith, *The Hippocratic Tradition* (n. 2), especially pp. 17 ff.
5. Vivian Nutton, 'Hippocrates in the Renaissance', in *Die Hippokratischen Epidemien: Theorie–Praxis–Tradition: Verhandlungen des Ve Colloque International Hippocratique, Sudhoffs Archiv* Beihefte 27, Stuttgart: Franz Steiner, 1989, pp. 420–39; also Iain M. Lonie, 'The "Paris Hippocratics": teaching and research in Paris in the second half of the sixteenth century', in Andrew Wear, R.K. French and I.M. Lonie (eds), *The Medical Renaissance of the Sixteenth Century*, Cambridge: Cambridge University Press, 1985, pp. 155–74 and 318–26.
6. Nutton, 'Hippocrates in the Renaissance' (n. 5), p. 435: 'Paracelsus can hardly be the cause, or even the catalyst, for his writings had little influence before the 1570s.'
7. Ibid., p. 421.
8. Smith, *The Hippocratic Tradition* (n. 2), p. 17.
9. See P.M. Rattansi, 'The Helmontian–Galenist controversy in Restoration England', *Ambix*, 12, 1964, pp. 1–23. Recent studies of Robert Boyle and his contemporaries have revealed the influence of van Helmont's theory on mid-century matter theory. See Barbara Beigun Kaplan, *'Divulging of Useful Truths in Physick.' The Medical Agenda of Robert Boyle*, Baltimore: Johns Hopkins University Press, 1993; William R. Newman, 'The corpuscular transmutational theory of Eirenaeus Philalethes', and Antonio Clericuzio, 'The internal laboratory. The chemical reinterpretation of medical spirits in England (1650–1680)', in P.M. Rattansi and Antonino Clericuzio (eds), *Alchemy and Chemistry in the 16th and 17th Centuries*, Dordrecht: Kluwer, 1994, pp. 161–82 and 51–83; and Nina Rattner Gelbart, 'The intellectual development of Walter Charleton', *Ambix*, 18, 1971, pp. 149–68.
10. Walter Pagel, *The Smiling Spleen: Paracelsianism in Storm and Stress*, Basel: Karger, 1984, pp. 17–27, summarised some of Severinus' key doctrines and indicated that Severinus was instrumental in creating a 'Paracelsian neo-Hippocratism', but he did not elaborate on Severinus' ideas or indicate the extent to which Severinus adapted Hippocrates to Paracelsus' philosophy.
11. Ibid., p. 23. Pagel must have suspected the influence of the *Idea medicinæ* on van Helmont's work when he wrote that van Helmont's praise of Hippocrates was 'not unlikely inspired' by Severinus. On van Helmont and Severinus, and on the importance of the *Idea medicinæ*, see Jole Shackelford, 'Paracelsianism in

Denmark and Norway in the 16th and 17th centuries', PhD Dissertation, University of Wisconsin, 1989. In a recent study, Antonio Clericuzio identified van Helmont's 'Eisagoge in Artem Medicam a Paracelso Restitutam' as a commentary on Severinus' *Idea medicinæ*. See Antonio Clericuzio, 'From van Helmont to Boyle. A study of the transmission of Helmontian chemical and medical theories in seventeenth-century England', *British Journal for the History of Science*, **26**, 1993, pp. 303–34 at p. 307, including n. 18. This suggests that van Helmont's view of Hippocrates may have been shaped by his early, close study of Severinus' work.

12. This is amply discussed in Allen G. Debus, *The French Paracelsians: The Chemical Challenge to Medical and Scientific Tradition in Early Modern France*, Cambridge: Cambridge University Press, 1991, and in the introduction to Allen G. Debus (ed.), *Science and Education in the Seventeenth Century. The Webster Ward Debate*, London: Macdonald, 1970.

13. Johannes Albertus Wimpenæus, *De concordia Hippocraticorum et Paracelsistarum libri magni excursiones defensiuæ, cum appendice, quid medico sit faciendum*, Munich: Adamus Berg, 1569; also Johannes Guinterius von Andernach, *De medicina veteri et nova tum cognoscendi tum facienda commentarij duo*, 2 vols, Basel: Henricpetri, 1571. On these early efforts to reconcile Paracelsian and Galenic medicine, see Debus, *The French Paracelsians* (n. 12), pp. 19–20.

14. One might also translate *idea medicinæ philosophicæ* as a 'brief outline of philosophical medicine', inasmuch as the 'idea' is the general form or outline, much as a footprint provides the general form or outline of the foot. However, I have chosen to retain the Platonic sense of form by rendering the title as *Ideal of Philosophical Medicine*.

15. Severinus, *Idea medicinæ* (n. 1), p. ix:

> I deserve your indulgence ... because I have often attempted unusual ways of interpretation. ... Following in the footsteps of the philosophers, I have imparted much that was neglected by others. ... We are neither reciters nor mere transcribers. We have caused streams of thought to flow from those same sources that have been tapped by ancient and more recent interpreters of nature concealed.

Tycho Brahe's programme is evident in the title of his book *Astronomiæ instauratæ mechanica*, Wandsbeck, 1598. In the preface dedicating the book to Emperor Rudolph II, Brahe expresses the hope that astronomy 'might finally be restored to wholeness and handed down to posterity more correct than at any time before'. See Tycho Brahe, *Instruments of the Renewed Astronomy*, ed. Alena Hadravova, Petr Hadrava and Jole Shackelford, Prague: Koniasch Latin Press, 1996, p. 10.

16. Severinus, *Idea medicinæ* (n. 1), p. 1. Paracelsus wrote in the preface to *Sieben defensiones* that God had revealed medicine through Apollo, Machaon, Podalyrius and Hippocrates. See Smith, *The Hippocratic Tradition* (n. 2), p. 15.

17. Severinus, *Idea medicinæ* (n. 1), p. 95, said that Hippocrates was following ancient precepts. On the Hermetic tradition and ancient theology see D.P. Walker, *The Ancient Theology: Studies in Christian Platonism from the Fifteenth to the Eighteenth Century*, Ithaca, NY: Cornell Univ. Press, 1972, and Frances Yates, *Giordano Bruno and the Hermetic Tradition*, Chicago: University of Chicago Press, 1964.

18. Recent efforts to restrict historians' use of the term 'Hermetic' to refer only to

the teachings of the *Corpus Hermeticum* fail to take into consideration the more general use of the term in the early modern world.
19. Severinus, *Idea medicinæ* (n. 1), p. iii.
20. Ibid., p. 1. On the rejection of 'hypotheses' in *Ancient Medicine*, see W.H.S. Jones, *Hippocrates*, Loeb. Vol. 1, London: Heinemann, 1923, pp. 6–8.
21. Severinus, *Idea medicinæ* (n. 1), p. iv:

> But then, little by little, true medicine began to change into speeches, abandoning the phenomena themselves and reliance on observations, and they began to seek hypotheses that were suited to geometrical demonstrations. Thus their clientelle of heats, coldnesses, wetnesses, and drynesses, and their retinue of degrees, defined by distinct numbers, were introduced into medicine: from these, convenient explanations for diseases and remedies could be deduced.

22. Ibid., p. 94:

> Passages of this sort, occuring here and there in the writings of Hippocrates, if they are compared by the mind's careful judgement ... make it clear that the foundations of Hippocratic medicine either had not been understood by Galen, or were impiously altered by virtue of inhuman envy.

23. Ibid., p. v. Also p. 385: 'Galen himself also will scarcely point out one specific and legitimate medicament not taken from the Empirics.'
24. Ibid., p. 366: 'Today's physicians have turned out to be heaters and bathers instead of healers.'
25. Ibid., p. 4. Presumably, Severinus is referring to the alchemists and their notorious practice of deliberately hiding their meanings in texts. On this principle of dispersion, see William R. Newman, *Gehennical Fire: The Lives of George Starkey, an American Alchemist in the Scientific Revolution*, Cambridge, Mass.: Harvard University Press, 1994, pp. 116–17
26. Severinus, *Idea medicinæ* (n. 1), p. v. Severinus realised that Hippocrates did not have a perfect medicine and that times change, bringing with them new conditions. However, he clearly viewed Galenic theory as having paralysed medicine, rendering it unable to respond to new diseases and accommodate new remedies, which were discovered by empirical physicians.
27. Ibid., p. 4.
28. Smith, *The Hippocratic Tradition* (n. 2), p. 20, noted that, for Sydenham and others, Hippocrates 'was a spirit and a method rather than a body of doctrine'.
29. Severinus, *Idea medicinæ* (n. 1), p. 73:

> Ite filij, uendite agros, ædes, uestes, annulos, comburite libros, emite calceos, montes accedite, ualles, solitudines, littora maris, terræ profundos sinus inquirite: animalium discrimina, plantarum differentias, mineralium ordines, omnium proprietates, nascendi modos notate: rusticorum Astronomiam & terrestrem Philosophiam diligenter ediscite, nec uos pudeat: tandem carbones emite, fornaces construite, uigilate & coquite sine tædio. Ita enim peruenietis ad corporum proprietatumque cognitionem, alias non.

30. At ibid., p. 374, Severinus noted that Hippocrates wrote nothing about preparing and exalting remedies – that is, about the methods of the chemists. Nevertheless,

he credited the ancient sage with establishing principles of chemical philosophy that are still valid.
31. Lonie, 'The "Paris Hippocratics"' (n. 5), p. 162: 'The Hippocratic text, *Coan Prognoses*, is of great importance for an understanding of the aims of the Parisians and an appreciation of the kind of medicine which they thought valuable. Both the text itself, and their work upon it, were at the very heart of their endeavor.' On p. 156 he says that, as a result of the Parisians' change in attitude toward restoring ancient Greek medicine, there 'were actual changes in therapy and a new interest in observation which was prompted by the reading of Hippocrates' *Epidemics*'.
32. It is generally recognised that Paracelsus left his methods and ideas in a form that was difficult to digest. The task of creating a coherent Paracelsian chemical philosophy therefore fell to his followers, among whom Severinus was an early and influential member.
33. On Augustine's *rationes seminales* see Michael J. McKeough, 'The meaning of rationes seminales in St. Augustine', PhD dissertation, Catholic University of America (Washington), 1926; Christopher J. O'Toole, 'The philosophy of creation in the writings of St. Augustine', PhD dissertation, Catholic University of America (Washington), 1944; and Jules M. Brady, 'St. Augustine's Theory of Seminal Reasons', *New Scholasticism*, 38, 1964, pp. 141–58.
34. Norma E. Emerton, 'Creation in the thought of J.B. van Helmont and Robert Fludd', in P. Rattansi and A. Clericuzio (eds), *Alchemy and Chemistry* (n. 9), pp. 85–101 at p. 85, has recently drawn attention to the importance of Genesis I as 'a crucial battleground on which the chemical interpretation of creation was defended and attacked in the contest to establish or defeat the chemical philosophy'.
35. Presumably this would reconcile the appearance of new diseases with the divine creation of all things in the beginning.
36. Jole Shackelford, 'Erastus and Severinus: the early reception of Paracelsian theory', *Sixteenth Century Journal*, 26, 1995, pp. 123–35, esp. pp. 129–30.
37. Severinus, *Idea medicinæ* (n. 1), p. 98:

> The nature of the mechanical spirits and seminal principles is far different. They are the chains [linking] the visible and invisible, the temporal and the eternal, the corruptible and the uncorruptible, the higher and the lower. Therefore, they ought to reveal the properties of both kinds of nature, yet so that they reflect the conditions of neither, purely and accurately.

Also p. 101:

> And these chains waver, in a way, between a corporeal and incorporeal nature. Nevertheless, they are bodies, but spiritual. And on the other hand, they are spirits, but corporeal.

38. Severinus relates the Paracelsian idea of predestinations to the apparent cyclical nature of phenomena, which reflect the 'risings and settings' of the stars that are internal to their *semina*.
39. See Jasper Hopkins, *A Concise Introduction to the Philosophy of Nicholas of Cusa*, 2nd edn, Minneapolis: University of Minnesota, 1980.
40. See, for example, Severinus, *Idea medicinæ* (n. 1), pp. 78, 96. Although Severinus used the term *lithurgia* in the *Idea medicinæ*, which might be interpreted as 'stone cutting', I believe he meant it to be an analogy to 'liturgy' as a routine or

mechanical process. This conclusion is supported by the fact that Mauritz Køning and William Davidson, scholars who adopted Severinus' ideas, spelt it *liturgia*.
41. On the seventeenth-century legacy of Severinus' view of 'mechanical' action, see Jole Shackelford, 'Seeds with a mechanical purpose: Severinus' *semina* and seventeenth-century matter theory', in Allen G. Debus and Michael T. Walton (eds), *Reading the Book of Nature: The Other Side of the Scientific Revolution*, Sixteenth Century Essays and Studies, Vol. 41, Kirksville, Mo.: Sixteenth Century Journal Publishers Inc., 1998, pp. 15–44.
42. Severinus, *Idea medicinæ* (n. 1), p. 141:

> Thus we have observed that *sysimbrium* has degenerated into mint, the turnip into the radish, *imperatoria* into angelica, wheat into darnel, basil into thyme, and many transplantations of this kind. ... Thus in the seed of wheat, the form of darnel lies hidden, but as an attendant, equivocal and accidental. This, if it obtains external assistance, ... will govern all things according to its predestination and knowledge and will introduce its characteristics.

43. This was a point of importance for Severinus, since he did not want his theory to be construed as Manichæan, which it was anyway.
44. The Paracelsian tradition did not recognise a clear professional distinction between surgery, medicine, and pharmacy, but rather taught that the true healer must be adept at all three. Although it is both practically difficult and methodologically unsound to link medical practice to medical results in the early modern period, I believe that this requirement enabled physicians to achieve greater success in post-operative care, which augmented the reputation of Paracelsian healers. Harold J. Cook, *Trials of an Ordinary Doctor: Johannes Groenevelt in Seventeenth-Century London*, Baltimore: Johns Hopkins, 1994, shows us that Groenevelt, an MD and successful lithotomist, did not consider himself to be merely a surgeon, prescribed internal medicines that he prepared himself and took great care to treat surgical wounds to prevent infection.
45. Severinus understood that the new chemical drugs could succeed where the old methods failed. For example, he wrote that physicians were not excused from treating epilepsies that struck patients over 25 years of age on the authority of Hippocrates, who had said that such cases were incurable. The Paracelsians revered ancient wisdom, but were not slaves to it.
46. Severinus gave horticultural transplantation a wide definition that included grafting and other techniques by which a plant might be made to violate its natural laws of development, as for example when roses are made to bloom in winter.
47. Severinus often recommended diaphoretics, purgatives, vomitives and sudorifics. Chemical drugs that cause what he called 'insensible transpirations' were also an important part of his therapeutic armoury.
48. This is the sort of 'Elizabethan compromise' that Allen Debus has written about. See Allen Debus, *The English Paracelsians*, London: Oldbourne, 1965, chapter 2.
49. Again, Severinus did not eschew everything Galenic – one finds in the *Idea medicinæ* vestiges of a human physiology based on the primacy of the liver, heart and brain, for example. But he rejected Aristotelian and Galenic embryology.
50. Severinus quotes from *On the Places in Man, Regimen, On the Nature of the Child, On the Nature of Man, Ancient Medicine, Diseases, Dreams (Regimen IV), Humours*, and *Breaths*, and refers otherwise to *Nutriments, Fleshes, On Birth, Affections, Regimen in Health, Epidemics, On Sacred Diseases, Airs, Waters, and Places*, and *Aphorisms*.

51. Passages that I have sampled agree well, but not verbatim, with the Loeb editions of Hippocrates' treatises. I have not yet matched up Severinus' quotations with a sixteenth-century Greek edition.
52. Severinus' dedication of the *Idea medicinæ* to King Frederik II is dated 1 November 1570, and I presume the book was finished by that date.
53. I doubt that Severinus would have put these passages on public display unless he was confident of his paraphrases and translations, for surely they were intended to exhibit his erudition. However, since he quotes mostly from books that were not considered to be 'Hippocratic' in content by Galen, it may be that he wished to establish that there were Greek texts behind his paraphrases, which he knew Galenists would find objectionable. Moreover, quotation of an exotic original had rhetorical value, which was preserved in the anonymous English translation of the *Idea medicinæ* (British Library, London. Sloane ms. 11, 'A Mappe of Medicyne or Philosophicall Path containinge the groundes of all the doctrines of Paracelsus, Hippocrates & Galen compiled by Peter Severine a Dane, philosopher & physician to Fredericke the II King of Denmarke & the Northerne partes'), where the Greek was rendered in Latin, which preserved the distance between the quotations and the surrounding English text.
54. Severinus, *Idea medicinæ* (n. 1), pp. 369–70. Ole Worm, a prominent physician in seventeenth-century Copenhagen, reported seeing a *Paraphrasis in libros Hippocratis de antiqua medicina* among Severinus' manuscripts.
55. Jones, *Hippocrates* (n. 20), p. lxii, referred to *Ancient Medicine* as one of 'the most important of the Hippocratic treatises not mentioned by Galen', but Wesley Smith, *The Hippocratic Tradition* (n. 2) pp. 209–10, noted that Galen knew of *Ancient Medicine* but did not agree with its message. He also pointed out that Severinus' contemporary, Mercurialis, the editor of the 1588 facing-page edition of Hippocrates' works, did not think *Ancient Medicine* was genuine.
56. Jones, *Hippocrates* (n. 20), Loeb, Vol. 4, p. xxxviii writes that Galen was 'not an enthusiastic admirer' of *Regimen*, the first book of which he considered to be 'entirely divorced' from the Hippocratic mind-set.
57. Severinus, *Idea medicinæ* (n. 1), p. 94.
58. Ibid., p. 5–6.
59. Ibid., p. 43.
60. Ibid., p. 204.
61. Ibid., p. 85.
62. Ibid., p. 65.
63. Ibid., p. 94.
64. Ibid.
65. Ibid., p. 406.
66. Ibid., p. 42.
67. Ibid., p. 43.
68. Ibid., p. 44.
69. Since Severinus elsewhere claimed that *The Nature of Man* was accepted as written by Hippocrates, I presume that he is intentionally placing a distance between the humoralism in *The Nature of Man* and the dynamism in some of the other books by questioning the authenticity here.
70. Severinus, *Idea medicinæ* (n. 1), p. 44.
71. Ibid., pp. 16, 246.
72. Ibid., p. 128. The quotations are from *Aphorisms* III.v (Vol. 4 of the Jones Loeb series, pp. 122–23, lines 1–2, 3–5.) On pp. 283–84 Severinus equates 'southern' qualities with chemical characteristics.

73. Severinus, *Idea medicinæ* (n. 1), p. 283.
74. Ibid., p. 151.
75. Ibid.
76. Ibid.
77. Ibid., p. 111: 'Hippocrates himself, and Aristotle, too, acknowledge that matter to be the container of the seed, and that when the spirits are beginning to be moved, it is thickened into skins, shells, and coverings.'
78. Ibid., p. 204.
79. Ibid., p. 205.
80. Ibid., p. 194.
81. Ibid., pp. 16, 138, Severinus specifically connects *dynameis* to *chærionia* and, on p. 345, he refers to 'dead and relollacean qualities' '*mortuis Relollaceisque qualitatibus*. *Relollacean* is a Paracelsian term referring to the dead, virtueless parts of nature. See A.E. Waite, *The Hermetic and Alchemical Writings of ... Paracelsus*, Vol. 2, London: James Elliott, 1894, p. 181.
82. Severinus, *Idea medicinæ* (n. 1), p. 19. Also, p. 23:

    Hippocrates attributed the functioning of the whole living being to [innate heat]. He declared that all faculties, even the most diverse, are completed at the proper places and times by virtue of this. He firmly asserted that crises and also the healthful concoctions of diseases proceed from the same source.

83. Ibid., p. 17.
84. Ibid.
85. Ibid.
86. Ibid., p. 152.
87. Ibid., pp. 110–11:

    Great knowledge lies concealed in the mechanical spirits and principles of generation. For they know how to form the heart, brain, liver, nerves, veins, arteries, and bones from the same elements, just as from the same bread a dog produces canine parts and a man produces human parts.

88. Ibid., p. 154.
89. Ibid., p. 149.
90. Ibid., pp. 104, 151.
91. Ibid., pp. 162–63. The quotation is from *Regimen I*, xxvi (Loeb, Vol. 4, pp. 262–64, lines 3–7):

    And all the limbs are separated and grow simultaneously, none before or after another; although those by nature larger become visible before the smaller, yet they are formed none the earlier.
    (Jones' translation)

92. Severinus, *Idea medicinæ* (n. 1), p. 86. I wonder if Paracelsus had understood the Hippocratic 'coction' as an alchemical process separating the pure from the impure – an idea that underlies his and Severinus' conception of what the *archei* do.
93. Ibid., p. 87. Severinus also interpreted Hippocrates' statement in *Nutriment* that nutriment is what nourishes, what exists as nourishment, and what will be nourished to mean that there is an identity or continuity between potential and actual (ibid., p. 88).

94. Ibid., pp. 89–90. The Paracelsians did not consider the celestial or supralunary world to be a realm of perfection, as did the Aristotelians. It was in this intellectual frame that Tycho Brahe, Severinus' friend, was to interpret the nova of 1572 as a newly generated, 'fixed' star.
95. Ibid., pp. 97, 121.
96. Ibid., pp. 88–89.
97. Ibid., p. 120.
98. Ibid., p. 157.
99. Ibid., pp. 237–38.
100. I do not mean to suggest that there were no differences between Galenic and Paracelsian therapy, merely that chemical physicians did not use chemically prepared drugs exclusively, but presumably interpreted traditional therapies in terms of their chemical paradigm.
101. Severinus, *Idea medicinæ* (n. 1), p. 365.
102. Ibid.
103. Ibid., p. 401. Severinus also maintained that Paracelsus called 'seed' what Hippocrates had called 'aliment'. See Severinus, *Idea medicinæ* (n. 1), p. 184.
104. Ibid., p. 366.
105. Ibid.
106. Paracelsus also considered *semina* to be astral. On spirit and astral body, see Walter Pagel, *Paracelsus: An Introduction to Philosophical Medicine in the Era of the Renaissance*, 2nd ed., Basel:Karger, 1982, pp. 117–20.
107. Severinus, *Idea medicinæ* (n. 1), p. 200.
108. Ibid., p. 201. Severinus quoted from *Regimen I*, x, (Loeb IV, p. 248, lines 15–26).
109. The illustration is in Robert Fludd, *Utriusque cosmi ... historia*, Vol. 2, Oppenheim: J.T. De Bry, 1619, p. 105, and is reproduced in William H. Huffman, *Robert Fludd and the End of The Renaissance*, London: Routledge, 1988, illustration 8. An association between the seven planets and the seven major organs was commonplace among students of Hermetic philosophy, including Tycho Brahe. See Jole Shackelford, 'Paracelsianism and patronage in early modern Denmark', in Bruce Moran (ed.), *Patronage and Institutions: Science, Technology, and Medicine at the European Court 1500–1750*, Woodbridge: Boydell, 1991, pp. 85–109 at p. 100.
110. Severinus, *Idea medicinæ* (n. 1), p. 330.
111. Ibid., p. 281.
112. Ibid., p. 269. The quotation is from *Humors* XVIII (Loeb IV, p. 90, lines 12–15). Tycho Brahe, who shared Severinus' belief in these correlations, maintained a meteorological journal at Hven during the last quarter of the century, presumably with the aim of discovering the correspondences between what he called the celestial and terrestrial astronomies.
113. Ibid., p. 283.
114. Ibid., p. 158. The quotation is from *Regimen I*, viii (Loeb IV, p. 242, line 7).
115. Ibid., p. 92.
116. This doctrine is an important part of the agreement between Severinus' natural philosophy and his interpretation of Genesis I.
117. Severinus, *Idea medicinæ* (n. 1), p. 276.
118. One of the manuscripts mentioned in the *Idea medicinæ*, and reported by Ole Worm, was *Liber de nominibus et rebus*.
119. Severinus, *Idea medicinæ* (n. 1), p. 212.
120. Ibid., p. 232.
121. Ibid., p. 81.

122. Ibid., p. 406.
123. Thomas Moffet, *De iure et præstantia chymicorum medicamentorum dialogus apologeticus*, Frankfurt: Wechel, 1584.
124. Nutton, 'Hippocrates in the Renaissance' (n. 5), p. 431, notes that 'Only at Ingolstadt, Freiburg and the London College of Physicians is Hippocratism given an equal standing with Galen'.
125. Five letters from Severinus to Zwinger survive in the university library at Basel, dated from February 1583 to August 1587, and have been translated into Danish by Hans Skov in Eyvind Bastholm, *Petrus Severinus og hans Idea medicinae philosophicae*, Odense: Odense Universitetsforlag, 1979. Zwinger died in 1588. The tone of Severinus' first letter suggests that it is a response to an initial letter from Zwinger and that the two were not previously acquainted. The chronology implies that Zwinger first wrote to Severinus while he was defending Moffet's thesis, the acceptance of which had been held up since 1578 because of its harsh criticism of the anti-Paracelsian, Thomas Erastus. See Charles Webster, 'Alchemical and Paracelsian medicine', in Charles Webster (ed.), *Health, Medicine and Mortality in the Sixteenth Century*, Cambridge: Cambridge University Press, 1979, chapter 9, p. 328.
126. Severinus' ideas were used in this context by Tycho Brahe's former assistant and, later, by theologian, Kort Aslakssøn. I discuss Aslakssøn in Jole Shackelford, 'Paracelsianism in Denmark and Norway', doctoral dissertation, University of Wisconsin, 1989 and in idem, 'Unification and the Chemistry of the Reformation', in Max Reinhart (ed.), *Infinite Boundaries: Order, Disorder, and Reorder in Early Modern Culture*, Sixteenth Century Essays and Studies, Vol. 40, Kirksville, Mo.: Sixteenth Century Journal Publishers Inc., 1998, pp. 291–32.

Part II

The Transformations of Hippocratism in Seventeenth- and Eighteenth-century Britain

CHAPTER FIVE

The Transformation of Hippocrates in Seventeenth-century Britain

Andrew Cunningham

Introduction: transforming Hippocrates

As other contributions to this volume will also be showing, it is a matter of consensus amongst historians of medicine today that the perception of historical figures and their achievements is usually made in a way which meets needs in the present in which that perception is created or current. In other words, with respect to Hippocrates, the image(s) and reputation(s) of Hippocrates created or current in any particular age meets the demands of that age, and may have little if anything to do with the historical figure him-, her- or (in the case of a multi-authored text such as the Hippocratic works) themselves.[1] This means, of course, that there are many possible Hippocrateses, even in one generation and one locale, serving different, and sometimes opposed, purposes.

The gist of what I am going to say about the transformation of Hippocrates in seventeenth-century Britain has already been briefly stated by Hal Cook, building primarily on the work of Wesley Smith, in the following terms:

> In the later part of the seventeenth century, the name of Hippocrates rather than Galen conjured up intellectual excitement and an aura of the frontiers of knowledge. The change is significant, for Galen's reputation had come to rest on his medical rationalism, while that of Hippocrates stemmed from his empiricism. At least that is how Paracelsus, Francis Bacon, Van Helmont, and others portrayed Hippocrates, and by the middle of the seventeenth century that is how most people thought of him: the collector of case studies, the compiler of medical details, the inductivist, the early founder of the true methods of natural history whose achievements had been devalued by the rationalist practitioners following him.
> Moreover, the man who was gaining a reputation as the true English Hippocrates was Thomas Sydenham ... [who] had strong antiacademic sentiments, believing that medicine ought to be taught by apprenticeship, not by books ...[2]

Cook then relates the famous anecdote in which the young Richard Blackmore asked the mature Sydenham 'to advise me what Books I should read to qualify me for practice'. Sydenham replied 'Read *Don Quixot*, it is a very good Book, I read it still'. Blackmore quoted this as an instance of Sydenham's contempt for medicine in books. Ludwig Edelstein has interpreted this sally as Sydenham saying that if you build your learning out of books you will be as misled, as unable to distinguish facts from phantasies, as was Don Quixote when he mistook windmills for armed men.[3] What is perhaps striking about this anecdote, if true, is that Sydenham did not say, 'Read Hippocrates', if that is what he meant.

This change, from the glorification of the rational and academic in medicine, to the foregrounding of the empirical and practical, is what Cook means by the title of his book, *The Decline of the Old Medical Regime* in seventeenth-century English medicine. In particular, the claim of the members of the College of Physicians to speak with authority on medical matters because of their possession of *scientia* and *theoria*, came to be dismissed by those unlearned or anti-learned persons who professed empiricism, quackery and trial-and-error.

This change may not have been unique to England in the seventeenth century, and its full explanation would require something more than concentrating on events in just one island, as I shall be doing here. But we can rest assured that in England, this change – this decline – like everything else there, was about class as much as it was about knowledge. Also, in Britain, the old order is always declining, learning is always being despised, and the barbarians are always already within the gates. But in Britain the old order always manages to adapt and survive and to outwit the challenges to its dominance, usually by adopting the weapons of the challengers themselves. This is what happened to the London College of Physicians, which survives still today, notwithstanding all the attacks on it in the seventeenth century and its state of all but total schism in the last decades of that century; as one of its strategies of survival, the members of the College adopted the empirical Hippocrates as one of their own forefathers.

To properly make the case about the transformation of Hippocrates in seventeenth-century Britain it would be desirable to review the opinion of Hippocrates held and expressed in print and manuscript by all those who wrote on medicine in Britain during the course of that century. In default of such a review, I shall proceed here by looking at a number of moments, from the 1660s to the 1740s, using the term 'moments' in two senses (as a still point in time, and as an instant of time when force is bringing about change), in order to see something of how the old team of Hippocrates and his interpreter Galen became separated and how Hippocrates thrived on the separation while Galen became dismissed. My 'moments' are mostly points of conflict, where the differences of opinion are most starkly evident, and I give greater space here to events that I have not previously dealt with in earlier publications.

The 'class' issue (as I referred to it above) that is evident throughout these disputes is that, essentially, between those who went to university for their medical education and those who didn't. And that means that it is revealed as conflicts between the learned and the unlearned, between elite and popular social and intellectual forms, between theoretical and manual, between rational and empirical, and between Latin and English. In particular, it appears at the level of practice as a conflict between Colleges of Physicians and 'lesser' grades of medical practitioner, especially the *apothecaries* in England and *surgeon-apothecaries* in Scotland. After the work of Charles Webster, Piyo Rattansi, Hal Cook and others, the terms and course of this conflict, at least in England, is quite familiar.[4]

Hippocrates the Scottish physician

We turn first to Scotland. Here there had never been a College of Physicians, although there had been a few failed attempts to create one in the early seventeenth century. Although there was one medical professor at a university (Aberdeen), and the universities claimed the right to award medical degrees, Scotsmen seeking to become physicians left Scotland for their education, going especially to France and Italy. While the absence of a College of Physicians meant that physicians were not an object of attack by lesser medical practitioners as they were in London, it also meant there was no uniting body for physicians as such. However, for surgeons, apothecaries and the distinctively Edinburgh combination of 'surgeon-apothecary', the major burghs had guilds which trained and regulated these trades. In Edinburgh the surgeon-apothecaries were an important guild and had representation on the Town Council, and in the mid-seventeenth century they felt that their rights of practice were being threatened by simple apothecaries. It was at a moment when they were defending their rights of practice that the physicians were able to step in and claim the kinds of authority and pre-eminence in medicine enjoyed by the London College.

After the Restoration of 1660, a group of continental-educated elite Scottish physicians in Edinburgh took advantage of royal patronage to go on the offensive against what they saw as the 'insupportable' pretensions of the Edinburgh surgeon-apothecaries. In particular, for the physicians this led to the need for them to create a College of Physicians. A Royal College epitomised all the differences between the learned, elite, Latin, classical-based medicine of the physicians and the unlearned, manual, empirical and vernacular medicine of the lesser types of practitioner. The Restoration meant a return to court culture, to the world of patronage; he with the best patrons always won the day. Luckily for others, the patrons themselves were often unstable and at the mercy of national politics. The physicians had patrons who were close to the king (especially to the Duke of York, later James VII of Scotland and II of England), and were more powerful than the patron of the surgeon-apothecaries, which was the Edinburgh Town Council. The Duke of Lauderdale, Scottish Secretary from 1661 to 1680, and the Earl of Perth, Chancellor of Scotland from 1684 to 1689, to whom they were personal physicians, were the physicians' best patrons.

Hippocrates formed a significant part of the physicians' scheme, in specific ways that were additional to his role as father of medicine in the classical tradition to which all the physicians looked back with respect. Robert (later Sir Robert) Sibbald (1641–1722) was at the centre of many of the physicians' Hippocrates-inspired initiatives, together with his friend Andrew (later Sir Andrew) Balfour (1630–1694). They had each acquired their medical education abroad – Sibbald in Leyden and Paris, and Balfour in Paris, Montpellier, Caen and Padua. For each of them their stay in Paris, frequenting the Jardin Royal, was of great importance. Sibbald wrote in a memoir of Balfour that Balfour:

> ... remained in Paris for many years because there was the greatest opportunity of learning medicine properly, if you reckon the numbers of learned men, the frequency of anatomical dissections, the number of hospitals, the Jardin Royal very well stocked with plants, and finally the *methodus medendi*, as perfectly simple as it is safe.[5]

Sibbald himself, in his autobiography, recalled that his Paris experiences had turned him toward the study of the natural productions of Scotland:

> ... for I had learned at Paris that the simplest method of Physick was the best, and these [natural products] that the country affoorded came neerest to our temper, and agreed best with us, so I resolved to make it a part of my studie to know what animalls, vegetables, mineralls, metalls, and substances cast up by the sea, were found in this country, yt might be of use in medicine, or other artes usefull to human lyfe, and I began to be curious in searching after ym and collecting ym.[6]

This general attitude, that the plants and other natural productions of a region are best suited for medicinal use there, since localities have their particular diseases, was taken in the seventeenth century to be essentially 'Hippocratic', although it is not (as far as I can determine) built on any one particular text in the Hippocratic *Corpus*. It is a sort of combination of the general doctrine of *Airs, Waters and Places* (with regard to every region having its own diseases), accompanied by a belief that God has placed cures near diseases.

In the case of Sibbald and Balfour, this 'Hippocratic' view led them, in the 1670s, to engage in the laborious and controversial founding of physic/botanic gardens in and around Edinburgh, and to establish a young man as, jointly, gardener and 'professor of botany' with an annual stipend. The money for this was wrung out of the town council. Several physicians were persuaded to contribute annual sums for the culture and importation of foreign plants but, Sibbald recorded, 'Some of the Chirurgeon Apothecaryes, who then had much power in the town, opposed us, dreading that it might usher in a Coledge of Physitians'.[7]

They were right: it did. When the surgeon-apothecaries were faced with a particularly obtuse surgeon, one Cuninghame, who had sided with the apothecaries, challenging the physicians' rights through the law courts, the physicians took the opportunity of using their powerful patrons to create a Royal College 'to secure our priviledges belonged to us as doctors, and defend us against the incroachments of the Chirurgion Apothecaries, which were insupportable', as Sibbald recorded.[8] It was an institution conceived in conflict, and which suffered conflict from both without and within for decades. Sibbald and his friends continued to use it to promote the classical ideals of medicine, and as a base from which to develop proper medical teaching in Scotland.

Hippocrates featured as one of the ways in which Sibbald tried to develop medical teaching in the 1680s. Dr Thomas Burnet (brother of Gilbert, the bishop of Salisbury) published a little work, *Hippocrates Contractus* in 1685. When he had been in London, Burnet, a charter fellow of the RCPE, had written in Latin a laborious 'Treasury of Practical Medicine, from the observations etc of the most outstanding physicians, both ancient and modern ...', which appeared in 1673, and which was dedicated to the Earl of Lauderdale, that fervent cultivator of the muses and polite literature (as Burnet called him).[9] Intended for the use of the medical student, it brought together, under disease names, the cures of virtually all diseases and symptoms, both internal and external, with some cures even taken from the chemists.

This commitment to providing materials for medical students to guide them through the morass of medical authors and opinions is shown also in Burnet's *Hippocrates Contractus*.[10] Here Burnet styled himself Royal Physician, and Fellow of the RCPE and dedicates the work to the Earl of Perth, the Chancellor of Scotland, 'patrono suo eminentissimo'. This contracted Hippocrates is very much a product of the group of physicians around Sibbald. Not only did it appear with their explicit approval and was dedicated to the members of the College (as well as to Perth), but it had also been produced at Sibbald's insistence. By chance, Sibbald had seen the little book that Burnet had prepared for his own use years before, and was still using, and in which he had excerpted what he regarded as the most important and useful sentiments from the Hippocratic books 'so that he might always have Hippocrates portable in his hands when he was out seeking the causes of diseases'. Rapidly reading it through, Sibbald urged Burnet to publish it for the use of medical students ('in Philiatrorum gratiam'). Burnet let himself be persuaded since (as he wrote), although Hippocrates ought to be as familiar to every physician as his own home is, he was nonetheless hardly known by many physicians; hence such people could be incited, having read this little book, towards reading Hippocrates diligently.[11]

The publication of *Hippocrates Contractus* may have been directly connected with the promotion of medical teaching in Edinburgh in the classic mode, for in 1685 Sibbald and his allies used the pressure of their patrons to insist that the town council create in their college three 'professorships' of medicine (without stipend). This was intended to both defend the newly won rights of the Royal College against the universities of Scotland and ensure that unqualified graduates of Scottish universities could not become members of the Royal College. Unless some remedy was found, Sibbald wrote, 'all the Apothecaries and Surgeons wee have will goe and be graduat at Aberdeen'. What was needed, he argued, was a proper medical faculty, which 'cannot consist of lesse than three professors who ought to be constant residentes and teachers of the several pairts of Medicin for the instructing of youth in that study'.[12] Three professors were appointed, including Sibbald himself, and one could presume that he would have taught a curriculum based on Hippocrates. However, this experiment was short-lived, probably because Sibbald himself had to withdraw from the scene shortly after this, because his patron, the Earl of Perth, converted him to Roman Catholicism in September 1685 and he had to flee the mob and take refuge for a few months in London. There he thought better of his conversion, and returned to Edinburgh a sober Presbyterian again.

In later life, aged over 60, Sibbald made a further attempt to provide proper and suitable education for prospective physicians, again with Hippocrates as its model,[13] offering to teach 'both natural history and the medical art which he has with God's help successfully practised for forty-three years'. This teaching, which he advertised in the local newspaper, was to be directed only at those who had Latin and Greek, 'the whole of philosophy' and the basics of mathematics. In response to criticism directed towards this offer, Sibbald published, in Latin, 'Commentaries on the Law of Hippocrates, in which is shown what things are necessary for the future physician'.[14] Here he arranged everything he had to say about what proper training for medicine involves and laid this out in the context of Hippocrates's teachings.

Sibbald took the *Law*, one of the *Letters* (to Hippocrates's son Thessalus), and the *Oath*, and commented on them as showing the basis of a proper physician's outlook, moral position and education. He also quoted *Decorum* liberally, praised Hippocrates and wrote that his reader would recognise that 'the Hippocratic method is the most excellent of all as it was born from the observations which Hippocrates made in practice and it has been confirmed by an amazing success'.[15] But, he announced, he was not going to be limited to Hippocrates's words:

> My intention is far different, for many things have been discovered by most excellent men in later ages and especially in this one just past, which pertain both to the theory of medicine and its practice ... I will show who they are who have best carried on successfully the torch of observations inherited from Hippocrates and passed it on to later generations; and those who have greatly advanced medicine through chemical experiments; and those who have in our age further illustrated and increased natural history (without which, according to Plato, the nature of man cannot be properly explained).[16]

In short, Sibbald claimed, his intention was to teach 'an "old-new" medicine', one built on the solid observations of the Ancients, augmented by the findings – but not the hypotheses – of more recent investigators.

The centrality of Hippocrates in the many schemes of Sibbald and his allies in Edinburgh is striking. It was a Hippocrates who was historically the basis of medicine and who served as a model both in natural history and in observation in medicine. He was also, as Sibbald's 1706 booklet made clear, a moral example to the young physicians of the time, not only in his selflessness and commitment, but also in his application to learning throughout life. It was a Hippocrates who was also linked directly to the profession, learning and dignity of the physician, taking his rightful (if embattled) place over the lesser medical practitioners (apparently, appealing to Hippocrates was not something that the surgeon-apothecaries or the apothecaries engaged in, at least in these contests). The Scottish Hippocrates was a physician, not a surgeon-apothecary.

Hippocrates the dreamer

We now turn to the capital of the southern kingdom, London, to look at some events roughly contemporaneous with what we have seen happening in Scotland, and which similarly involve the role of Hippocrates as underwriting the claims to dignity and power of the establishment physicians, epitomised by their Royal College.

Hippocrates came to be the centrepiece of a conflict between the Royal College of Physicians in London and its chemical – in particular its Helmontian – rivals in 1665. In that year Marchamont Nedham (1620–1678) published under his initials, but not his name, a long tirade against the College, claiming to offer 'the cure of medicine'. This was his *Medela Medicinae. A Plea for the Free Profession, and a Renovation of the Art of Physick ... .*[17] The work caused quite a stir in the College, and Nedham claimed that the College had to put four people up to answer him in print,[18] three of whose defences can still be identified. Nedham was an early journalist, and his pen was for hire. One of his contemporaries called him 'a Jack of all sides, transcendently gifted in opprobrious and treasonable droll', and Anthony à Wood called him 'this most seditious, mutable and railing author'.[19] At the beginning of the Civil War Nedham supported the parliamentary cause and produced the news-sheet *Mercurius Britanicus* (1643) to attack royalists; in 1647 he changed sides, and produced *Mercurius Pragmaticus* to promote the royalist cause; in 1650 he changed back and supported the Commonwealth government with *Mercurius Politicus*. Having thus made enemies all round with his mercurial changes of allegiance, he wisely left England for Holland for a short while at the Restoration. But as well as being a political scribbler, Nedham was also a physician, having been educated at Oxford in medicine, and, for some years, having earned his living in London as a medical practitioner when no-one was prepared to hire his pen.

The *Medela Medicinae* took as its primary target the physicians of the London College, the defectiveness of their education, the undesirability of their control over medical practice in London, and the need to end their dominion over the apothecaries. Nedham was, of course, a Helmontian (whether genuine or faking for money it is impossible now to tell), promoting the virtues and superiority of chemical medicines. Part of his argument to this end was that, in the modern world, diseases had changed, not only from what they were in antiquity, but also from what they were two centuries earlier. Not only were there two significant new 'modern' diseases, the French pox and scurvy, which had become very widespread by infection, but these two diseases 'having gotten dominion inwardly'[20] in the bodies of everyone, had distorted and corrupted other diseases.

> In a word, for the right understanding of my Drift in this Discourse, consider, that I distinguish betwixt the Tinctures or *Ferments* of those two grand Diseases, and the Diseases themselves: The Diseases sometimes appear like themselves, when they are gotten in the common way; but when the *Ferments* propagate themselves, either by *Lactation*, or *Hereditary Propagation* or by *Contagion*, they seldom or never appear like branches of such a Stock ... [and are cured] by such Remedies only, as either totally alter or extirpate the *Ferments*, which are complicated with, or Tinctured in them.[21]

That diseases had changed in recent centuries, and that they could be transmitted at a distance, seems to have been part of Helmontian doctrine. To the pox and the scurvy of the Helmontian tradition Nedham added his own pet modern disease, worms, whose presence at the subvisible level in all corrupting disease was (he claimed) being revealed every day by the microscope and whose presence in invisible form could therefore be inferred in many other diseases. Part of Nedham's evidence for these changes in the incidence and virulence of diseases came from the London *Bills of Mortality* published and analysed by John Graunt.

Diseases had changed, Nedham claimed, and could not therefore be cured, like the old ones, with the methods of Hippocrates and Galen. But, fortunately, effective medicines had been developed to meet this change, and the last few decades had brought better and more powerful medicines than were known to antiquity, largely through Helmontian chemistry. For the progress of medicine it was therefore necessary to give up the old way of medicine:

> Vain therefore is that Learning which ties men up to a general set Method in curing, and inables them to excuse themselves for any thing they do, if they can but produce an od [sic] Aphorism, or Text of *Hippocrates* or *Galen*, for a justification, and thereby prove (as *Balzac*'s Italian Doctor did at *Padua*) that the *Patient died with the fairest Method in the world*; whereas that ancient Prince of the Faculty [i.e. Hippocrates], and *Galen*

> the Usurper, being no Prophets, and little able to divine what Alterations of things would fall out in our days, could never foresee how to frame Precepts and Rules to guide Us in our Concernments. There are many things admitted and enjoyned by them in the *Methodus Medendi*, which may by no means be allowed in ours, as the Case now stands.[22]

He continued: we should look at the knowledge of wisewomen and empirics; as Robert Boyle advises, we should not disdain to take our medical knowledge from any person. We must resort to experiment, we must learn from van Helmont. We must jettison the doctrines of Galen, whom van Helmont called 'the great Corrupter of so much as was tolerable in *Hippocrates*'.[23] So away (Nedham cried) with the frigid notion of the four elements, in favour of the five principles of the chemists; away with the four qualities, away with the doctrine of temperaments, away with the four humours. We need to jettison the doctrines of critical days, pulses and urines, phlebotomy and current medicines. In their place we should introduce the much superior Helmontian doctrines. In particular, we should recognise that each disease is 'a *real substantial thing*, inherent in that which they call the *Archeus* or *Vital Spirit* ...', rather than a mere excess of quality, as the Schools teach.

> And truly, in this matter, *Hippocrates* was wiser than his Successors, in aiming at the essence of Diseases, while he ascribes so much to that which he calls *Spiritus Impetum Faciens*, or the *Active forcible Spirit*, as including the essentials of a Disease; for in that Vital Spirit (which we call the *Archeus*) implanted in any part of the Body, lurk the difficult sort of Diseases; and till that Spirit be pacified, or rectified, by a proper Remedy, or by some extraordinary beningnity of Nature, it is, in such Cases impossible to attain a recovery ....[24]

Nedham's attitude towards Hippocrates was remarkably hostile, to an extent I have not seen elsewhere. He spoke of him as someone who dreamed things up. He described university-educated physicians as paying money 'as a test of their being lawful Sons of those two great Dreamers, *Hippocrates* and *Galen*'.[25] However, he was also keen, when possible, to claim Hippocrates for his own position. Not only did he try to equate his own *archeus* with Hippocrates's *spiritus impetum faciens*, but he also claimed, for instance, that his view that there is infection at a distance was supported by Hippocrates who said that, in diseases, there is '*quid divinum*, which I translate *somewhat of a more occult nature, of a more sublime, Spirituous, subtile, finer consideration*, than what comes from Discourse upon Tempers and distempers arising from First and Second Qualities'.[26] And Nedham professed, as might be expected, that 'I would not willingly detract from the Antients; *Amicus Hippocrates, Amicus Galenus, sed Magis Amica Veritas*'.[27] It is interesting (but not necessarily trustworthy) that he claimed that his criticism of the value and verity of Hippocrates's *Prognostics* was built on his own experience of them in practice:

> For, perceiving in the course of Practise, that many of them, and of the *Coacae Praenotiones*, did fail me, I could not, at first, tell what to think of the rest; but afterwards, having the summ of them reduced into order under certain Heads Alphabetically, after the manner of *Common Places*, ready to be produced, I began to compare them upon occasion in visiting the Sick, and by this means I am the better able to advise others to be wary how they trust them, because they have so often deceived me.[28]

But the nub of Nedham's criticism of Hippocrates, and the reason why he made it, was that collegiate practitioners were obsessed with defending Hippocrates's reputation, 'as if the credit of Physick must needs fall to the ground, if that man were detected of Error, who in an ignorant Age, imposed upon the world his own *Dreams*, as matters of *Eternal Verity*'.[29] So it is not surprising to find that one particular defence against Nedham consisted in trying to defend Hippocrates and hence restore the structure of learned medicine, including the College of Physicians of London and the universities as nurseries of the best medical learning.

The defender of Hippocrates in this case was Robert Sprackling, one of the 'Whifling Novices' who, according to Nedham, were put up to it by the senior members of the College of Physicians, who 'standing behind the Curtain, reckoned it enough for them, to cry up in private everywhere, that I had four Answers given which confuted me'.[30] Sprackling's *Medela Ignorantiae* ('The Cure of Ignorance') was published in 1665[31] and was dedicated to Francis Glisson, anatomical leading light of the College of Physicians. Sprackling devoted his whole book to countering Nedham's critique of Hippocrates. His argument against Nedham had two strands. The first was that Nedham's criticisms were based on ignorance: either the text of Hippocrates doesn't say what Nedham claimed it says, or it means something other than what Nedham claimed, or it applies to different persons or occasions than Nedham claimed. Sprackling quoted the Greek text of Hippocrates in the course of his refutation. At all points he was at pains to point out that Hippocrates is *rational* and *empirical* – the two things that Nedham had claimed he was not, and for which faults he should not be followed or held in esteem. Here, for instance, is Sprackling's defence of one of the *Prognostics*. Nedham's criticism had been that:

> In the second Book of Prognosticks, after three Texts spent about Dropsies (the second whereof is oraculous, because a Riddle) he tells us in the fourth, If the head, hands, and feet grow cold, while the middle parts burn, 'tis ill, and that it is best, that the whole body be warm and moist.[32]

Sprackling responds:

> Indeed all the Aphorisms and Prognostiques of *Hippocrates* are Riddles (though some of them as evident as the dictates of nature and common sense) to this unintelligent Animadverter, who would cast down *Hippocrates* as a monstrous *Sphinx*, not because he can explain any obscure

Sentence in him, but because he cannot apprehend the clearest and most intelligible, as may be seen in this Prognostique for example [then he gives the text in Greek, which he then translates thus:] *Those in whom Dropsies arise from the Liver, Coughs and endevours of Coughing befall. Notwithstanding they spit forth little considerable, and their feet swell, and nothing is evacuated from the Intestines, but tough excrements, and those with extreme difficulty. Withal, swellings arise about the Belly, (as well such as are settled, as those by intervals changing) sometimes on the right otherwile on the left side.* What Riddle is there in this true and plain Prognostique? Coughs in the Hydropical proceed from the oppression of the *Diaphragm*, and other Organs of respiration; The breast then being thus compress'd, little matter is in coughing evacuated; the feet swell, from that *aqueous* matter which is there congested from the Arteries; the Belly is commonly bound, in defect of that humor (now cast into other parts) which before served as a vehicle for the *Faeces*: Tumors beset the *abdomen*, sometimes constant, as where the Tympany is greater, other while changing, the tension being lessned on the removal of the waterish matter, which sufficient flatulency is not conjoyned to continue it. Doth not evident experience demonstrate all this, as well as evident reason?[33]

Experience and reason, those contested virtues, were thus shown to be on Hippocrates's side, and typical of his practice, rather than on that of Nedham and his crazed chemists. But these virtues were typical, too, of Hippocrates's modern followers, the members of the College of Physicians – 'the industrious Physicians of this Age' – whose investigations were daily improving on the work of the ancients and correcting their errors. This was Sprackling's other line of argument to refute Nedham: that the College of Physicians were perfect, improving Hippocratics. He wrote:

> ... what clear reason, and continued experience of succeeding Ages hath approved, they are content to receive as from them [i.e. from the Ancients], with honor and gratitude to their memories. But it must be withal acknowledged that the late eminent discoveries have in many things corrected the unanimous errings of Antiquity, and in other things produced *de novo* doctrines of singular use and importance. Who can compare the Treatise of *Hippocrates* [The Heart] to that of Doctor *Harvey de motu Cordis*, or the one [The Seed] to the other *de Generatione*? what is there in his Tractate [Fleshes] of such able and happy invention, as the nourishment of the solid parts cleared by Doctor *Glisson* and Doctor *Ent*? and who seeth not a difference between *Hippocrates* his imperfect discourse [Glands] and Doctor *Wharton*'s most accurate *Adenographia*? But because others by their learning and industry correct and add to the Coacal [i.e. Coan; that is, Hippocratic] Doctrine, therefore this Pleader [Nedham] presumeth, without either, to deprave and vitiate it.[34]

This second line of argument was also typical of another of the responses to Nedham, that by George Castle, *The Chymical Galenist: A Treatise wherein the Practice of the Ancients is reconcil'd to the new Discoveries in the Theory of Physick*, which appeared in 1667, its publication having been delayed by Castle's flight from the plague, 'so dismall a Disease, against which, flight is the onely infallible preservative'.³⁵ Despite its title, this work conceded virtually nothing to Nedham's chemical position. Rather, it claimed that 'the improvement which *Physick* has receiv'd in this latter Age, ought to be ascrib'd to the learned *Physicians*, and men bred up in *Universities* and *Colledges*', of which the members of the College of Physicians were (Castle claimed) universally acknowledged to be the greatest examples. Harvey, Glisson, Ent, Highmore, Wharton and Willis were enlisted in evidence, and Willis on fevers³⁶ was used extensively to refute Nedham's points. Castle wrote that:

> The modern Discoveries in Anatomy and Chymistry, are so far from destroying the Practice and Method of the Ancients, that they very firmly corroborate, and establish their Doctrines, by furnishing us with the true reasons of those Processes and Methods which were delivered down to us from them, only upon their experience and knowledge of the matter of Fact, though they were ignorant of the true causes ... Wherefore in the reforming of Physick, and suiting an Institution to the late Discoveries in *Anatomy* and *Chymistry*, care must be taken, that we imitate wise and thrifty Builders, who, in raising a new House in the place of an old one which they have pull'd down, make use of many of the old substantial Materials, some of which are often much the better for their age.³⁷

Again, the moderns were shown to be empirical, rational, concerned with matter of fact, and thus in no way in dispute with Hippocrates, as they went about building modern advances on the foundations established by the ancients – or at least using the materials of the ancients.

Hippocrates the Sydenhamian

The greatest transformation on the British scene that Hippocrates underwent occurred at the hands of Thomas Sydenham, as he researched epidemics and their cures in Restoration London. More than anyone else he represented Hippocrates as having been empirical and averse to theory, as a practitioner who observed, who built cures on what he could see and not on what he could not, who considered the effects of the environment on the appearance and nature of diseases. In particular, Sydenham celebrated Hippocrates as the *historian of diseases*.

In his writings Sydenham did not seek to justify the wisdom of Hippocrates: this was a given. For Sydenham, Hippocrates was 'the Romulus of medicine'. His most extensive passage on Hippocrates was straightforward assertion about the virtues of Hippocrates that we need to emulate. Sydenham talked about the need for an exact history of diseases:

> A Physician may as certainly take the curative Indications from the smallest Circumstances of the Disease, as he does the Diagnostick from them: And therefore I have often thought, if we had an exact History of every Disease, we should never want a Remedy suitable to it, the various

Phaenomena of it plainly shewing the way we ought to proceed in; which *Phaenomena*, if they were carefully compared one with another, would lead us to those obvious Indications, which are taken truly from Nature, and not from the Errors of Fancy.

And by these Means and Helps, the excellent *Hippocrates* arriv'd at the top of Physick, who laid this solid Foundation for building the Art of Physick upon, *viz. Nature cures Diseases*. And he delivered plainly the *Phaenomena* of every Disease, without pressing any Hypothesis for his Service, as may be seen in his Books of Diseases, Affections, and the like. He also delivered some Rules gathered from the Observation of that Method that Nature uses in promoting and removing Diseases; such are his *Praenotationes*, his *Aphorisms*, and the like: And of these things consisted the Theory of the Divine Old Man, which was not drawn from a vain and lascivious Fancy, like the Dreams of sick Men, but it exhibited a legitimate History of those Operations of Nature, which she produces in the Diseases of Men. And now seeing this Theory was nothing else but an exquisite Description of Nature, it was very reasonable, that in practice, his only aim should be to relieve her when she was oppressed, by the best means he could; and therefore he allowed no other Province for Art, than the succouring of Nature when she was weak, the restraining her when she was outragious, and the reducing her to order, and to do all this in that way and manner whereby Nature endeavours to expel Diseases; for the sagacious Man [i.e. Hippocrates] perceives that Nature judges Diseases, and does in all, being help'd by a few simple Forms of Remedies, and sometimes without any.[38]

The above passage is from the celebrated Preface to the third edition of the *Observationes Medicae*, published in Latin in 1676; the first edition, *Methodus curandi febres, propriis observationibus superstructa*, had been published in 1666. The title of this work, in both its versions, is significant, for it calls on *observation*, and in particular *one's own* observation, as the basis of medical improvement. This Hippocrates is none other than Sydenham himself. I do not mean to imply by this that Sydenham simply created a version of Hippocrates out of his own brain: on the contrary, Sydenham certainly knew the Hippocratic texts. What I do mean is that the Hippocrates that Sydenham perceived in those works was the Hippocrates most like himself. It is customary for us to speak of Sydenham as having been 'influenced' by Hippocrates. However, it is difficult to be actively influenced by a dead person: in any act of so-called 'influence' from a book by a dead writer, it is the *reader* who is the active party, who constructs – or perhaps selects – an image of that dead person or his or her 'message' by which to be (as we say) influenced.

In his published writings Sydenham claimed to be following both Bacon and Hippocrates in his medical procedures, and historians have customarily taken this assertion at face value, as if adopting the Hippocrates of the *Epidemics* was a self-evidently desirable thing to do, and as if Bacon's advice to build case histories of diseases as a first step towards improving therapies was an equally self-evidently good line to follow.[39] But, as Charles Webster has shown in *The*

Great Instauration, Bacon was adopted in different ways as an ideological mentor during the course of the seventeenth century, and Baconianism was highly political in all its different historical guises, whether at the hands of the Puritans of the 1620s to the end of the Commonwealth, or at the hands of the latitudinarians of the Royal Society who favoured the Restoration settlement of the 1660s.[40] I have argued elsewhere[41] that Thomas Sydenham was the product of a typical gentry family on the parliamentary side in the Civil War, committed to the Puritan programme of preparing for the Apocalypse. I have tried to show that his medical practice after the Restoration was that of a disgruntled relic of the Commonwealth period and that his medicine was one which met the ideals of that period including those of working to improve medicine and extending the benefits of medical care to the poor, especially with respect to the diseases which most affect them – epidemic diseases. I have argued also that Sydenham's association with Robert Boyle and John Locke convinced him that only *phenomena*, not theory, can constitute the essential *matter of fact* which is required to build true medical histories. If this argument is valid, then it would mean that Sydenham saw, in the Hippocrates that he read, the same ideals about making histories of diseases and of building, hand-in-hand with nature, new modes of cure experimentally, and that he ascribed these to Hippocrates, as the core Hippocratic doctrines, interpreting the rest of the Hippocratic writings through this lens. The case-histories of epidemics, in a generalized form, which Sydenham presented in *Observationes Medicae* and in *Methodus curandi Febres*, may be considered as elaborated versions of the case-histories of Hippocrates's *Epidemics* added to the doctrine of *Airs, Waters and Places*. As Sydenham wrote, equating his own practice and epistemology with that of Hippocrates: 'That practice, and that alone, will do good which elicits the indications of cure out of the phenomena of the disease itself. This made Hippocrates divine.'[42]

Hippocrates transformed

For Sydenham to be favourably called 'the English Hippocrates', as he was after his death, required *his* version of Hippocrates to have caught on and be seen as the 'true' Hippocrates.[43] As we have seen, it was the Hippocrates of the *Epidemics* whom Sydenham promoted. Was this version of Hippocrates – empirical rather than theoretical, expectant rather than intervening, busy making case histories – taken up widely in Britain? Although Sydenham's approach had some early British followers, it was not universally adopted: according to Sydenham himself it was not only controversial but also very unpopular amongst other physicians; moreover, Sydenham's own position in the College of Physicians was only marginal as a licentiate.[44] However, this version became widely popular in the early eighteenth century as a result of its adoption by that great maker of medical peace, Hermann Boerhaave in Leyden, and, later, as a consequence of its importation into Britain by Boerhaave's English, Scottish and Irish students.[45]

Our last dispute takes us back to the College of Physicians – that bastion of conservatism – and to the promotion there of precisely the Hippocrates of the *Epidemics*, with the shade of Sydenham called on in support. Here, we have a dispute between two collegiate physicians over both Hippocrates and Sydenham, and over the question of who is the best follower of both. It is an argument also about the centrality of observation, experiment and induction in theorising, with both parties believing themselves to be observers, experimenters and inductivists, but their opponent not to be.

In 1717 John Freind issued his volume of the text of Books I and III of the *Epidemics*, in both Greek and Latin, announcing on the title page that 'to these he has accommodated nine commentaries on fevers'.[46] Freind was one of the most accomplished classicists of his generation of physicians and, later, when he was imprisoned in the Tower of London, he was to write, virtually from memory, the first volume of a history of physick 'chiefly with regard to practice', which was intended to run from the time of Galen to the beginning of the sixteenth century.[47] Here, he urged modern physicians to become acquainted with the Ancients:

> It is an arrogance peculiar to some of our age and nation, to despise the most learned and celebrated Writers in their own Profession: and the darling notion of free-thinking carried beyond its bounds, has done a great deal of mischief in Physick, as well as in Divinity ... I am apt to believe, upon an impartial inquiry it will appear, that it was upon very good grounds that *Hippocrates*, and *Galen*, and their successors, have been all along reckon'd the great lights and fathers of the faculty, and that such an universal deference has been paid to their Writings thro' an uninterrupted succession of many centuries....[48]

But, while Freind was a friend of the ancients, he was also an adherent of the iatromechanical school. His first work *Emmenologia* (on the menses), published in 1703, was written in the 'mathematical' way of Archibald Pitcairne, itself built upon Newtonian fluid dynamics. In addition, he had lectured at Oxford on chemistry, equally explained by mechanist arguments, and he also uses such arguments here in his commentaries on Hippocrates to argue for the great efficacy of cuticular evacuation.[49] The particular points that Freind developed in his commentaries were that:

- 'Whoever reads this work [the *Epidemics*] with any skill of judging, will find nothing missing either about the signs of diagnosing diseases, or the method of healing'[50]
- Hippocrates showed that fevers have constant characters wherever they occur in the world (and that Sydenham confirmed this)

- purging should be administered in smallpox
- we can build on Hippocrates's practice to develop methods of cure in acute fevers.

Freind claimed that, in all the cases that Hippocrates gives where the patient survived (25 out of 42), they all had some kind of *evacuation*. This therefore showed which way the physician's art should follow nature in these diseases. Freind then went on to classify the seven different kinds of evacuation promoted by Hippocrates (breaking out of blood, sweats, vomits, abscesses, excreting of sputum, urine flow and flux of the bowels), and explored them by means of experience (*usus*) and observation.

Exception to Freind's commentaries was taken by John Woodward, Professor of Physic at Gresham College, as well as a Fellow of the College of Physicians and of the Royal Society. He was the author of the celebrated *An Essay Toward a Natural History of the Earth* (1695),[51] and was highly addicted to public disputes. In a recent joint consultation on a patient in London, Woodward and Freind had disagreed on the treatment of smallpox. Woodward had his own view about the treatment of smallpox, which he saw as a disease increasing in its incidence. Because the peccant matter of all diseases was centred on the stomach (Woodward argued), what one needed to do in the second fever in smallpox was not purge, as Freind recommended, but vomit the patient. He wrote:

> Dr. *Freind* has now set forth an Edition of two excellent Books of *Hippocrates*: and pays a great Deference to him, very justly. Few Ages have shewn a Man of so high a Genius, Penetration, and Capacity, as he had. Nor were his Vertues, his good Nature, and Humanity, less considerable. Then his Diligence, and Observation, were so great, and accurate, that 'tis no small Pleasure to me to find so close a Conformity, of what he has deliver'd with what I here offer simply from the Contemplation of Nature ....[52]

And this great Hippocrates did not only correctly maintain that 'there ought not, by any Means, to be given Purges to those that are seiz'd with high Fevers until the Fever remitts',[53] even though he had never seen a case of the smallpox, but this great Hippocrates also maintained that a knowledge of *cause* in disease is essential to good treatment. This Freind seemed to have denied:

> Nor will I be brought to believe that a Gentleman of the Learning of Dr. *Freind*, can be in the Dark as to this Affair. Which makes me somewhat wonder that he should openly give out that the *Causes of Diseases are hid to us, and will probably ever be so*. This is, indeed, inconsistent with what he had formerly written: and a *Theory in Physick*, that takes not in the Causes of Diseases, cannot carry with it much Demonstration or Mathematical Certainty. Then he [Freind] is much in the wrong, where he asserts that *Hippocrates has not a Word concerning the Causes of Diseases*. So much, that, in almost all his Works, that sagacious Writer is

searching into, and pointing forth those Causes. Particularly in the two very Books that Dr. *Freind* has here publish'd ...[54]

It is extraordinary, from a modern point of view, to see Woodward accusing Freind of evading issues of cause in physic, given that Freind was a principal advocate of the mathematical form of reasoning in medicine. However, what Freind was attempting to do here was first build on and generalize from Hippocrates's modes of cure, and then seek to introduce causal explanations for why it worked. In other words, his Hippocrates is a judicious empirical practitioner under whose practice lay an unspoken, and even unconscious, theory which we can elicit. Woodward read this as Freind absurdly dismissing the role of causal explanation – especially of the kind that had led Woodward himself to his understanding of the role of the stomach and digestion in the cause of most diseases.

Woodward was particularly incensed that Freind had called Sydenham to his support: 'Indeed, upon the whole, I am not able to find out why they will have Dr. *Sydenham* to be a Patron and Voucher of this Practise'.[55] For Sydenham's practice in the smallpox was quite otherwise, and even though he was wrong for a while (Woodward wrote) he was nevertheless someone able to learn astutely from nature and change his treatment accordingly.[56]

This dispute – this 'smallpox war', as it has been called – was far from concluded at this point, and it led to a paper battle between Freind and his allies, including Dr Mead on the one side and Woodward on the other. It climaxed in a famous real-life battle – an impromptu duel between Woodward and Mead in Gresham College. In the duel, Mead had Woodward at his mercy and then (according to one version) said, 'Take your life!', to which Woodward replied, 'Anything but your physic!'[57]

Conclusion: Hippocrates the model empiric?

Throughout the disputes that I have been looking at, *reason* and *experience* are constantly argued over. Everyone is on the side of both reason and experience, and reason and experience are on the side of everyone, but they mean different things to different people. The experience of a collegiate physician is worthless in the eyes of a Helmontian chemical physician; the reason of a Helmontian is unreason in the eyes of a university-educated physician. And vice versa. The terms are important because they are, in all cases, believed to be the basis of whatever medical practice is in question, and proper medical practice is a matter of life and death. However, they are probably not very useful categories, either in the seventeenth or the twentieth centuries, by which to explore the historic Hippocrates, whoever he was.

But another contrasted pair of terms is also in dispute in all these controversies – *youth* and *old age*. Were the ancient physicians and, of course, most especially Hippocrates, wiser than us? Are their doctrines to be valued because they are ancient and have the guarantee of centuries of successful implementation? Or were they living only in the childhood and youth of medicine, and thus does their knowledge need to be confirmed by the experience of later ages before it can be trusted? Francis Bacon raised this question, concluding that the ancients lived in the youth of knowledge. My impression is that the radicals and chemists tended to say that Hippocrates lived during the childhood of medicine, and hence his teachings needed to be supplemented by modern experience. The more conservative, collegiate, physicians said that the oldest is best, wisest and most safe. The conservatives also claimed that a virtue of Hippocratic medicine was that it was most generalized – highlighting the importance of Hippocratic oracular and aphoristic sayings, such as the *Epidemics* and *Aphorisms* respectively. Marchamont Nedham urged people to throw out the concept of critical days in diseases as being:

> ... as childish a Conceit as ever was owned by any Long Beards called the Children of men; for, truly it is like the Children's game called *Ludere Par Impar, Even and odd*, and yet the Antients are all very grave at it. ... The establishment of them was by *Hippocrates* in his *Aphorisms* and *Prognosticks*; and from him, *Galen*, and all the rest of the Commentators have borrowed the Phantasie.[58]

Did Hippocrates (with or without Galen) lay the foundations of medicine, to which we can judiciously add? Or should we, with our greater maturity in medicine, be rejecting their structure for the immature and inexperienced work that it really is?

Finally I turn to William Heberden the elder (1710–1801), in the hope of indicating that at least some of the most forward-looking and research-oriented of establishment physicians in Britain had by the early decades of the eighteenth century, accepted a view of Hippocrates which is primarily the 'Epidemics' view that Sydenham promoted – though with a twist. Heberden – a Fellow of the College of Physicians from 1746, rising to become an Elect – was a third generation follower of Sydenham but, unlike Sydenham, he thought that anatomy and other such disciplines had much to offer the physician. Dr Johnson famously called him 'Ultimus Romanorum, the last of our learned physicians', while Samuel Thomas von Soemmerring in Germany was to call him 'Medicus vere Hippocraticus' (and, to confuse the issue, William Osler later called him 'the English Celsus'!).

In 1741, while still at Cambridge teaching and practising medicine, Heberden contributed to the curious work, published anonymously and coordinated by the Earl of Hardwick, called *Athenian Letters*.[59] This piece of moral entertainment purported to be a series of recently discovered letters from a Persian royal agent, a certain Cleanthes, in Athens during the Peloponnesian War. It was a way of giving an accessible account of classical Greece to a lay readership, and also, of course, of highlighting the concerns of modern Englishmen by relating them to the conditions of ancient Greece and vice versa. Cleanthes witnesses the war, he goes to the Olympic games, he reports on the advantages of Athenian political arrangements, he discusses the state of Greek philosophy, he chats with Socrates, he hears a lecture on fossils as the evidences of a great flood (highly topical in the eighteenth century) and so on. He also writes a letter to his friend, the royal physician of Persia, describing Hippocratic medicine. It is this letter which Heberden penned. In it we can find, in this lightly fictionalized form, Heberden's long-term attitudes towards Hippocrates and discern, in his evaluation of it, something of his medical concerns, which he attributed to Hippocrates.

Hippocrates, descended from a long line of physicians, skilled in gymnastic physic, and familiar with the votive tablets in the temple of Aesculapius, has introduced a new practice, Cleanthes writes to his friend, that of constantly visiting the sick in their beds.

> By which careful attendance to the whole course of the distemper, he has not only been able to give a timely assistance against every inconvenient or dangerous accident, but is become superior to all other physicians in the knowledge of diseases, and in foretelling their events. From this practice he has got the name of a Clinic physician.

It is also to Hippocrates's credit that he resolved to take out of the hands of the philosophers those parts of philosophy relevant to physic. His knowledge of theory thus acquired, as well as his knowledge of practice from his application to the sick, put him in an ideal situation: 'On the one hand he is preserved from the useless refinements of theorists, as on the other from the gross errors and superstitions of vulgar empirics.' However, Hippocrates has gone too far. For he claims that the whole of physic is now found out, whereas it is really still in its infancy:

> In particular, he is not master of a sufficient number of simples for all the various purposes of physic; and does not perhaps fully understand the true uses and qualities of those he has; for too much stress seems to be laid on some ineffectual ones, while others more violent in their effects are used with too little caution. The study of anatomy is still less advanced; all that is known is derived, either comparatively from the animals, that are sacrificed, or from the Aegyptian embalmers of human bodies; and I much doubt, whether Hippocrates ever saw a human body dissected. However, he has endeavoured to supply, from fancy and conjecture, his imperfect knowledge of the structure and true use of the parts; but, as is usual, where this is done, his accounts are generally improbable, often ridiculous and inconsistent.[60]

These views of Hippocrates as an excellent empirical physician, but a misguided theoretical one, we find again in a work by Heberden, written in the mid-1740s, on the desirable form of education for a physician,[61] a work intended for his students or possibly his son. Here, Heberden praised Sydenham in the chapter 'Of the history of diseases and their cure':

> We are therefore come at last to the great business of the physician, to which all that has hitherto been said is only preparatory. In this pursuit he is to set himself no bounds, but must be perpetually adding either to his own observations by those of others, or enlarging what others have done by what he himself observes, nor must his study in this part end except with life. I shall point out some useful authors to him, by whom he may be initiated ... The first of those writers who have treated only of a few distempers (who are to be preferred to those who have built systems out of other people's observations and writings) is the admired Sydenham, whose merit is, that he is an original one, giving only what he himself observed in diseases he is judged to come nearer to the true idea of a practical writer than most other authors, as he has mixed but little of hypothesis and speculation with what he says, being generally contented with relating an exact history of the rise and progress of the disease, and of that method of treating the patient which was found most effectual in conducting him easily to a speedy recovery.[62]

Heberden modelled his own research on that of Sydenham. Believing that medicine could be improved by the systematic keeping of disease histories over the years, a project in which he sought to engage his fellow collegiate physicians, Heberden was, as a result, able to identify a number of new disease syndromes in the course of his years of medical practice in Cambridge and London, of which the most famous were probably *angina pectoris* (announced in 1768) and chicken-pox. But although, to us, this kind of medical research might seem to resemble that of Hippocrates in the *Epidemics* as much as it resembles that of Sydenham, Heberden was, as we have seen, far less enthusiastic about recommending Hippocrates than he was about Sydenham on the grounds that the ancients had no chemistry, their materia medica was not very good, they rarely dissected the human body, and their physiology was 'but a heap of wild notions'.[63] He continued:

> All these defects in the above mentioned branches of this study, which can hardly be disputed by any one, must therefore be abundantly compensated by their [i.e. the ancients'] merit in the history of diseases, which alone remains to support their character. Hippocrates in particular is represented as excelling all others upon this head. He was indebted to nature for a sound understanding, & applied himself to the schools of the philosophers for all the learning of the age. Fortune conspired with his own industry to furnish him with several uncommon opportunities of improving himself in his particular profession ... Thus qualified for making observations, he was happily for us remarkably faithful & ingenuous in reporting them. If this great man was not perfect, it was owing to the imperfection of human nature, & some disadvantages that necessarily attended the times in which he lived.[64]

But even though Hippocrates was gifted and ingenious, his writings could not be accepted without further ado, according to Heberden. For Hippocrates was (of all things!) a great system-maker, leaping to conclusions without adequate facts. This is an unexpected accusation, and one that could probably only be made if Sydenham was taken as the model in terms of recording case histories and seeking cures. Heberden writes:

> Knowledge in nature is justly called the daughter of Time & Experience, & indeed of much longer time & experience than we are apt to imagine after the discovery has been made. It is a great while before men are capable of making any use of what passes before them unless they are put upon the observing of it. When they first enter upon a new field of knowledge, they are struck with many insignificant appearances & pass over others of the greatest importance: they are too impatient to wait for the slow production of nature for the formation of their system, & so help it forward by the warmth of their fancy: they are too hasty in coming to general conclusions & aphorisms from too small a number of facts; which sort of knowledge, like the ill-gotten possessions of those who haste to make themselves to be rich, seldom thrives, moulders, & comes to nothing with their posterity. All which is exemplified in Hippocrates & all other principal writers of antiquity. These then are the disadvantages Hippocrates laboured under from the condition of physic & natural philosophy, & were the faults of the age. He would be more than human if he did not add to them by his own.[65]

Thus, since Hippocrates lived in the youth of medicine, 'We can never therefore safely practise upon any of his aphorisms that have not been confirmed & made probable by later experience'. Even when Hippocrates writes on diseases, we must check what he says against nature itself.

The model physician himself, the divine old man, whose writings were built on observation and experience, and which had been the foundation for all medicine for 2000 years, had now been turned into someone whose statements need to be tested, just like anyone else.

Notes

1. The most blatant example of this that I have found with respect to Hippocrates is a work of 1821 called *Le Magnetisme Animal Retrouvé dans l'Antiquité, ou Dissertation Historique, Etymologique et Mythologique sur Esculape, Hippocrate et Galien*, by Etienne Félix Hénin de Cuvillers, Paris, Chez Barrios l'aîné etc., but this may be so blatant to us only because animal magnetism is *passé*.
2. Harold J. Cook, *The Decline of the Old Medical Regime in Stuart London*, Ithaca, NY: Cornell University Press, 1986, p. 185. The significance of Sydenham's anti-academic sentiments here is that Cook is writing about the College of Physicians, of which Sydenham was not a vocal supporter.
3. Ludwig Edelstein, 'Sydenham and Cervantes', in Ludwig Edelstein, *Ancient Medicine*, ed. Owsei Temkin and C. Lilian Temkin, Baltimore: Johns Hopkins University Press, 1967, pp. 455–61.
4. Charles Webster, *The Great Instauration: Science, Medicine and Reform, 1626–*

1660, London: Duckworth, 1975; P.M. Rattansi, 'The Helmontian–Galenist Controversy in Restoration England', *Ambix*, **11**, 1963, pp. 1–23.

5. Sir Robert Sibbald, *Memoria Balfouriana, Sive Historia Rerum, Pro Literis Promovendis, Gestarum a Clarissimis Fratribus Balfouriis, D.D. Jacobo, Barone de Kinaird, Equite, Leone, Rege Armorium: et D.D. Andrea, M.D., Equite Aurato*, Edinburgh: Heirs of Anderson, 1699, p. 49.
6. Francis P. Hett (ed.), *The Memoirs of Sir Robert Sibbald, Knt., M.D. Oxford: Oxford University Press*, 1932, pp. 64–65.
7. Ibid., p. 66.
8. Ibid., p. 78.
9. Thomas Burnet, *Thesaurus Medicinae Practicae, ex Praestantissimorum tum Veterum tum Recentiorum Medicorum, Observationibus, Consultationibus Consiliis & Epistolis, summa Diligentia collectus ordineque alphabetico dispositus, Studio et opera Thomae Burnet Scoto-Britanni, M.D. & medici regis ordinarii*, London: G.R. for Robert Boulter, 1673.
10. Thomas Burnet, *Hippocrates Contractus. In quo Magni Hippocrates Medicorum Principis Opera Omnia, in brevem Epitomen, summa diligentia redacta habentur*, Edinburgh: Mosman, 1685.
11. *Praefatio Ad Lectorem* (not paginated).
12. As quoted in W.S. Craig, *History of the Royal College of Physicians of Edinburgh*, Oxford: Blackwell Scientific Publishing, 1976, pp. 385–86.
13. The following section is based on Andrew Cunningham, 'Sir Robert Sibbald and Medical Education, Edinburgh, 1706', *Clio Medica*, **13**, 1978, pp. 135–61.
14. Sir Robert Sibbald, *In Hippocratis Legem, et in ejus Epistolam ad Thessalum Filium, Commentarii: in quibus Ostenditur, quae Medico Futuro, Necessaria Sunt*, Edinburgh: Symson, 1706.
15. Cunningham, 'Sir Robert Sibbald' (n. 13), p. 10.
16. Ibid., pp. 10–12.
17. Marchamont Nedham, *Medela Medicinae. A Plea for the Free Profession, and a Renovation of the Art of Physick, out of the Noblest and most Authentick Writers. Shewing The Publick Advantage of its Liberty; The Disadvantage that comes to the Publick by any sort of Physicians, imposing upon the Studies and Practise of others; The Alteration of Diseases from their old State and Condition; The Causes of that Alteration; The Insufficiency and Uselessness of meer Scholastick Methods and Medicines, with a necessity of new. Tending to the Rescue of Mankind from the Tyranny of Diseases; and of Physicians themselves, from the Pedantism of old Authors and present Dictators*, The Author, M.N. Med. Londinens. London: For Richard Lowndes, 1665.
18. See Nedham's Preface to Marchamont Nedham, *A New Idea of the Practice of Physic; Written by that Famous Franciscus de le Boe, Sylvius ... All Cleard by Anatomical Experients and Chymical Demonstrations; As also their Cures. Whereto is prefixed a Preface written by Dr. Mar. Nedham. Translated faithfully by Richard Gower, formerly Student under the Author*, London, 1675.
19. Both in Anthony à Wood, *Athenae Oxoniensis. An Exact History of All the Writers and Bishops who have had their Education in the University of Oxford. Edited by Philip Bliss*, 4 vols London: F.C. and J. Rivington, 1817, Vol. 3, cols. 1185, 1189.
20. Nedham, *Medela Medicinae* (n. 17), p. 40.
21. Ibid., pp. 173–74.
22. Ibid., p. 232.
23. Ibid., p. 240.

24. Ibid., pp. 294–95.
25. Edward Bolness, *Medicina Instaurata, or; a Brief Account of the True Grounds and Principles of the Art of Physick. With the Insufficiency of the Vulgar Way of Preparing Medicines, and the Excellency of such as are made by Chymical Operation ... Also an Epistolary Discourse upon the whole, by the Author of Medula Medicinae*, London: Starkey, 1665; see Nedham's Epistolary Discourse.
26. Nedham, *Medela Medicinae* (n. 17), pp. 120–21.
27. Ibid., p. 351.
28. Ibid., p. 353.
29. Ibid., p. 351.
30. See Nedham's Preface to *New Idea* (n. 18).
31. Robert Sprackling, *Medela Ignorantiae*, London: R. Crofts, 1665.
32. Ibid., p. 85.
33. Ibid., pp. 85–87.
34. Ibid., pp. 50–51.
35. George Castle, *The Chymical Galenist: A treatise, wherein the practice of the Ancients is reconcil'd to the new discoveries in the theory of physick; shewing, that many of their rules, methods, and medicins, are useful for the curing of diseases in this age, and in the northern parts of the world. In which are some reflections upon a book, intituled, Medela Medicinae. By George Castle, Dr. of Physick, lately Fellow of All-souls Colledge in Oxon*, London: Printed by Sarah Griffin for Henry Twyford, 1667.
36. Thomas Willis, *Diatribae Duae Medico-philosophicae, Quarum Prior agit De Fermentatione, Altera De Febribus*, London: J. Martin, 1659.
37. Castle, *The Chymical Galenist* (n. 35), p. 196.
38. I use the first and best translation: Thomas Sydenham, *The Whole Works of that excellent practical physician, Dr Thomas Sydenham. Wherein not only the History and Cures of Acute Diseases are treated of, after a New and Accurate Method; But also the Shortest and Safest Way of Curing most Chronical Diseases*, trans. John Pechey, London: R. Wellington, third edition, 1701 (First published 1695). The quote is at A4v–A5r.
39. The most important passage where Bacon speaks of Hippocrates is Francis Bacon, *The Advancement of Learning*, London: Dent, 1965 (first published 1605) Book 2, X, section 4:

> The first [deficiency of medicine] is the discontinuance of the ancient and serious diligence of Hippocrates, which used to set down a narrative of the special cases of his patients and how they proceeded, and how they were judged by recovery or death. Therefore having an example proper in the father of the art, I shall not need to allege an example foreign, of the wisdom of the lawyers, who are careful to report new cases and decisions for the direction of future judgements.

40. Webster, *Great Instauration* (n. 4).
41. See Andrew Cunningham, 'Thomas Sydenham: Epidemics, Experiment and the "Good Old Cause"', in Roger French and Andrew Wear (eds), *The Medical Revolution of the Seventeenth Century*, Cambridge: Cambridge University Press, 1989, pp. 164–90.
42. Sydenham's 'Epistle to Dr Brady', sec. 51, in his *Whole Works* (n. 38).
43. On this title, see F.N.L. Poynter, 'Sydenham's Influence Abroad', *Medical History*, **17**, 1973, pp. 223–34.

44. On the primarily political reasons for its unpopularity, see Andrew Cunningham, 'Sydenham versus Newton: the Edinburgh fever dispute between Andrew Brown and Archibald Pitcairne', in W.F. Bynum and V. Nutton (eds), *Theories of Fever from Antiquity to the Enlightenment*, London: Wellcome Institute for the History of Medicine, 1981, pp. 71–98.
45. On Boerhaave's eclectic and eirenic medical doctrine, see Andrew Cunningham, 'Medicine to calm the mind: Boerhaave's medical system and why it was adopted in Edinburgh', in Andrew Cunningham and Roger French (eds), *The Medical Enlightenment of the Eighteenth Century*, Cambridge: Cambridge University Press, 1990, pp. 40–66.
46. John Freind, *Hippocratis de Morbis Popularibus liber primus, et tertius. His accommodavit Novem De Febribus commentarios Johannes Freind, M.D., Coll. Med. Londin. & Soc. Reg. Socius*, London: William Innys, 1717.
47. On Freind and the writing of this history, see Julian Martin, 'Explaining John Freind's *History of Physick*', *Studies in History and Philosophy of Science*, 19, 1988, pp. 399–418.
48. John Freind, *The History of Physick; from the Time of Galen, to the Beginning of the Sixteenth Century. Chiefly with Regard to Practice. In a Discourse written to Doctor Mead. Part I. Containing All the Greek Writers*, London: Walthoe, 1725, pp. 305–6.
49. See Theodore M. Brown, *The Mechanical Philosophy and the "Animal Oeconomy". A Study in the Development of English Physiology in the Seventeenth and Early Eighteenth Century*, reprint of 1968 Princeton University PhD thesis) New York: Arno Press, 1981, esp. pp. 280–81.
50. My translation from p.5 of Freind (n. 48).
51. John Woodward, *An Essay Toward a Natural History of the Earth: and Terrestial Bodies, especially Minerals ...*, London: R. Wilkin, 1695.
52. John Woodward, *The State of Physick: and of Diseases; with an Inquiry into the Causes of the Late Increase in Them: But More Particularly of the Small-pox. With Some Considerations Upon the New Practice of Purgeing [sic] in that Disease*, London: Home, 1718, p. 90.
53. Ibid., pp. 142–43.
54. Ibid., pp. 60–61.
55. Ibid., p. 75.
56. See ibid., pp. 78–79:

> Dr. *Sydenham*, takeing Notice of the Inconveniencyes that attended the Hot Method [in smallpox], fell, over hastily, into the other extreme: and recommended the Cooling. Reason and Nature give realy [sic] not Countenance to either ... Nor will it be thought strange that a Man, of Diligence and good Sense of Dr. *Sydenham*, should, after some Time, and further Experience, again quit that, as he had before rejected the hot Method: and fall finaly into the temperate. For he gave Acids, Small Beer, and other cooling Things, but very sparingly, in the latter Times of his Practise. This I learn from Mr. *Malthus*, his Apothecary, and intimate Friend: and I am the more forward to note it because, by Dr. *Sydenham*'s Writeings, Some, who attend more to Authority, and what they read, than to Nature and Things, have in this Article, however right he may have been in others, been led into a not slight Error.

57. The story is told in Joseph M. Levine, *Dr Woodward's Shield. History, Science,*

and Satire in Augustan England (first published 1977), Ithaca, NY: Cornell University Press, 1991, chapter 1.
58. Nedham, *Medela Medicinae* (n. 17), pp. 306–7.
59. [Philip Yorke, 2nd Earl of Hardwicke], *Athenian Letters: or, The Epistolary Correspondence of an Agent of the King of Persia, residing at Athens during the Peloponnesian War. Containing the History of the Times, in Dispatches to the Ministers of State at the Persian Court. Besides Letters on various Subjects between Him and His Friends*, 4 vols, London: Bettenham, 1741–43.
60. Ibid., p. 198.
61. William Heberden, *An Introduction to the Study of Physic, with a Prefatory Essay by Leroy Crummer*, New York: Hoeber, 1929.
62. Ibid., pp. 108–10.
63. Ibid., p. 132.
64. Ibid., pp. 132–33.
65. Ibid., pp. 133–34.

CHAPTER SIX

Hippocrates and the Politics of Medical Knowledge in Early Modern England

Robert L. Martensen

Introduction

When seventeenth-century natural philosophers put forward their views, many routinely cited classical Greek and Roman sources as well as their contemporaries and near-contemporaries either in a supportive context or to debunk their opinion. Occasionally they mused on the general merits of 'ancients' versus 'moderns' as cognitive guides. Subsequently, many historians and others who have explored early modern natural philosophy – what has come to be known as the 'scientific revolution' of Western Europe – have commented on various aspects of this 'ancients and moderns' theme, generally in the context of the decline of scholasticism that occurred during the period.[1] Indeed, the subject occurs regularly in university courses dealing with the intellectual history of early modern Europe.

In this essay I propose to use differences among early modern views of Hippocrates as a cognitive authority in order to briefly examine some issues that until now have been largely obscured in the historiography of the 'ancients versus moderns' story. My focus is on a period of extended social, religious and political crises in England, mainly the decades 1640–1690 that encompassed its Revolution, Restoration, and Glorious Revolution. My intention is to show how religious and political factors helped shape responses made by some influential medical knowledge-makers to Hippocrates, Galen and their seventeenth-century contemporaries.[2] I am particularly interested in exploring tensions that developed between those who cited Hippocrates and those who did not, and some ways in which these reflected their divergent political and religious affiliations in the turbulent decades of the mid- to late seventeenth century. In such a way I hope to open up the question as to why they felt they had to choose between Galen and Hippocrates when earlier practitioners had not felt compelled to make such a choice. The essay's first three sections deal with some intellectual differences between those who chose Hippocrates as their 'ancient' and those who did not in three contexts:

1. Harvey's intellectual disciples at Oxford;
2. some of their critics;
3. the emergence of Thomas Sydenham as a medical authority in the later part of the century.

The fourth section explores why the choice became important.

Hippocrates, Galen, and the Oxford physiologists

In trying to make sense of the status of Hippocratic knowledge in early modern England, consider the following: In 1628 William Harvey published *De motu cordis et sanguinis*, an exposition on the structure and function of the heart and blood vessels that led mid-century almanac writers, not to mention eminent learned physicians, to call him 'immortal' in his lifetime. While Harvey's other principal works – the anatomical lecture notes of 1616 and his 1653 work on animal reproduction – contained several references to Hippocrates (as Thomas Rütten observes in this volume), each, as did *De motu*, referred much more to Galen and Aristotle than Hippocrates as ancient authorities. *De motu* itself contained one reference to Hippocrates, which occurred in chapter 17, when Harvey noted him as the author of a brief, 800 word, text, *De corde*, which Harvey interpreted as Hippocrates's affirmation of the heart as a muscle.[3] However, Thomas Willis, leader of the experimentalists who assembled at Oxford in the 1640s and 1650s to take up issues suggested by Harvey's work, made no reference to Hippocrates in his 1664 *Cerebri anatome*, England's other enduring anatomical book from its 'scientific revolution'. Indeed, the post-Harvean experimentalists who established early modern England as an influential centre of scientific medicine from the 1650s to 1680s – for example, Willis, William Petty, Robert Hooke, Richard Lower, John Mayow, Robert Boyle, Francis Glisson and Thomas Wharton – seldom referred to Hippocrates.

Instead, when the Oxford physiologists – to use Robert Frank's phrase for the group of medical natural philosophers active in Oxford from the mid-1640s through the mid-1660s – referred to ancient authority, they referred mainly to Aristotle, Galen, Democritus and Eristratus; when they referred to moderns, they did so most frequently to their contemporaries and near contemporaries. For example, among the near moderns, Harvey in *De motu* refers to Fabricius of Aquapente, Realdo Columbo, Andreas Laurentius, Casper Bauhin, Jean Riolan the younger, Jacob Silvius, Andreas Vesalius and Daniel Fernel. He limited the ancients to Eristratus and Galen. Willis, attempting in 1664 in *Cerebri anatome* to do for the brain and nerves what Harvey accomplished for the heart and vessels a generation earlier, acknowledged Descartes, Gassendi, Malpighi, Fernel, Hooghelande and Henricius as moderns, while his ancients included Aristotle, Plato, Pythagoras and Galen.

Why did the Oxford physiologists pay so little attention to Hippocrates? Early in his career, Willis provided a straightforward reason why investigative physicians of his era – the generation that came to maturity in the 1640s and early 1650s – made most of their references to contemporaries and near-contemporaries: it was because Harvey's theory of the circulation of the blood had completely upset conventional wisdom on disease causation and treatment. As Willis expressed the issue in his treatise of fevers, originally published in the mid-1650s:

> ... because the Antients relying on a false Position concerning the Motion of the Blood ... often fell foully and dangerously: wherefore it is no wonder ... for the thorough Instauration of Physick, and for the re-Edifying the Building ... on that which our most Famous Harvey hath laid, the Circulation of the Blood ... and it is granted us to know the Causes of things before hidden.[4]

Not only did the specific contents of Harvey's circulation theory stimulate a reconceptualisation of diseases and treatments, his reliance on anatomical methods showed that

> ... naked Experience, without the helps of Method and Reason, avails little, yea very often doth much hurt. ... He seems to have hit the mark, who joyns both together, that reason may not pervert Experiments, and Nature itself, not that this may remove Reason from its place.[5]

If the foregoing sets out the predominant attitude toward medical knowledge among those English experimentalists who followed Harvey, what might explain Harvey's preferential use of Galen and Aristotle, rather than Hippocrates, in constructing his physiological narrative of the human body? Several reasons come to mind, but the most important is that Hippocrates, by which I mean the Hippocratic authors, did not perform human dissections.[6] In fact, their writings forbade experimentation and emphasised instead close superficial observation of patients in their social and environmental contexts.[7] Eristratus and Hierophilus performed dissections in Ptolemaic Egypt, but investigations into human anatomy then stopped for approximately 1500 years in the Christian West. Furthermore, no non-Western medical system ever developed an anatomical tradition.

Hippocratic knowledge, particularly that expressed in the texts common in the high Renaissance and early modern period – the *Epidemics*, *Airs, Waters, and Places*, and *Fevers* – did not concern the inner workings of the body. Nor did the Hippocratics pay much attention to aetiology. But to anatomically inclined physicians, structure, function and cause mattered greatly. Anecdotal evidence suggests that Harvey planned to write a final work that integrated his anatomical knowledge of healthy and sick bodies with diagnostic and therapeutic approaches, but abandoned the project when his records were destroyed late in his life.[8] Willis, the most influential physician to work in his shadow, did write such a book, which was published posthumously and titled (in its English translation), *Rational Therapeutics*.[9] In short, for Harvey as well as his followers, Hippocrates seemed irrelevant. By contrast, Galen, whom many of the Oxford physiologists cited, was a consummate anatomist who, like them, was committed to a 'rational' medicine based on knowledge of the structure and function of deep bodily structures.

Hippocrates and the counter-anatomists

Hippocrates merited high praise, though, for his accessible and practical knowledge from several mid-century English healers who published inexpensive medical self-help books. For example, Nicholas Culpeper, the populariser most noted for his inexpensive texts on herbals published during the 1630s and the Civil War, favoured the Levellers – that is, the Puritan sect with pronounced egalitarian outlooks.[10] Fed up with expensive medicine and arcane medical advice, Culpeper argued in 1649 that professional hierarchies should be eliminated – 'priests, physicians, lawyers, all of them monopolists'.[11]

During the 1650s and 1660s conservative humoralists, such as Edmund O'Meara,[12] as well as some alchemical and empirical healers, attacked the Oxford group for their belief in the value of anatomical arguments. In 1654 John Webster, who earned his living practising medicine and surgery, published (in English) his *Academiarum examen*, a critique of university curricula, particularly in medicine.[13] Webster, who earlier studied religion and alchemy, had served as a chaplain and surgeon in the parliamentary army. Within a few months of Webster's publication, John Wilkins, an early sponsor of the Oxford physiologists, and Seth Ward, then Savilian Professor of Astronomy at Oxford (and subsequently Bishop of Salisbury), published a response, the *Vindiciae academiarum, containing some briefe animadeversions upon Mr. Webster's book*.[14]

Here, I want to concentrate on those aspects of the controversy that dealt with bodily investigation, for a brief examination of the debate will help convey the extent of incommensurability that characterised mid-seventeenth-century disputes about what constituted proper medical knowledge.

Paradoxically, Webster's curricular reforms contained many of the same elements as those encouraged by Wilkins and Ward in the extra-curricular clubs that nurtured the Oxford physiologists. According to Webster, students must 'learn to inure their hands to labour' through a chemical work.[15] They were to have 'Laboratories as well as Libraries'.[16] Not only should students study Plato's *Republic*, Thomas More's *Utopia*, and Bacon's *New Atlantis*, they should also read the moderns – Pierre Gassendi, the French priest who helped revive Epicurean atomism, and Réné Descartes. Webster's recommendation for ocular inspection and 'handwork' (hands on experimentation) was not substantively different – at least on the surface – from Ward's for 'observation and experiment'.[17]

These nominal similarities are superficial, however, as a brief look at the participants' respective ideas of anatomy reveals. Whereas the 'ocular demonstrations' of interregnum Oxford club anatomy claimed to provide precise demonstrations of the structure and function of (formerly) living humans, Webster's anatomy was explicitly 'mystical'. Although he praised the contributions of 'our never-sufficiently honoured countryman Doctor Harvey', understanding the 'wonderful secret' of the blood's circulation was of 'small advantage' in curing diseases. Harvey's kind of anatomy, while it could 'bring great satisfaction to a speculative understanding', did little 'to remove dolor, danger, or death'.[18]

According to Webster, the true anatomy was 'Mystical Anatomy'.[19] This process, which Webster did not define, actually discovered the 'true Schematism' of 'that invisible Archeus' that was the true 'opisex' (*sic*) of all 'salutary and morbifict' bodily experiences. Approved authorities included Paracelsus, J.B. van Helmont – both of whom approved of Hippocrates but not Galen – and Robert Fludd.[20] In common with these alchemists, Webster also loathed Aristotle. Interestingly, Ward did not criticise Aristotelian learning directly, but in his Savilian lectures he ignored the sponsor's stipulation that they comment exclusively on Aristotelian texts.[21] Willis later did likewise in his Sedleian lectures of the 1660s.

Another indication that Webster's programme of hands-on experiment was quite different from that of Wilkins and Ward was their differing use of the term 'natural magic'. After describing the virtues of 'mystical anatomy', Webster then proceeded to recommend for curricular inclusion the 'science of physiognomy'. Such a recommendation was based on the Renaissance doctrine of signatures: external features revealed inner qualities. Behind that lay the tradition of reasoning by analogy with microcosm and macrocosm. The goal of the universities should be to train 'true Natural Magicians'.[22]

But, then, what was true natural magic? In refuting Webster on his discussion of natural magic, I think it telling that Ward did not argue that natural magic did not exist, but rather that Webster followed a false path. According to Ward, students learned 'true naturall Magick' not by the 'pretence of specificall vertues' in things, but by 'applying agent and Materiall causes to produce effects'. Harvey's discovery of the circulation of the blood, as well as all the attendant discoveries it had inspired, had improved both the theory and practice of physic. Just consider, Ward wrote, a recent instance: two physicians were among a group witnessing the judicial hanging of a young woman for infanticide. After 'she had been hanged at least half an hower', they participated in 'recovering the Wench'.[23] This reference could only be to the hanging of Anne Green, a servant convicted of infanticide in Oxford in 1651. Willis, the anatomist William Petty and Willis's partner, the surgeon William

Day, attended the execution with a plan to dissect Green's corpse subsequently. When they removed the body to Day's lodgings, however, they noticed a movement. Willis and Petty then thumped her chest and otherwise attempted to revive her, and Green subsequently woke up. Granted clemency, she continued to live in Oxford and the three men received substantial credit for the 'resurrection'.[24] For Ward, Green's revival by learned physicians was 'naturall magick', a category that also included the learning represented in the membership of the College of Physicians.[25]

Coming after Culpeper, O'Meara, and Webster in 1664, when the Interregnum dust may have settled but professional rivalries between elitist physicians and their competitors continued unabated, the anonymous author of *The Method of Chemical Philosophy and Physick* revered Hippocrates for recognising that 'Nature (is) the governor of Man'.[26] But he or she expended more effort on trashing Galen, who 'hath never attained unto the secrets of Hippocrates, whereby he hath left the essence of Nature untouched and uncomprehended'.[27]

Sydenham, Hippocrates, and the rise of the natural history method

Thomas Sydenham's (1623–1689) work reveals additional differences between those who cited Hippocrates and those who did not. Ironically, although the 'English Hippocrates', as Sydenham came to be known in the eighteenth century, and the Oxford physiologists were contemporaries and Sydenham studied in Oxford when the latter were active young investigators, his attitude towards medical knowledge could not be more opposed to theirs. According to Sydenham, whose published works contained references only to Hippocrates and no other medical authorities, God had designed man so as to be capable of perceiving only the superficial aspects of reality, the 'outer husk of things'.[28] The metaphor for true knowledge was not mathematics, as Galen, Willis and other rationalists imagined, but botany: 'It is necessary that all diseases be reduced to definite and certain species and that, with the same care which we see exhibited by botanists in their phytologies.'[29] Furthermore, Sydenham considered nature 'an abyss of cause'.[30] For instance, anatomists were incapable of achieving an understanding of the brain because, although it displayed the 'method of the Supreme Artificer in his wondrous and wise machinery', the brain was 'so coarse a substance (a mere pulp, and that not over-nicely wrought)' that 'no diligent contemplation of its structure will tell us how [it] should subserve so noble an end'.[31]

Importantly, Sydenham thought that cause was not only unknowable by definition, but also that such knowledge was not useful in the practice of medicine. Two years after Willis's *Cerebri anatome* (1664), Sydenham first published his *Methodus* (1666). In a passage from this edition that may have referred directly to Willis, then Oxford's Sedleian Professor of Natural Philosophy, Sydenham explicitly eschewed interest in medical philosophy or aetiology:

> For my own part, I am not ambitious of the name of a Philosopher, and those who think themselves so, may, perhaps consider me blamable on the score of my not having attempted to pierce into these mysteries. Now writers like these I would just recommend, before they blame others, to try their hand upon some common phenomena of Nature that meet us at every turn .... Aetiology is a difficult, and perhaps, an inexplicable affair; and I chose to keep my hands clear of it.[32]

For Sydenham the overarching biological and medical concepts became the 'species' and the 'constitution' and he used both terms heuristically (and often loosely) to categorise fevers and their effects on humans. The physician's diagnostic task was one of recognising patterns of interaction between kinds of fever, local environmental factors and individual bodies. Taken together, these formed an 'epidemic constitution'. Although Sydenham did not use the term 'species' until his later work, the *Observationes medicae* of 1676, already in 1666 he was describing fevers – particularly the frequency of fits in tertian or quartian fevers – in species-like terms. The differentiating factors of a particular fever might be unknown and among nature's secrets, but they possessed stable differences of timing, phases and stages.[33] Although Sydenham sometimes used the term 'constitution' in a limited way to refer to an individual's conformation, age, sex and general health, he more commonly used it to refer to those interactions between people and the environment that made fevers appear in large numbers at certain times from year to year.[34]

When describing fevers, Sydenham often resorted to portrayals of febrile diseases as being the consequence of the interaction between an alien 'something' with the blood. In these dramas, the blood behaved very much like a molested *Archeus* in Helmontian and Paracelsian conceptions.[35] Writing in 1666 in the *Methodus*, Sydenham described an initial encounter between fever and blood as follows:

> ... the febrile matter which ... has been imperfectly assimilated dilated with the volume of the blood, has become, not only useless, but inimical to Nature whom it frets and vexes. She, on her part, stirred up by what we may call a natural sense, and planning, as it were, an escape, creates a shivering and a shaking throughout the body, as the evidence and the measure of her aversion.[36]

Descended from a landowning family of religious dissenters who were hostile to the Stuarts, Sydenham remained on the fringes of the medical elites of his day. But he was hardly alone in his attitude towards medical knowledge, for, from the late 1660s onwards, Sydenham closely associated himself with John Locke and Locke's patron, Anthony Ashley Cooper, later first Earl of Shaftesbury and an influential early Whig. Indeed, Locke may have written some lines attributed to Sydenham.[37] For the mature Locke, who had been interested in iatrochemistry and anatomical dissection while a student at Oxford and a lecture student of Willis, Sydenham's emphasis on 'observ[ation] of History of Diseases' formed a 'better Way' than 'that Romance Way of Physick' that had been practised by Galenists, Helmontians or chemists.[38]

Eventually, Locke despaired that medicine could achieve a reliably certain or scientific knowledge of 'natural bodies', a category that included all forms of unprocessed matter. Try as one might, he wrote in the *Essay on Human Understanding* (1692), one could not even know 'so much as their very outward shapes, or the sensible and grosser parts of their constitutions'.[39] Some Restoration empiricists argued that medicine should be content to remain an art and not aspire to be a science. Sydenham's extant writings, incidentally, used the term 'science' only once in reference to medicine; Locke's made no mention of the word.[40]

Robert Boyle who, like many clerics and members of the gentry, practised medicine occasionally as an amateur, also doubted that medicine was a science. Like a number of other influential people in the mid-seventeenth century, Boyle had doubts about the practical value to physicians of the rationalist anatomical method. Although Boyle experimented chemically and performed anatomical experiments, he directed his medical efforts towards improving therapy through chemical medicines. And, in therapy, knowledge of cause counted for little. What mattered was effect:

> Why should we hastily conclude against the efficacy of specifics, taken into the body, upon the bare account of their not operating by any obvious quality, if they be recommended unto us upon their own experience by sober and faithful persons?[41]

Behind this preoccupation with improvement in therapy as the main goal of medical research lay the premise that efforts that were not immediately directed towards therapy were of lesser importance in medicine. Chief among these was the study of anatomy, which Boyle believed would require a 'process of time' before its '*historia facti*' would be 'fully and indisputably made out' so that the resulting 'theories' would have sufficient form to 'highly conduce to the improvement of the therapeutical part of physick'.[42]

Boyle was a landed aristocrat, and Locke, who came from prosperous yeoman stock, was the confidante of highly placed Whigs. Clearly, with regard to the epistemic status of anatomy and the natural history method more than class was at stake, an opinion supported by the fashion in early Georgian genteel Whig circles for Locke's and Sydenham's approach to medical knowledge. By the closing decades of the seventeenth century, and continuing through the eighteenth century, Hippocrates, thanks largely to his singular prominence in Sydenham's writings, likewise ascended to prominence among orthodox learned physicians while Galen (and Aristotle) went into eclipse. Nonetheless, during the mid-eighteenth century, London's fashionable elite crowded to watch William Hunter's anatomy demonstrations at Great Windmill Street[43] as Georgian printers reissued Culpeper's herbals in deluxe hand-coloured formats with their author now designated as Nicholas Culpeper, Gent'.

Interpretations

Understanding early modern shifts in attitude to medical knowledge has engaged a number of historians in recent decades. In his influential study of 1986, *The Decline of the Old Medical Regime in Stuart London*, Harold Cook used records of London's College of Physicians (now the Royal College of Physicians) as a basis for exploring rivalries between the elite members of the College and competitors outside of it in order to explain both the decline in influence that the College experienced towards the end of the seventeenth century and the general shift from Galenic to Hippocratic standards for medical knowledge. In this present book, Andrew Cunningham (Chapter 5) has extended Cook's work into Scotland to look at the uses that elitist Scottish physicians made of Hippocrates during the Restoration as they sought to form a Royal College of Physicians in Edinburgh and marginalise their surgeon-apothecary rivals.[44] Cunningham also revisits the Restoration attempt by English Helmontian (alchemical) physicians to gain a royal charter for their own medical college and its opposition by the established College. He reminds us, quite rightly, that class issues suffused these struggles, in the sense that they pitted those who went to university for their medical education against those who did not. The extensive and valuable work by Cunningham, Cook and their colleagues on Hippocratic medicine in the context of early modern professional rivalries permits my comments to touch on related, but distinct, themes.

What interests me most is not so much why early Georgian Britain jettisoned the anatomical or Galenic tradition and its emphasis on aetiology and structure/function relationships to 'go Hippocratic' but, rather, why influential physicians and others during the Restoration felt that they had to choose between Hippocrates and Galen – that is, between the 'natural history method' and the anatomical approach. Their predecessors do not seem to have felt such pressure. With the exception of the alchemists, Paracelsus and J.B. van Helmont and their followers who favoured Hippocrates, no significant medical figures from the Renaissance expressed a strong preference for Hippocrates at the expense of Galen or vice versa. Instead, they tended to lump them together as luminaries confirming the writer's opinion at hand. Furthermore, with the exception of the alchemists, continental medical writers active in the mid-seventeenth century tended not to divide themselves into Hippocratic and Galenic camps in terms of their attitude to medical knowledge-making. But they did in England. Why?

An important part of the answer lies in the prominence of religious dispute in seventeenth-century England.[45] As I have argued elsewhere, I think it is impossible to understand the investigative programme of the Oxford physiologists, as well as their critics, without careful consideration of their religious contexts.[46] For example, the young men who became most involved in Harveian physiology at Oxford came from predominantly formalist or High Church backgrounds. Moreover, several of them entered Oxford intending a priestly vocation. However, during the Civil War, major figures, such as Thomas Willis, as well as minor but significant contributors, such as Ralph Bathurst, changed their academic emphasis from religion to medicine when a career as an Anglican divine seemed impossible.[47] As did Bathurst, others earned part or all of their incomes practising natural philosophy (Seth Ward, for example, became Savilian Professor of Astronomy at Oxford in 1649) until the Restoration settlement made a High Church religious vocation possible once more. In terms of family background, five of the 13 investigators whom Robert Frank considered 'major' had fathers following Anglican religious vocations.[48] They also tended to come from established families, some of whom owned considerable property and enjoyed a high social status.

Significantly, the most influential member of the Oxford group after Harvey – Thomas Willis – consistently glossed his anatomical work with religious terms. Not only did he present his work as an examination of God's handiwork – the brain was described as the 'Chapel of the Deity' – he also presented the investigative physician in Christ-like terms: 'There should be an Entrance into the Church thorow the Spittle; for all it appears, our Saviour to have used almost this method.'[49] I doubt that Willis used this type of language (and there is lots of it in his prefaces and introductions) cynically – that is, to gain approval from censors for the otherwise dubious activity of cutting open dead bodies. For one thing, Gilbert Sheldon, Archbishop of Canterbury during most of the Restoration, was Willis's principal patron as well as a patient. Also, Sheldon sponsored Willis's colleagues, most of whom achieved substantial professional success. Furthermore, Willis's private life was centred among Royalists who were religiously orthodox: Willis's first wife was a devout High Church woman who defied parliamentary soldiers during the Civil War and his close friends included Richard Allestree, Provost of Eton, and John Fell, his brother-in-law and Bishop of Oxford.

By way of contrast, those who identified themselves as Hippocratic during the seventeenth century (but not necessarily during the eighteenth) tended to dissent from formalist groups within the Church of England. Some of them, notably the early Quakers, embraced Christian mysticism in a manner that had profound implications for investigative natural philosophy, including medical philosophy. For example, the notable 'Friend', Viscountess Anne Conway (1631–1679), chronically ill with headaches but an accomplished philosopher, believed that 'every Body is a Spirit, and nothing else ... so that this distinction is only modal and gradual, not essential or substantial'.[50] Furthermore, matter was not only interconvertible with spirit, it was also interconnected. Indeed, the 'Reasons and Causes of Things' depended on the fact that 'all Creatures from the highest to the lowest are inseparably united one with another'.[51] Once that was understood, one might 'easily see into the most secret and hidden Causes of Things, which ignorant Men call occult Qualities'.[52] The anonymous author of *The Method of Chemical Philosophy and Physick* cited earlier, far from advocating invasive approaches, believed that no one could know nature unless they 'thorought seeth the nature of this undefiled Virgin ... unless they kiss this Virgin with a sweet kiss'.[53] Conway – who consulted both Harvey and Willis on her headaches, incidentally – believed that the essence of the body was in the blood. Her belief in the fundamental unity of spirit and matter did not lead her to devalue reason, but she believed that access to the highest consciousness was through attention to an 'inner light'.[54] When the Oxford physiologists made reference to light, however, it was most often to 'ocular demonstrations', by which they meant post-mortem examinations, vivisections, chemical experiments and other manipulations of the tangible.

During the Restoration, a fundamental tension existed between empiricist and mystical approaches that acknowledged Hippocratic authority and the rationalist anatomical approach of the Oxford physiologists over the place of enthusiasm and spirit in civil, religious, professional and philosophical life, none of which existed as distinct domains in seventeenth-century Europe. To some degree, all contemporary English people, except those loyal to the Roman Church, were inheritors of Calvinist doctrines that gave pride of place to an individual's unmediated experience of God. Was one saved or irredeemably fallen, and therefore damned? Earlier in the century a majority of Puritans had argued that one could not know one's estate in this regard through the operations of reason and humane learning alone. The key was faith, and faith was a function of submitting one's guiding spirit, or 'inner light', to God.

Believers looked for some sign of God's providence. Hence, an essential human experience was the experience of conversion, a numinous religious ecstasy that virtually required some manifestation of enthusiasm. As John Winthrop, an early Puritan leader of Massachusetts, recalled his illumination, he noted that he had been 'filled with joy unspeakable, and glorious and with a spirit of Adoption'.[55] Speaking in tongues and other manifestations of possession by the Holy Spirit were received in this formulation as signs (believers hoped) of the extension of Divine Grace.

It was so, too, for medical practitioners with a wholehearted faith in alchemical approaches: 'spirit' and 'inner light' were valued over characterisations of the body as a 'machine' that was governed by the brain and its Rational Soul and whose 'secrets' could be known by anatomical investigations. But the empiricists and alchemists (many practitioners were both) believed that only rudimentary knowledge of anatomy was needed for wise medical practice.

Hippocratic texts common in the early modern period – notably *Airs, Waters, Places* and the *Epidemics* – generally expressed a secular outlook on illness and its treatment; thus, they might not be expected to be a resource for avowedly Christian mystical healers. However, their emphasis on observation and their reticence concerning anatomy served to buttress the opinions of all those who opposed the rationalist philosophy, religious orthodoxy and Royalist politics of most of the Oxford physiologists, their genteel patients and their patrons.

Comprehending early modern tensions concerning the place of spirit and enthusiasm is not simple. Allegiances to one or another camp were often contingent. For example, the alchemical healer George Starkey, who supported a Leveller political agenda in the Revolutionary years, nonetheless managed to recouch his theories in Royalist terms during the Restoration. John Wilkins, a leader of 'latitudinarians' during the Restoration, managed to make the transition from being Oliver Cromwell's brother-in-law (as of 1656) to becoming the Bishop of Chester (1668). These examples are not isolated instances, for the position of various groups concerning the relative importance of spirit, enthusiasm, rationality and learned investigation changed as the century progressed.[56]

Finding a sustainable balance between these factors preoccupied mid-seventeenth-century thinkers not only in medicine and natural philosophy, but also in religion and politics. Indeed, I would argue that the physiological task for the Oxford physiologists was similar to the theological task of the High Church divines with whom they prayed – the proper composition of the orthodox English body. If the emphasis by the religious, political and healing sects on enthusiasm threatened orthodox claims for the need for episcopacy in the polity and a supreme rational cerebral cortex in the body, constructions of nature and the Church as essentially material and civil raised the spectre of atheism. In this sense, the formulations of the Cartesians and of Thomas Hobbes were never far from orthodox theological concern, just as they also exerted intellectual pressure on Oxford physiological theory. The goal was to find the proper balance. If this post-Restoration balance led to what historian Richard Westfall has termed a late-century 'spiritual mediocrity', nonetheless it satisfied High Church desire for an episcopally controlled piety that excluded significant religious and political dissent.[57]

The Willisians' ability to use anatomical arguments and textual representations to 'naturalise' their patrons' ideological commitments took advantage of anatomy's venerable prestige in the hierarchy of medical knowledge. Although performance of human anatomy as a juridical activity, as well as a medical subject, barely occurred during the classical period (probably only for a 50-year period in authoritarian Ptolemaic Alexandria), it formed an important element of medical curricula early in the development of university medical faculties that began during the late twelfth century in Italy. Scholarly clerics there rediscovered and translated Galen; numerous pseudo-Galenic texts circulated as well. According to Nancy Siraisi, by the end of the twelfth century more than 40 'Hippocratic' treatises circulated as well as a much larger number attributed to Galen.[58] Medical writers such as Mondino de Liuzzi (d. 1326) promoted the anatomical study of humans as both dignified and intellectually worthwhile. Using reason to understand the body's order and the 'very causes of the diseases of our bodies' was a more noble university subject than law, which established itself earlier in the universities, according to Bartolomeo Fazio, or Facio (d. 1457).[59]

An important reason why many English seventeenth-century healers felt that they needed to take a stand concerning medical knowledge, I speculate, was that they experienced an extended period of major religious, professional and political unrest – the Revolution, Protectorate and Restoration – during which no plurality of healers (or political or religious leaders) succeeded in achieving a lasting hegemony concerning the meaning and relative value of order and spirit in any context. Instead, persistent and serious conflicts made slippages visible in what previously seemed relatively seamless: the coexistence of vernacular (read Hippocratic in medicine) and universalist (read Galen and rationalist anatomy) approaches. Consider one layperson's voice, albeit a privileged one: Margaret Cavendish (1623–1673), Duchess of Newcastle, wrote extensively on natural philosophy in the 1660s. For her, patient dissection was a matter-of-fact necessity in learned medicine. She did not want to see learned physicians criticised because they could not 'restore every Patient to his former health ... [when] they have only outward signs of inward distempers'.[60] Even when Cavendish expressed scepticism concerning techniques of the new natural philosophy, such as the microscope ('deluding glasses' to the Duchess), she supported learned versus popular medicine. To do otherwise, she believed, would be to support 'Herreticks'.[61]

Furthermore, disputes among medical writers about the value of learned experimentalist approaches versus simple vernacular methods parallel a venerable fault line in Western Christianity that also became active in seventeenth-century England. Unlike every other major religious tradition (that is, Judaism, Islam, Hinduism and Buddhism), theology – in its meaning as the study of God in relation to the world – and disputes about it have occupied a central place in Christianity.[62] One need read only the direct and simple language of Jesus of the Gospels and compare it with the rest of the New Testament, redolent of Greek philosophy, to have a sense of the divided legacy. In short, the historical origins of Christianity left the West with two quite distinct versions of being Christian, not to mention a propensity to dispute between them: a simple and direct way for ordinary people to find spiritual comfort in a harsh world, and an intellectually demanding set of issues concerning God's relation to nature and man. If this is so, drawing parallels between dissenting religious sects that favoured scriptural authority, plain religious service and an absence of Church hierarchy and the emergence of empiricist medical sects and their rivals, clerical apologists for episcopal order and physicians advocating rationalist anatomy (the primacy of the cerebral cortex over the rest of the body) seem plausible, at least during the Restoration.

But this interpretation leaves at least one important question unanswered: how and why did the tables turn so that England entered the eighteenth century with empirical 'Hippocratics' in the ascendant? By the late 1680s, almost all the Oxford physiologists had died, although I doubt whether those natural events explain the Hippocratic 'turn' among the orthodox that then began in earnest. I want to suggest that any account of the rise in intellectual prestige of empirical approaches (and the decline of the physiological/anatomical tradition) that occurred during the eighteenth century, for which Hippocrates and Sydenham served as ancient and modern Enlightenment embodiments, might do well to consider the emergence of the word 'constitution' and its cognates in many contexts, not only medical, during late seventeenth-century England.

In the late 1680s the increasingly brittle Restoration political and religious settlement finally fell apart in a bloodless revolution. At the same time Sydenham's refurbishment of the old Hippocratic notion of 'constitution' began to gain credence among the same social and intellectual circles that favoured relaxation of Church disciplinary zeal and the exchange of the absolutist James II for the more 'constitutional' monarchy of William and Mary. In natural philosophy and medicine, the 'natural history' method for determining 'constitutions' and a fondness for nosology – nicely explored in Chapter Six of this book by Andrea Rusnock – supplanted the 'ocular demonstrations' of mid-century Oxford. Some late seventeenth- and early eighteenth-century medical theorists, notably Archibald Pitcairn and James Keill, glossed their histories and observations with Newtonian rhetoric,[63] but few British physicians in the first half of the eighteenth century carried out the kind of rigorous investigations that earned Harvey and the Oxford physiologists extensive international influence. Instead, around the 1690s the centre of gravity in substantive medical knowledge-making that deflected conventional wisdom shifted from England to continental Europe.

Furthermore, anecdotal evidence suggests that the basis of professional success among elite physicians also shifted. English anatomical knowledge, backward in every respect compared to that on the continent at the beginning of the seventeenth century, improved dramatically with Harvey. But it took several decades for a physician's investigative reputation to enhance his medical practice. The later Harvey enjoyed a bountiful practice among elite social strata, but he did once complain that the dissemination of his views in *De motu cordis* harmed his practice financially during the 1620s and 1630s.[64] His intellectual successors, particularly Willis and his followers, earned large sums partly because of their reputations for experimental accomplishment, but, by the 1690s, John Radcliffe, then England's most prosperous elite physician, boasted that he did not experiment and that he read few medical books other than, ironically, Willis's.[65]

If pressed to explain these changes with one phrase, I would invoke, without being able to prove it here, 'exhaustion with the search for cause'. In other words, Sydenham's characterisation of nature as an 'abyss of cause' and denigration of anatomy in favour of aphorisms based on superficial observations, which I mentioned earlier, reflected (and perhaps helped shape) a widely held sentiment among the late-century literate to give up any hope of achieving consensus concerning reliably certain knowledge – literally *scientia* – of what constituted *the* English healer, individual body, religious dogma or body politic. Instead, a majority probably embraced a 'constitutional' model made up of several factors that related dynamically to each other. Importantly, the model permitted considerable latitude in private behaviour, professional approach and political arrangements.

The increasing acceptability of empirical approaches suited the general relaxation of professional standards characteristic of British medicine in the eighteenth century. Also, it may have suited early Georgian attitudes among the genteel toward learning. According to sociologist Nicholas Jewson, professional success in the eighteenth-century medical marketplace turned increasingly on one's success in passing as a gentleman.[66] Attention to superficial appearance, as it were, displaced mid-seventeenth-century preoccupation with cause and mechanism. Interestingly, Oxford and Cambridge enrolments, which peaked just before the mid-century, did not approach their early- to mid-seventeenth-century levels again until the 1880s.[67] The sons of the well-placed who had flooded the universities in the 1630s and 1640s were sending an increasing proportion of their sons and grandsons from the 1680s onwards to London to study finance and law.

With regard to religion, tactics used by Archbishop Sheldon and his allies to assure tight control of forms of worship in the 1660s and 1670s gave way to 'latitudinarian' relaxation and the natural theology espoused in the Boyle lecturers of the 1690s.[68] In broad terms, early eighteenth-century England achieved closure of its seventeenth-century schisms through a broad-scale, if occasionally testy, toleration of plurality in many areas of civic, religious and professional life.[69] Taken together, these developments suggest the philosopher of science, Ludwik Fleck's, words, written in 1935 concerning the genesis and development of scientific facts and thought collectives: 'In science, just as in art and in life, only that which is true to culture is true to nature.'[70]

An important difference between Civil War Hippocratics, such as the egalitarian Culpeper, and Sydenham and his Whiggish eighteenth-century followers lay in their respective attitudes towards what we might term 'social justice'. The reservations of the latter group, unlike those of seventeenth-century radical empirics, did not fundamentally concern the social injustice of the professional medical (and religious and legal) hierarchy. Indeed, both

Sydenham and Locke found their medical – and occasionally literal – homes in caring for the nascent Whig aristocracy and gentry. Sydenham *wanted* full entry into the College of Physicians; Locke manoeuvred for lucrative government posts and investment opportunities.[71] This shift in the political content of late seventeenth-century Hippocratism reflected a broader cultural shift among literate Englishman of diverse religious beliefs away from a desire for broad-scale political reform to a quest for modest private improvements. For example, unlike the millenarian Puritan reformers of the 1640s and 1650s, latitudinarians like the later Wilkins did not intend the prospect of a Final Judgement to hasten the reform of social injustices.[72] Their millenarianism provoked only limited social ambition.

Although Sydenham characterised himself in terms that Culpeper might have used in a self-description – as 'dedicated to the welfare of the public'[73] – he made it clear that he was not writing popular texts for a lay audience. While complaining about the practice of prescribing 'heating' medicines for pleurisy in the *Methodus*, Sydenham criticised 'certain women' for the practice. Instead of providing medical care, such women 'would be better employed in feeding the poor than in physicking them'.[74] Furthermore, he followed learned medical convention by publishing in Latin (with the help of Locke), joining the College of Physicians, and attempting to merge with (and deflect) the mainstream of elite medical thought.

Nor did the revitalised Hippocratism of Sydenham and his eighteenth-century followers necessarily imply mild treatments. For example, phlebotomy, a practice whose value Willis minimised,[75] remained a persistent mainstay of Sydenham's therapeutics. Given that the goal of his fever treatment was to return the blood from 'ebullition' to its normal state, he argued that one must bleed as much as necessary.[76] One administered vomitives and cathartics as needed, depending on the patient's history of evacuations, but one almost always bled, and generously. Describing the appropriate treatment for pleurisy, for example, Sydenham recounted that he 'seldom abstain[ed]' from drawing blood until the amount equalled 'forty-two ounces or thereabouts'.[77] Given that the normal human blood volume is approximately 12 pints (192 ounces), such phlebotomies must have produced a significant physiological effect. Sydenham acknowledged as much by cautioning the physician to ascertain in advance of treatment 'the patient's strength'.

My point in recounting this anecdote on therapeutics is not to indict Sydenham but to suggest that the uncoupling of learned medicine from its venerable core discipline of anatomy had significant implications for therapy. In the case of treatment for pleurisy, for example, what mattered finally was not the patient's body as such, but only the blood as it was affected by fever. In this sense, a significant check on therapeutic aggressiveness – intellectual commitment to the apprehension of the body's inner structure and function – had been lost. Paradoxically, Sydenham's version of Hippocratic medicine elided the ancient Hippocratic cautionary to healers – *primum non noccere* – thereby becoming the first of numerous Enlightenment 'Hippocratic' texts that recommended the heroic therapies that nineteenth-century anatomists and physiologists later sought so diligently to debunk.

Notes:

1. For example, see the works of Herbert Butterfield, the historian who coined the phrase 'scientific revolution'. See in particular, Herbert Butterfield, *Origins of Modern Science*, London: Bell, 1957.
2. James Jacob and Margaret Jacob, 'The Anglican origins of modern science: the metaphysical foundations of the Whig constitution', *Isis*, **71**, 1980, pp. 251–267.
3. For the only extant translation of *De corde* of which I am aware, see Frank Hurlbutt jr, 'Peri kardies: a treatise on the heart from the Hippocratic Corpus', *Bulletin of the History of Medicine*, **7** (9), 1939, pp. 1104–13.
4. Thomas Willis, 'Preface', *Dr. Willis's Practice of Physick, Being the Whole Works of that Renowned Physician*, trans. Samuel Pordage, London: T. Dring, C.Harper, J. Leigh. 1684.
5. For a recent view on the limits of using 'epistemology' and its cognates in reference to early modern medical knowledge, see Andrew Wear, 'Epistemology and learned medicine in early modern England', in Don Bates (ed.), *Knowledge and the Scholarly Medical Traditions*, Cambridge: Cambridge University Press, 1995, pp. 151–75.
6. Heinrich von Staden, 'The discovery of the body: human dissection and its cultural contexts in ancient Greece', *Yale Journal of Biology & Medicine*, **65**, 1992, pp. 223–41.
7. James Longrigg, *Greek Rational Medicine*, London: Routledge, 1993.
8. Samuel Hartlib, *Ephemerides*, London, 1652.
9. Thomas Willis, *Pharmaceutice rationalis*, in 2 Parts, London, James Allestry, 1674 and 1675.
10. Christopher Hill, *The World Turned Upside Down*, Oxford: Oxford University Press, 1972.
11. Nicolas Culpeper, *A Physical Directory*, London, 1649, p. 23.
12. Edmund O'Meara, *Examen Diatribae Thomae Willisii*, London: 1665. See also Richard Lower's defence of Willis and the Oxford approach in Richard Lower, *Vindicatio*, London, 1665, available in facsimile with an introduction by Kenneth Dewhurst, Oxford: Tempest, 1983.
13. John Webster, *Academiarum Examen, or the Examination of Academies*, London, 1654. Facsimile in Allen Debus, *Science and Education in the Seventeenth Century*, New York: Science History Publications, 1970.
14. Seth Ward, *Vindicae Academiarum*. London, 1654. Facsimile in Allen Debus, *Science and Education* (n. 13).
15. Webster, *Academiarum* (n. 13), p. 106.
16. Ibid.
17. Ward, *Vindicae* (n.14) p. 34.
18. Webster, *Academiarum* (n. 13), p. 74.
19. Ibid.

20. Ibid.
21. For an extended discussion of early Puritan attitudes towards formal education, see John Morgan, *Godly Learning: Puritan Attitudes Towards Reason, Learning and Education, 1560–1640*. Cambridge: Cambridge University Press, 1986.
22. Ibid., p. 106.
23. Ward, *Vindicae* (n. 14) pp. 34–35.
24. Anonymous, 'News from the dead, or a tru and exact narration of the miraculous deliverance of Anne Greene', Oxford, 1651 in *Phoenix Britannicus*, London, 1732, Vol. 1, pp. 23–40.
25. Ward, *Vindicae* (n.14), p. 50.
26. Anonymous, *The Method of Chemical Philosophy and Physick*, London: 1664. Huntington Library #474249.
27. Ibid., p. 21.
28. Thomas Sydenham, *Works*, 2 vols, ed. R.G. Latham, London: Sydenham Society, 1848, Vol. 1, p. 171.
   Interestingly, although Sydenham never exhibited enthusiasm for alchemy, 'husk' was a contemporary trope for the notion that alchemical fire would burn through the nature's 'husk' to reveal the 'kernal' of truth. See J.A. Mendelsohn, 'Alchemy and politics in England 1649–1655', *Past & Present*, **135**, 1992, pp. 30–79 at pp. 46–47.
29. Sydenham, *Works* (n. 28), Vol. 1, p.13.
30. Ibid., Vol. 1, p.102.
31. Ibid., Vol. 1, p.84.
32. Thomas Sydenham, *Methodus Curandi Febres Propriis Observationibus Superstructuras*, London, 1666, III.1.5.5. in Sydenham, *Works* (n. 28).
33. On the inchoate notion of species, see Sydenham, *Methodus* (n. 32), I.5.5. and I.5.27. For its development in Sydenham's mature work see Don Bates, 'Thomas Sydenham: the development of his thought, 1666–1676', unpublished PhD dissertation, Johns Hopkins University, 1975, 'Part III: Sydenham's Species Concept', esp. chapters 7–9.
34. Don Bates, 'Thomas Sydenham' (n. 33), p. 63.
35. Walter Pagel, *The Smiling Spleen*, Basel: Karger, 1984; idem, 'The religious and philosophical aspects of van Helmont's science and medicine', supplement to the *Bulletin of the History of Medicine*, (2), 1944; idem, 'Van Helmont's concept of disease – to be or not to be? The influence of Paracelsus', *Bulletin of the History of Medicine*, **46**, 1972, pp. 419–54. See also Alan Debus, *The Chemical Philosophy*, 2 vols, New York: Science History, 1977.
36. Sydenham, *Methodus* (n. 32), English translation from Latham's edition of the works in 1848, Folkestone: Winterdown Books, 1987, 'Section Three: of intermittent fevers', p. 99.
37. See John Locke 'Anatomie', 1668, Public Record Office (London) 30/24/47/2.
38. John Locke, *Familiar Letters between Mr. John Locke and Several of his Friends*, 4th edn, London, 1742, pp. 223–24.
39. John Locke, *An Essay Concerning Human Understanding*, 1692, reprinted New York: Dover, 1959, Bk IV, 'Extent of Human Knowledge', ch. III, sect. 25–27.
40. Sydenham *Works* (n. 28).
41. Robert Boyle, 'On the usefulness of natural philosophy', in Thomas Birch (ed.), *The Works of the Honourable Robert Boyle*, London, 1772, Vol. II, p. 183.
42. Ibid., pp. 163–64. See also Lester S. King, 'Robert Boyle as an amateur physician', in *Medical Investigation in Seventeenth Century England*, Los Angeles: UCLA, Clark Library, 1968, pp. 29–49.

43. W.F. Bynum and Roy Porter (eds), *William Hunter and the Eighteenth-Century Medical World*, Cambridge: Cambridge University Press, 1985.
44. See also, Piyo Rattansi, 'The Helmontian–Galenist controversy in Restoration England', *Ambix*, **12**, 1964, pp. 1–23; Charles Webster, 'English medical reformers of the Puritan revolution: A background to the Society of Chymical Physitians', *Ambix*, **14**, 1964, pp. 16–41.
45. For recent work, see O.P. Grell and Andrew Cunningham (eds), *Medicine and the Reformation*, London: Routledge, 1993; and O.P. Grell and Andrew Cunningham (eds), *Religio Medici: Medicine and Religion in Seventeenth-century England*, Aldershot: Scolar Press, 1996.
46. Robert Martensen, ' "Habit of reason": anatomy and anglicanism in Restoration England", *Bulletin of the History of Medicine*, **66**, 1992, pp. 511–35; idem, 'Alienation and the production of strangers', *Culture, Medicine & Psychiatry*, **19**, 1995, pp. 141–82.
47. On Willis, see J. Trevor Hughes, *Thomas Willis 1621–1675*, London: Royal Society of Medicine, 1991.
48. Robert Frank, *Harvey and the Oxford Physiologists*, Berkeley: University of California Press, 1980.
49. Thomas Willis, 'Epistolary Dedicatory', *Pathology of the Brain and Nervous Stock*, Trans. S. Pordage, 1667.
50. Ann Conway, *Principles of the Most Ancient and Modern Philosophy* (1692), ed. Peter Loptson, The Hague: Martinus Nijhoff, 1982.
51. Ibid., p. 193.
52. Ibid., p. 164.
53. Anonymous, *Method* (n.26), 'Introduction'.
54. Conway, *Principles* (n. 50).
55. Winthrop Papers, Boston: Massachusetts Historical Society., Vol. 1, pp. 1498–1628.
56. It is worthwhile remembering that, despite their ambivalence about the value of elaborate learning and social hierarchy, in the early seventeenth century influential Puritans actively supported the expansion of the universities at Oxford and Cambridge, as well as the founding of Harvard along lines that preserved traditional curricula. Numerous Royalist Anglicans were ejected from Oxford and Cambridge during the Interregnum, but many were not. Neither was the curriculum sustantially altered. See John Morgan, *Godly Learning* (n. 21), as well as Michael Heyd, *'Be Sober and Reasonable': The Critique of Enthusiasm in the Seventeenth and Early Eighteenth Centuries*, Leiden: E.J. Brill, 1995.
57. Richard Westfall, *Science and Religion in Seventeenth-Century England*, New Haven, Conn.: Yale University Press, 1958.
58. Nancy Siraisi, *Medieval and Early Renaissance Medicine*, Chicago: University of Chicago Press, 1990.
59. Bartolomeo Fazio, *De Viribus Illustribus Liber Bartholomei Facii*, ed. L Mehus, Florence, 1745, p. 35. Cited by Siraisi, *Medieval* (n. 58) p. 78, n. 2.
60. Duchess of Newcastle, *Philosophical Letters or Modest Reflections upon Some Opinions in Natural Philosophy*, London, 1664, p. 352.
61. Ibid., p. 377.
62. John Polkinhorne, *Belief in God in an Age of Science*, New Haven, Conn.: Yale University Press, 1998.
63. See, for example, James Keill, *Medicina Statica Britannica*, 3rd edn, ed. J. Quincy, London: J. Newton, 1723.
64. John Aubrey, *Lives and Letters of Eminent Persons*, London, 1813.

65. John Radcliffe, *Memoirs of the Life of John Radcliffe*, London, 1715.
66. Nicolas D. Jewson, 'Medical knowledge and the patronage system in 18th century England', *Sociology*, **8**, 1974, pp. 369–85.
67. Lawrence Stone, *The Crisis of the Aristocracy, 1558–1641*, Oxford: Oxford University Press, 1976, chapter 12.
68. John Spurr, *The Restoration Church of England, 1646–1689*, New Haven, Conn.: Yale University Press, 1991.
69. Westfall, *Science and Religion* (n. 57).
70. Ludwik Fleck, *Genesis and Development of a Scientific Fact*, Originally published in German in 1935, trans. F. Bradley and T.J. Trenn, Chicago: University of Chicago Press, 1979, p. 35.
71. Despite its hagiographic tone, Fox-Bourne's nineteenth-century biography of Locke provides a full narrative of the latter's career moves and worldly ambitions. See Henry Fox-Bourne, *The Life of John Locke*, London, 1876.
72. Jacob, and Jacob, 'Anglican origins' (n. 2).
73. Thomas Sydenham, 'Epistolary dissertation to Dr. Cole', in *Works* (n. 28), Vol. 1, p. 57.
74. Sydenham, *Methodus* (n. 32), II.VI.3.3.
75. Thomas Willis, *Affectionum Quae Dicuntur Hystericae et Hypochondriacae*, London: J. Allestry, 1670.
76. Sydenham, *Methodus* (n. 32), 'Of continued fevers', VI.3.4., p. 75.
77. Sydenham, *Methodus* (n. 32), 'Of symptoms', VI.3.4., p. 75.

CHAPTER SEVEN

Hippocrates, Bacon, and Medical Meteorology at the Royal Society, 1700–1750

Andrea Rusnock

No stranger to medical schools, Hippocrates made a surprising appearance at the Royal Society of London during the first half of the eighteenth century. Although a bit down at the heels during this period, the Royal Society nevertheless remained the most significant institution dedicated to the pursuit of the new natural philosophy.[1] Its members met on a weekly basis to discuss a range of topics associated with natural philosophy, natural history and, to some extent, medicine. Domestic and foreign correspondents eagerly offered observations and reports in the hope of a public reading at a meeting and possibly publication in the Society's journal, the *Philosophical Transactions*. Fellowship was sought after not only by aspiring philosophers and physicians, but by noblemen as well. To members, correspondents and aspirants, the Royal Society represented modernity and civility, and fellowship meant precisely that: a community of shared tastes and interests, among gentlemanly scholars who embraced new, useful knowledge and challenged ancient authority.[2]

So what was the ancient Hippocrates doing at the home of the moderns? He most frequently appeared during discussions of medical meteorology, the study of the effects of air and climate on human health[3] which formed part of the wider agenda of environmental medicine – the study of how the environment (climate, geography, living and working conditions) affected health. Throughout the eighteenth century, environmental considerations assumed an increasing importance in the work of natural philosophers. Voyages of exploration to distant lands and colonial experiences in the New World brought accounts which dramatically highlighted differences in climate, health and disease. Closer to home, growing urbanisation, especially during the second half of the eighteenth century, transformed city landscapes, and new methods of manufacturing altered working and living conditions. Contemporary observers were keenly aware of these changes, and they sought to develop methods to describe and evaluate the effects of the environment on the health of various populations.

Medical meteorology was one approach and it became very fashionable during the eighteenth century, especially at the Royal Society which played a central role in its advancement. The Society's interest dated back to the early 1660s, when explorations in meteorology were initiated by Christopher Wren, Robert Hooke and other founding fellows. These men invented instruments such as the hygroscope, wind gauge, rain gauge and barometer, which allowed for more precise measurement of meteorological phenomena. Their improvements to instrumentation encouraged others to take up the systematic recording of meteorological observations, and many individuals both inside and outside the Society kept meteorological diaries.[4] During the first half of the eighteenth century, several physicians who were fellows of the Society, including John Arbuthnot (1667–1735), Francis Clifton (d. 1736), John Huxham (1692–1768) and James Jurin (1684–1750) continued to promote meteorology and combined medicine with observations on the weather. Through their work, medical meteorology became a major research focus in the Royal Society.

Hippocratic writings provided the framework for inquiries regarding the connections between health and the weather. Three texts from the *Corpus* became especially influential: *Airs, Waters, and Places* and *Epidemics I* and *III*. *Airs, Waters and Places* provided observations on prevailing environmental conditions in different locales, which aided the healer in making more accurate prognoses. Of particular importance were the direction of winds, the location of spring waters and seasonal variations in weather. In *Epidemics I* and *III* observations about the weather and climate preceded individual case histories. In all three texts, disease incidence and outcome were linked with prevailing meteorological conditions.

It is no accident that writings in the Hippocratic *Corpus* informed Royal Society inquiries, despite the fellows' ostensible insistence on the rejection of classical authorities. Physicians made up 16 per cent of the membership for the period 1735 through 1780, and surgeons accounted for an additional 9 per cent.[5] Thus one-quarter of the fellows were medically trained, and familiarity with ancient medical writings was an essential part of a physician's education throughout most of the eighteenth century.[6] Furthermore, several physicians served in the influential position of secretary to the Royal Society for much of the eighteenth century – namely, James Jurin (1721–1727), William Rutty (1728–1730), Cromwell Mortimer (1730–1752) and Matthew Maty (1765–1784).

Another reason for the presence of Hippocrates at Royal Society meetings was the continued interest in classical learning, a benchmark of gentleman-scholar status, particularly during the first half of the eighteenth century. The discussion of antiquities was an essential part of the Royal Society's agenda, and only with the formal establishment of the Society of Antiquaries during the 1750s did a gradual separation of antiquarian and natural historical topics begin.[7] Most of the antiquities presented to the Royal Society concerned inscriptions found at archaeological sites; hence knowledge of classical authors and texts was key to interpretation.

Finally, Hippocrates appeared at meetings of the Royal Society in discussions of scientific method. During the seventeenth and eighteenth centuries, emphasis on observation and the collection of facts was typically associated with Francis Bacon's new philosophy and fellows actively promoted this approach to knowledge. In his book, *The Advancement of Learning*, Bacon had admired Hippocrates for his close attention to detail and his careful observations of nature,[8] yet in other writings he held Hippocrates as an example of the barrenness of observation when it did not lead to theory or synthesis, as Helen King points out in her essay in this volume (see Chapter Two). However, physicians tended to seize on Bacon's favourable comments about Hippocrates, and, over the course of the eighteenth century, the view emerged that Hippocratic–Baconian methodology constituted a single approach to science – namely, that the compilation of carefully recorded observations would yield new and useful knowledge about the natural world.[9] One particularly influential advocate of this methodology was the Dutch physician Hermann Boerhaave (1668–1738) who emphasised an empirical Hippocrates – that is, Hippocrates as an astute observer of nature. As one of the most popular medical teachers of the eighteenth century, Boerhaave helped boost Hippocrates into the canon of the new natural philosophy and medicine. His impact on the Royal Society was direct: many fellows had studied medicine with Boerhaave and his followers in Leiden, including secretaries Jurin, Mortimer and Maty.[10]

Thus it is not difficult to account for the presence of Hippocrates at the Royal Society in a general sense. However, understanding the uses of Hippocrates, both methodological and theoretical, and his value to fellows of the Royal Society during the first half of the eighteenth century requires further explanation. The first section of this essay addresses medical meteorology and details the various plans presented to the Society to improve observations of disease and weather. Its purpose is to show how those who promoted these endeavours employed Hippocratic ideas and methods. The second section discusses attempts to develop Hippocratic theories about the effects of weather and climate on health and disease by examining the work of several fellows of the Royal Society who wrote influential treatises on human physiology. It highlights the use of new mechanical explanations – the reigning natural philosophy at the Royal Society during this period – to explain the effects of climate on health and disease. In short, the essay attempts to explain the role Hippocrates played at the Royal Society and how an ancient was accommodated to the new modern natural philosophy.

An observant Hippocrates: developing a natural history of weather and disease

At the weekly meeting of the Royal Society on 29 April 1733, the physician Cromwell Mortimer, secretary to the Society, reviewed a pamphlet by the physician and fellow Francis Clifton, entitled *Tabular Observations Recommended as the Plainest and Surest way of Practising and Improving Physick in a Letter to a Friend* (1731). Clifton took as his major theme the revival of the Hippocratic method, by which he meant careful observations recorded in detailed case histories in order to advance the understanding of disease. In his review of the book, Mortimer emphasised Clifton's Hippocratic leanings. 'The Design of this Place is to revive, recommend, facilitate, and improve the ancient Method of Clinick Observations & to bring Hippocrates's Observations to the Test,' Mortimer asserted, at once invoking the ancient Hippocrates, as well as echoing the modern methodological approach of the Royal Society – to verify reports by observation and experiment.

Clifton's pamphlet, like Mortimer's review, signalled another intellectual debt, that to Francis Bacon. 'The great *Lord Bacon* has judiciously inculcated the *Hippocratical* method of improving Physick, by observation,' proclaimed Clifton.

> The Words of this Author are so expressive of the thing I aim at, that I cannot forbear transcribing them. In setting down the *Deficiencies of Physick*; 'The first is (says he [Bacon]) the Discontinuance of that useful Method of *Hippocrates*, in writing *Narratives* of particular Cases; with diligence and exactness; containing the Nature, Cure, and event of Distempers. – This Continuation therefore of *Medicinal Reports*, we find deficient, especially in the Form of an entire Body, digested with proper Care and Judgement.'[11]

By introducing Hippocratic ideas through the words of Bacon, Clifton brought an ancient approach in line with the precepts of the new natural philosophy promoted by the Royal Society, whose publicists (if not members) hailed Bacon as the founder of methods for certain knowledge.[12]

Such a rhetorical move was not unique to Clifton nor to the Royal Society. The Royal College of Physicians in the latter half of the seventeenth century trumpeted Hippocrates over Galen in order to bolster their public image, as Andrew Cunningham discusses in his essay in this volume (see Chapter Five). Bacon, among others, had rehabilitated Hippocrates as a model of empiricism and the College was keen to align themselves with the new natural philosophy.[13] Hippocrates occupied a special place among ancient philosophers. His reputation as an observer of nature, an empiricist rather than a rationalist, dovetailed nicely with the experiential epistemology advocated by English philosophers of the time.[14]

Francis Clifton and his reviewer, Cromwell Mortimer, were typical of these philosophically oriented doctors who were active in the Royal Society. Both had studied with Boerhaave and received medical degrees from Leiden in 1724, and both became fellows of the Royal College of Physicians in 1729. Clifton became a fellow of the Royal Society in 1727 and enjoyed a successful, although brief, career as a London physician from 1724 through 1734, when he left London abruptly for Jamaica where he died only two years later.[15] He was a skilled classicist and his translation and commentary of the Hippocratic text *Airs, Waters and Places* (1734) went through two editions.[16] Mortimer became a fellow of the Royal Society in 1730 and, in that same year, assumed the position of secretary, a post he held until 1752. He worked alongside Sir Hans Sloane (president of the Royal Society and the Royal College of Physicians) in Sloane's medical practice in Bloomsbury Square, and prescribed medicines for Sloane's patients.[17] Through their contributions to the Royal Society, both Clifton and Mortimer took on the task of developing the Hippocratic–Baconian method in medicine.

In his book, *The State of Physick, Ancient and Modern, Briefly Consider'd: with a Plan for the Improvement of It* (1732), Clifton expanded some of the ideas that he initially presented in his *Tabular Observations*. Of the moderns, Clifton considered Thomas Sydenham (1624–1689) the hero because he 'seems to have done more real service, than all the rest of the *English Physicians* together'.[18] Sydenham had carried out a study of London epidemics between 1661 and 1675 which tied observations about climate to disease patterns and which he modelled on the Hippocratic texts *Airs, Waters and Places* and *Epidemics I* and *III*.[19] Clifton applauded Sydenham's pursuit of the Hippocratic idea that certain diseases prevailed in different seasons and years because of the particular 'constitution' of that period of time.[20] He criticised Sydenham's contemporaries who had focused too narrowly on iatrophysical topics. 'The body has been survey'd inch by inch', Clifton remarked, 'and the supposed force of every fibre computed, with a shew of surprising exactness; the fluids have been examined by all the ways that could be thought of.' Despite these efforts, or perhaps because of them, Clifton concluded that 'Diseases are known much less than might reasonably be expected'.[21] He sought to redirect medical research and declared somewhat optimistically, 'The Structure of the Body is well known; the Materials we work with are known too; and nothing remains but a more perfect knowledge of Diseases.'[22]

With regard to the connection between disease and climate, Clifton was not simply interested in confirming Hippocratic observations, but in improving them. Like many of his contemporaries, he believed that Europeans faced new diseases that Hippocrates had never witnessed.[23] To improve knowledge of diseases, Clifton recommended the use of a table, thus adopting one of Bacon's key methodological innovations. Bacon had advocated the use of tables for the collection of natural histories, and Clifton utilised this method to develop a natural history of disease. While Hippocratic case histories had been written in prose form, Clifton thought the tabular form would simplify the record-keeping of physicians and, more important, facilitate comparison between cases. Clifton's table contained the following columns:

| Sex, Age Constitution Occupation Way of Life | Day of Illness | Disease Phenomenon | Day of Month | Remedy | Result |

The second column, 'Day of Illness', reveals Clifton's concern with establishing the course of the disease. The fourth column, 'Day of Month', reflects his interest in recording the season with the disease. Finally, the inclusion of a column on remedies marks a break with Hippocrates, since the majority of Hippocratic case histories did not mention treatment.[24] Clifton included two complete tables in his book in order to illustrate his new method and to encourage its dissemination among physicians.

In the initial design of his table, Clifton had tried to include a column for weather observations. The complexity of record-keeping, however, forced him to partition meteorological observations into a separate book. 'There was another column at first, for the *Weather*,' he wrote, 'but having since got a Book by it self for those observations, in which I every day set down the course of the wind, and the dryness or moistness of the air; I have long left this article out.'[25] He had discovered that it was logistically difficult to record detailed information on both weather and disease in one table.

The tabular form was a significant break from traditional medical writing, where case histories either took the form of the short, almost telegraphic, reports found in the Hippocratic *Corpus*, or the extended, somewhat detective-like, narratives characteristic of Galen's writings. Clifton's introduction of this methodological novelty caught Mortimer's eye. He observed:

> He [Clifton] intimates that the Difficulty of Writing exact Observations has been a principal Reason, why so little has been done of late in that way. In order to facilitate the business of Observation the Doctor has invented a new kind of Table wth separate Columns, to contain the several remarkable particulars that can happen in any Distemper. So that the Labour of the Physician is thus greatly eas'd and the Observations at once properly rang'd, or class'd, for Inspection and use.[26]

In fact, Mortimer was quite sanguine about the possible success of such a design: '... upon this footing Diseases might possibly, in time be found to be as regular in their Course as any other Phænomena, and are cur'd with as much ease as they are now contracted.'[27] Thus, according to Mortimer, using a tabular format fulfilled two purposes: first, it reduced the labour of the individual physician – filling in a table was presumably less time-consuming than writing case histories in prose; and, second, it promoted the nosological goals of classification and comparison. In this way, Clifton and Mortimer clothed the ancient Hippocrates in the fashionable attire of a Baconian investigator, observer and compiler of natural histories, which suited the methodological goals of the Royal Society.

Clifton's was one of many schemes presented to the Society during the first half of the eighteenth century, outlining plans for the collection of information on disease and weather. Several years earlier, in 1723, James Jurin had initiated a project to collect meteorological records from observers in Europe and colonial America.[28] Jurin announced his intent at a meeting of the fellows in December 1723. According to the minutes of this meeting, he 'first set forth the great advantages which would accrue to Mankind from having a compleat Theory of the Weather, and that especially in the improvement in the Medicinal art.'[29] He thus located his project within a Hippocratic framework that linked meteorology and disease.

Jurin's interest in medical meteorology had two sources – one in natural philosophy, the other in medicine. He had received his BA and MA from Trinity College, Cambridge, the college most closely associated with Newtonian natural philosophy. There he studied mathematics, hydrostatics and other aspects of natural philosophy with the Newtonians, William Whiston and Roger Cotes. In his first publication, an updated version of Bernhard Varenius's *Geographia Generalis*, Jurin applied the natural philosophical knowledge gained in his studies and added supplements on meteorology, tides and properties of the air. His medical training also contributed to his interest in meteorology. Like Clifton and Mortimer, Jurin studied medicine in Leiden in 1708 where Boerhaave was already lecturing, although Jurin received his MD from Cambridge in 1716. He became a fellow of the Royal Society in 1718 and served as secretary between 1721 and 1727.[30] From this position, Jurin was able to coordinate his meteorological project.

The project received full support from the Royal Society, and Jurin issued a formal invitation in Latin (printed in the *Philosophical Transactions* and separately), which contained specific instructions concerning the collection and recording of observations and included a sample table filled with entries.[31] In addition to making record-keeping uniform through the use of his table, Jurin took the further step of standardising measurements by advocating the use of particular meteorological instruments, specifically those manufactured by the London instrument-maker, Francis Hauksbee the younger. Jurin petitioned the Royal Society Council to send thermometers and glass tubes, from which to construct barometers, as gifts to far-flung observers. The request was granted for three consecutive years, thus indicating the importance of meteorology as a research topic at the Society.[32]

Jurin forwarded his invitation to learned men throughout Britain, the North American colonies and continental Europe, and engaged meteorological observers in Uppsala, St Petersburg, Berlin, Leiden, Naples, Luneville, Boston and many towns in Great Britain and Ireland.[33] Numerous physicians contributed to Jurin's project, including Edward Bayly who recommended that observations on diseases be included alongside the meteorological ones. 'I have ... added a Column for Diseases which I extracted from a log in which I keep of all the Distempers wch appear from time to time in & about this Town,' Bayly wrote to Jurin. He went on to confess: 'I don't know whether you may think it worth while to have such a Column inserted for the future & I find more difficulty in managing this part then I first imagin'd when I propos'd it to you.' The difficulty lay in 'reducing the several Species of Diseases to their proper Classes'. How was the physician to make sense of his encounters with sick individuals whose symptoms varied considerably and made disease classification difficult? In the abstract, nosology had an appeal, as Mortimer had noted, but at the level of individual cases it remained a daunting pursuit. Nonetheless, Bayly asserted that 'by nicely observing those that are most predominant one may be able in time to collect some Observations towards the forming a Natural History of Diseases.'[34]

Jurin agreed and added a column for diseases in his revised invitation for meteorological observations. 'Your acc^t of ye reigning diseases, tho' attended as you Say, with considerable difficulties, may however be of very good service, especially if ye same be done by other Observers in different parts,' Jurin replied to Bayly. 'Upon ye hint you gave me, I inserted that article into a Second Edition of my Invitation & have already had some Observations of that kind Sent me, & hope for more.' Here, Jurin offered a way to reduce the complexity of classifying individual illness by asking physicians to limit their observations only to the most widespread and prevalent diseases. Further, Jurin hoped that, through comparison of geographically distinct areas, a more concrete link between climate and disease might be established. In Jurin's words, 'Perhaps ye comparing them together may give us some light into ye obscure Theory of Epidemical Distempers.'[35]

The difficulties of record-keeping emerged as a central motif in medical meteorological projects of the first half of the eighteenth century. With regard to the weather, Jurin and his correspondent, Bayly, found that an additional column in their meteorological diaries was necessary in order to make notes on prevailing diseases. This was precisely opposite to the approach taken by Clifton, who began with case histories of illness and added a column for weather observations, which he later had to remove into a separate book. What Jurin, Bayly and Clifton shared was the frustration of trying to record disparate, individual observations in a concise and uniform manner.

They also encountered the difficulties in trying to standardise observers – that is, making individuals record observations consistently. Both Jurin and Clifton relied on the observations of individual physicians to establish disease patterns – basically an extension of the Hippocratic model – but the accuracy, precision and detail of the observations depended entirely on the physicians themselves. In his second book, Clifton suggested an alternative method:

> ... that three or four persons of proper qualifications shou'd be employ'd in the *Hospitals* ... to set down the cases of the Patients there from day to day, *candidly* and *judiciously*, without any regard to private opinions or publick systems, and at the year's end publish these facts just as they are, leaving every one to make the best use of 'em he can for himself. Wou'd not some such method as this let us more into the *Nature* of diseases in a few years, than all the books of *Theories*, or even the books of *Observations*, hitherto publish'd?[36]

Clifton thus recognised the limitations of the Hippocratic method in which individual doctors kept records, and he foresaw greater possibilities for more consistent record-keeping within an institutional setting.

Roger Pickering suggested another remedy for the vagaries of individual record-keeping when he presented a paper detailing 'A Scheme of a Diary of the Weather; together with Draughts and Descriptions of Machines subservient thereunto' at a meeting of the Royal Society on 3 May 1741.[37] In his introduction, Pickering referred to Hippocrates as the founder of this type of inquiry. 'A Sense of the Importance of observing the Weather induced Hippocrates, in his Remarks upon the Epidemic Diseases in Thasos, to premise a general History of the Weather preceding them,' Pickering explained. But modern instruments and methods of recording information had 'brought the Natural History of the Air to a surprising Degree of Perfection, beyond what the Antients ever could pretend to, or even thought of.'[38]

Pickering's paper introduced another method of record-keeping, as well as detailed descriptions of several instruments to measure moisture (a new hygrometer), the force of the wind (an anemoscope) and the quantity of rain (an ombrometer). His method of keeping meteorological observations consisted of nine horizontal columns drawn in a diary, which would record the following information: date of observation; time of observation; weight of air; temperature; moisture or dryness; wind direction; wind force; weather (rainy, cloudy, clear); and quantity of rain. Below this, Pickering added, 'the Space between the last Line and the End of the Paper, for the Bill of Mortality'.[39] Acute cases were to be written in the record as they depended upon the 'State of the Air'.

This last addition distinguished Pickering's proposal from Jurin's and Clifton's earlier schemes. Contributors to Jurin's project who had included notes on epidemic diseases had all been physicians and had based their observations on their own personal experience as healers. Similarly, Clifton's initial proposal for tabular observations on disease patterns had been directed to physicians. Pickering, by contrast, proposed that mortality figures for acute diseases be taken from the bills of mortality. He realised that he might encounter professional resistance to this idea because the bills were compiled from the testimony of searchers, generally old women who reported the cause of death to the local parish clerk. 'Perhaps the Ignorance of the Searchers, appointed to inspect dead Bodies, as to the precise Diseases People die of, may lay this

Method open to Objection,' he conceded. Nonetheless, he continued, 'we must be content to take our Advice on this Point from such Hands, rather than none.'[40] Thus, Pickering tried to avoid the difficulties of collecting disease observations from individual physicians by relying on an already somewhat standardised (but admittedly not accurate) source – the London bills of mortality.

By 1750 the combined efforts of Clifton, Pickering, and especially Jurin, had established medical meteorology as part of the Royal Society's research agenda. Medical meteorology fitted the Society's methodological goals because it relied on the collection of extensive observations in order to create a natural history of air and disease. Although only Jurin's project was in fact widely taken up, all the proposals sought to improve on the ancient Hippocratic observations on weather and disease. Improvement, for these physicians, literally took three forms: first, better record-keeping via standardised tables for both disease and weather as suggested by Clifton, Jurin and Pickering; second, a wider collection of observations including some from places unknown to Hippocrates (for example, the North American colonies); and, third, new techniques for correlating weather and disease which did not rely on the observations of individual doctors but instead looked to hospital records and bills of mortality. In short, medical meteorology epitomised the new Hippocratic–Baconian approach to the study of nature promoted by the Royal Society. Its practitioners regarded it as both Hippocratic and an improvement on Hippocrates.

A mechanical Hippocrates: explaining the effects of climate on health

Alongside initiatives to collect information relating climate to health and disease were theoretical treatises on how weather (especially qualities of the air) affected the body. The physicians John Arbuthnot and John Huxham, both fellows of the Royal Society, penned especially influential works that combined insights from contemporary physiology with the latest research on medical meteorology. These authors consistently referred to Hippocrates in their writings, but the types of explanation they offered –iatromechanical and iatrochemical – were intimately connected with the new sciences.[41] As with medical meteorology, the Royal Society provided the critical context for this work: iatromechanical and iatrochemical subjects were frequently discussed at weekly meetings, and important papers on these topics were published in the *Philosophical Transactions*.[42]

Both Arbuthnot and Huxham took Hippocrates as their starting point. 'The most famous Physicians have observ'd, with great Assiduity, the Effects of Air in the Oeconomy of Diseases, and none perhaps with so much Accuracy as the first Founder of our Art, the great Hippocrates,' commented Arbuthnot in his influential *An Essay Concerning the Effects of Air on Human Bodies* (1733).[43]

Arbuthnot credited Sydenham, 'endowed with the Genius of Hippocrates', with renewing this line of inquiry[44] and stated as his aim the elucidation of the effects of climate on the human body: 'I have ventur'd to explain the Philosophy of this Sagacious old Man [Hippocrates], by mechanical Causes arising from the Properties and Qualities of the Air.'[45] This goal, of course, was largely shaped by the natural philosophy promoted by the Royal Society – a philosophy that prized mechanical explanations above all others.

The first four chapters of Arbuthnot's book summarised the recent discoveries in meteorology brought about by the use of thermometers, barometers and hygroscopes. Chapter One, entitled 'Of the Contents of the Air', contained a discussion of chemical analyses of the air. The second chapter, 'Of the Properties of the Air', addressed the use of barometers to measure the weight of the air. Temperature, gauged primarily by Fahrenheit's mercury thermometer, formed the topic of the third chapter, 'On the Qualities of the Air', and, here, Arbuthnot referred to observations taken throughout Europe to establish the various degrees of heat. For example, Arbuthnot compared variations in temperature with different degrees of perspiration.

> Another great Effect of the Heat of the Air upon Human Bodies is, that by the Degrees of it the Quantity of Perspiration, sensible and insensible, is regulated. By Journals that have been kept it appears, that the Perspiration of *England* scarcely equals all the other excretions, and that the summer Perspiration is near double to that of winter; whereas in *Paduan* Air, the Perspiration the Year round is to all the other Excretions as 5 to 3, and perhaps in hotter Countries the Proportion is greater. This must occasion a greater Variety of Human Constitutions and Diseases, according to different Climates.[46]

In the same chapter, Arbuthnot drew on various studies, beginning with those of the Paduan physician Santorio Santorio (Sanctorius) (1561–1636), which measured the input and output of an individual body and delineated differences in human physiology according to climate. The fourth chapter, 'Of the Nature of Air in different Situations, Regions, and Seasons', linked geography with variations in climate, and Arbuthnot based some of his remarks on observations made about humidity levels measured by the hygroscope. Thus, in the first half of his book, Arbuthnot synthesised efforts to quantify different qualities of the atmosphere using new instruments and connected these observations with effects on the human body.

The approach to physiology initiated by Sanctorius continued during the first half of the eighteenth century, especially in the work of the well-known natural philosopher and fellow of the Royal Society, Stephen Hales (1677–1761).[47] A less well-known contributor was John Lining, a Scots physician who practised in Charleston, South Carolina and became renowned for his writings on yellow fever in colonial America. Following a roughly similar procedure to Sanctorius, Lining performed a set of 'statical experiments' on himself over the course of an entire year, measuring the intake and output of his body and recording these amounts alongside weather observations. His approach differed in one important respect. 'Sanctorius, it is true, lived in a warm Climate, and has deduced many useful Aphorisms from his Experiments', wrote Lining, 'but then he has not left us the Experiments themselves; Hence we are not only deprived of the Authorities from whence he deduced his Aphorisms, but likewise of a long-continued Series of Experiments; from whence the Changes induced upon the human Frame, in the different Seasons, might have experimentally appeared.'[48] Here, Lining was echoing the Hippocratic–Baconian method, advocated by the Royal Society, which emphasised the importance of detailed natural histories and included carefully recorded observations.

Lining, like Arbuthnot, was seeking to discover the intermediary mechanisms that caused changes in weather to give rise to different acute diseases. As he observed:

> From the Histories of the Air and epidemic Diseases, we learn what Constitutions of the Air are productive of certain Diseases. ... Were we, however, once furnished with a Course of Statical Experiments of one whole Year, together with the History of the Weather, we, probably, might have more distinct Views of the Nature of the Diseases themselves, by knowing experimentally the Changes produced in our Constitutions, disposing us to such and such Diseases, in certain periods of the Year.[49]

Lining argued that the increases and decreases of various excretions were the 'only Index of the Changes produced in the human Constitution, by the Vicissitudes of the Weather.'[50] In other words, he sought a method to quantify the effects of climate and weather on the body.

John Huxham, a highly regarded English physician who practised in Plymouth, took a different approach from that of Arbuthnot and Lining. In 1739 he published a book entitled *Observations on the Air and Epidemic Diseases from the Year 1727 to 1737 inclusive*, which was dedicated to Sir Hans Sloane, president of the Royal Society, and more generally to the 'illustrious Members' of the Society. Most of the book was devoted to annual meteorological observations, coupled with remarks on the prevailing epidemic diseases during the same period.[51] In his preface, Huxham reviewed the connections between air and health and disease discussed in *Epidemics I* and *III* of the Hippocratic *Corpus*. Like Arbuthnot, Huxham pulled together several independent research traditions and moulded them into a single project. First, he drew on the work of Newtonian philosophers and others who tried to explain various physiological processes mechanically – for example, the action of lungs in respiration and the effects of different types of air on respiration. Second, he continued the detailed, quantitative meteorological observations that he had initiated in 1724 on the encouragement of James Jurin. Finally, he provided descriptions of prevailing epidemics and suggested links between the quality of air, the season and disease patterns.

Moreover, rather than simply drawing correlations between types of air (hot, humid, cold, dry) and specific diseases, Huxham tried to explain how these various types of air rendered the human body more or less susceptible to certain diseases. So, for example, he connected atmospheric pressure, blood circulation and health:

> The Pressure of the Atmosphere much contributes to promote the Circulation of the Blood, its greater therefore increases, and a lesser diminishes it: Hence it happens that when the Air is dry and serene, that is when it is endued with a proper Gravity and Elasticity, we find ourselves more alert and strong; for, the Velocity of the Blood being increased, our natural Secretions and Excretions are increased also, especially Perspiration, which being duly carried on produces both Vigour of Mind and Body.[52]

He referred to the work of the famous chemist Robert Boyle (1627–1691), as well as to that of Stephen Hales and Sanctorius to support his arguments and, like Arbuthnot, related differences in human physiology to meteorological and climatological conditions. Throughout the eighteenth century Huxham's work remained a model for how an individual physician, through careful observations of the weather and his medical practice, could contribute to the understanding of the relationship between climate and disease.

Taken together, Arbuthnot, Lining and Huxham established a research tradition of combining detailed natural histories of air and disease with mechanical explanations to elucidate the effects of climate on human physiology. While these authors used Hippocratic ideas as their framework and, indeed, continued to situate their work within the Hippocratic tradition, they nevertheless went beyond correlating specific diseases with certain climates. They incorporated contemporary research on human physiology and observations taken from the growing number of meteorological records to construct entirely new types of explanation that were more characteristic of natural philosophy of the period. In sum, they offered mechanical explanations for how meteorological conditions affected the human body in different ways.

Conclusion

The Royal Society provided an important forum for discussions about, and contributions to, medical meteorology during the first half of the eighteenth century. Although the natural philosophy advocated by the Society typically distanced itself from classical authorities, British medical meteorologists uniformly invoked Hippocrates at the beginning of their writings. Theories linking climate and disease found in Hippocratic writings, especially *Airs, Waters and Places* and the *Epidemics I* and *III*, continued to serve as meaningful paradigms for medical meteorology. There were two reasons for making this exception. First, the majority of medical meteorologists were physicians who not only were familiar with Hippocratic writings by virtue of their education, but also played an influential role in Society affairs. Second, the Hippocratic emphasis on careful observation and detailed record-keeping fitted harmoniously with the Baconian methods advocated by the Society.

One of the most significant developments in medical meteorology during this period were the new methods of measurement and record-keeping. The Society's embrace of the Baconian programme to provide natural histories of various phenomena encouraged fellows to record observations on disease and weather. 'Journals of the Weather, Reigning Diseases, and Remedies successful, would be of great use to Mankind, and more especially to Physicians,' wrote Arbuthnot. 'From such Journals perhaps it might be possible to predict both the weather and the epidemical Diseases.'[53] The utility of journals would be enhanced by new methods of record-keeping. In Mortimer's words, tables, such as those suggested by Jurin and Clifton, when 'properly rang'd, or class'd' made observations available for 'Inspection and use'.

While the correlation between climate and health – a central theme in the Hippocratic *Corpus* – remained an important subject for eighteenth-century physicians, fellows of the Royal Society reshaped and redirected these old Hippocratic ideas. In the works of Arbuthnot, Lining and Huxham, the improved observations collected by medical meteorologists were extended through causal explanations of how changes in weather affected the human body and human health. From the perspective of eighteenth-century fellows of the Royal Society, the usefulness of Hippocratic writings only went so far; new findings in physiology and new natural histories of the weather and disease superseded Hippocratic texts. Thus there were limits to the extent to which a 'modern' could rely on ancient ideas. Clifton articulated as much in the preface to his second book, *The State of Physick*, in which he commented that he wrote the book partly to vindicate himself 'from a reflection that had been cast upon me, on account of my book of *Tabular Observations for the improvement of Physick*, publish'd last year; as if out of an over-fondness for the Ancients, I had slighted the Moderns too much'.[54] It seems that Hippocrates could attend meetings of the Royal Society, but only as an observer, not as an authority.

Acknowledgements

I would like to thank the participants of the Hippocrates and Modern Medicine Conference held at the College of Physicians of Philadelphia, 3–5 May 1996, for their stimulating questions on the first draft of this essay, especially David Cantor who has provided thoughtful and perceptive comments on subsequent drafts. Above all, I am indebted to Paul Lucier.

Notes

1. David Miller, ' "Into the Valley of Darkness": reflections on the Royal Society in the eighteenth century', *History of Science*, **27**, 1989, pp. 155–66; and Richard Sorrenson, 'Towards a History of the Royal Society in the Eighteenth Century', *Notes and Records of the Royal Society*, **50**, 1996, pp. 29–46.
2. Susan Lawrence discusses how natural philosophy and affiliation with the Royal Society enhanced an individual's status. See Susan C. Lawrence, *Charitable Knowledge: Hospital Pupils and Practitioners in Eighteenth-century London*, Cambridge: Cambridge University Press, 1996, pp. 227–34. For the classic treatment of the debate between ancients and moderns, see Richard Foster Jones, *Ancients and Moderns: A Study of the Rise of the Scientific Movement in Seventeenth-Century England*, St Louis: Washington University Press, 1961.
3. For a recent overview of medical meteorology see Caroline Hannaway, 'Environment and Miasmata', in W.F. Bynum and Roy Porter (eds), *Companion Encyclopedia of the History of Medicine*, London and New York: Routledge, 1993, Volume 1, pp. 292–308, esp. pp. 296–300. Environmental medicine is Ludmilla Jordanova's term. See L.J. Jordanova, 'Earth science and environmental medicine: the synthesis of the late Enlightenment', in L.J. Jordanova and Roy S. Porter (eds), *Images of the Earth – Essays in the History of the Environmental Sciences*, London: British Society for the History of Science, 1979, pp. 119–46. See also, Genevieve Miller, ' "Airs, Waters and Places" in history', *Journal of the History of Medicine and Allied Sciences*, **17**, 1962, pp. 129–140; James C. Riley, *The Eighteenth-Century Campaign to Avoid Disease*, London: Macmillan, 1987; and Clarence J. Glacken, *Traces on the Rhodian Shore: Nature and Culture in Western Thought from Ancient Times to the End of the Eighteenth Century*, Berkeley and Los Angeles: University of California Press, 1967, Chapters 12 and 13.
4. For general histories of meteorology, see Theodore S. Feldman, 'Late Enlightenment meteorology', in Tore Frängsmyr, J.L. Heilbron, and Robin E. Rider (eds), *The Quantifying Spirit in the 18th Century*, Berkeley, Los Angeles, and Oxford: University of California Press, 1990, pp. 143–78; H. Howard Frisinger, *The History of Meteorology to 1800*, New York: Science History Publications, 1977; Abraham Wolf, *A History of Science, Technology, and Philosophy in the 16th and 17th Centuries*, 2nd edn prepared by Douglas McKie, London: George Allen & Unwin, 1962, Volume I, pp. 306–24; and Abraham Wolf, *A History of Science, Technology, and Philosophy in the Eighteenth Century*, London: George Allen & Unwin, 1938, pp. 274–341.
5. Sorrenson, 'Towards a History of the Royal Society' (n. 1), p. 36.
6. Iain Lonie suggested that continued adherence to humoral theories of disease and treatment and an appreciation of craft knowledge demonstrated in, and perhaps learned from, the Hippocratic corpus are two possible explanations for the popularity of Hippocrates. See Iain Lonie, 'Hippocrates the Iatromechanist', *Medical History*, **25**, 1981, pp. 113–50, esp. pp. 118–20.
7. Miller, ' "Into the Valley of Darkness" ' (n. 1), p. 158.
8. Francis Bacon, *The Advancement of Learning* (1605), Book 2, in James Spedding, Robert Leslie Ellis, and Douglas Denon Heath (eds), *The Works of Francis Bacon*, New York: Hurd and Houghton, 1869, Volume VI, p. 246.
9. Lawrence, *Charitable Knowledge* (n. 2), p. 238.
10. G.A. Lindeboom, *Hermann Boerhaave – The Man and his Work*, London: Methuen & Co., Ltd, 1968, pp. 55, 69, 381; Wesley D. Smith, *The Hippocratic*

Tradition, Ithaca, NY and London: Cornell University Press, 1979, esp. pp. 23–27 on Boerhaave's Hippocratism.
11. Francis Clifton, *Tabular Observations Recommended as the Plainest and Surest Way of Practising and Improving Physick in a Letter to a Friend*, London, 1731, p. 4. Clifton cited the original Latin passage in a footnote, from Bacon, *de Augment. Scientiar*. Lib. IV. Cap. 2.
12. Thomas Sprat's history is the most well known in this regard. See Thomas Sprat, *History of the Royal Society*, ed. Jackson I. Cope and Harold Whitmore Jones, St Louis: Washington University Studies, 1958 [1667].
13. See Andrew Cunningham, Chapter Five, this volume. See also, Harold Cook, *The Decline of the Old Medical Regime in Stuart London*, Ithaca, NY and London: Cornell University Press, 1986, p. 185.
14. In France, too, especially at the medical school in Montpellier, Hippocrates was invoked as the founder of observational medicine, as Elizabeth Williams points out in Chapter Eight of this volume. See also, Elizabeth A. Williams, *The Physical and the Moral: Anthropology, Physiology, and Philosophical Medicine in France, 1750–1850*, Cambridge: Cambridge University Press, 1994.
15. In 1729 he was appointed physician to the Prince of Wales. For a laudatory, although brief, discussion of Clifton, see E. Ashworth Underwood, *Boerhaave's Men*, Edinburgh: Edinburgh University Press, 1977, p. 43.
16. Abbé Des Fontaines, who translated Clifton's second book, *The State of Physick, Ancient and Modern, Briefly Consider'd: with a plan for the Improvement of It* (1732), called Clifton 'le fameux Editeur de l'Hippocrate d'Angleterre'. Clifton's translation and notes on Hippocrates went through a second edition in 1752.
17. Underwood, *Boerhaave's Men* (n. 15), p. 55.
18. Clifton, *Tabular Observations* (n. 11), p. 5.
19. Kenneth Dewhurst, *Dr. Thomas Sydenham (1624–1689) – His Life and Original Writings*, Berkeley and Los Angeles: University of California Press, 1966, pp. 60–61.
20. For more on Sydenham's ideas see Oswei Temkin, 'Health and Disease', *The Double Face of Janus and Other Essays in the History of Medicine*, Baltimore and London: The Johns Hopkins University Press, 1977, pp. 419–40, esp. p. 427; and idem, 'An historical analysis of the concept of infection', *The Double Face of Janus and Other Essays in the History of Medicine*, pp. 456–71, esp. p. 463.
21. Clifton, *Tabular Observations* (n. 11), pp. 2–3.
22. Ibid., p. 16.
23. On diseases, Clifton wrote: 'Nay we have the same diseases among us, as he [Hippocrates] had in his countrey; besides some few that he knew nothing of; the Venereal Disease for instance, the Small Pox &c. How far his observations will hold good with us, is uncertain …' *Tabular Observations* (n. 11), p. 13. See also Lloyd G. Stevenson, ' "New diseases" in the seventeenth century', *Bulletin of the History of Medicine*, **39**, 1965, pp. 1–21.
24. Oswei Temkin, 'The scientific approach to disease: specific entity and individual sickness', in *The Double Face of Janus* (n. 20), pp. 441–55, esp. p. 451.
25. Clifton, *Tabular Observations* (n. 11), p. 18.
26. Register Book Copy of the Royal Society, RBC.15.344, Archives of the Royal Society, London.
27. Ibid.
28. James Jurin's meteorological project is discussed in the following works: Andrea Rusnock (ed.), *The Correspondence of James Jurin, Physician and Secretary to the Royal Society*, Amsterdam and Atlanta: Rodopi Press, 1996, pp. 27–31; John

Heilbron, *Physics at the Royal Society during Newton's Presidency*, Los Angeles: William Andrews Clark Memorial Library, 1983, pp. 104–9; James McClellan III, *Science Reorganized: Scientific Societies in the Eighteenth Century*, New York: Columbia University Press, 1985, pp. 161–62; and Gordon Manley, 'The weather and diseases: some 18th-century contributions to observational meteorology', *Notes and Records of the Royal Society of London*, **9**, 1952, pp. 300–7.
29. 12 December 1723, RS Journal Book XII, Archives of the Royal Society, London.
30. For a biography of Jurin, see Rusnock, *The Correspondence of James Jurin* (n. 28), pp. 8–61.
31. James Jurin, 'Invitatio ad Observationes Meteorologicas communi consilio instituendas', *Philosophical Transactions*, **32**, 1723, no. 379, pp. 422–27.
32. The Royal Society approved Jurin's initial request at the Council Meeting on 15 April 1725, with the proviso that no more than 12 instruments be sent abroad. One year later Jurin informed the Royal Society Council that the distribution of the instruments had improved the quality of observations and requested permission to distribute additional instruments. The Council granted this request and disbursed funds for an additional six instruments: RS Council Minutes, 12 May 1726. In 1727, an additional 6 instruments were allocated: RS Council Minutes, 20 April 1727, Archives of the Royal Society, London.
33. The Royal Society Archives contain 18 weather diaries spanning one or more years dating from Jurin's tenure, and many more from the following years. See Meteorological Archives, Archives of the Royal Society, London.
34. Edward Bayly to James Jurin, 21 June 1725, Royal Society Early Letters B.2.99, Archives of the Royal Society.
35. James Jurin to Edward Bayly, 29 January 1725/6, Jurin Correspondence, Library of the Wellcome Institute for the History of Medicine, London; reprinted in Rusnock, *The Correspondence of James Jurin* (n. 28), pp. 322–23.
36. Francis Clifton, *The State of Physick, Ancient and Modern, Briefly Consider'd: with a Plan for the Improvement of It*, London, 1732, p. 171.
37. Roger Pickering, 'A Scheme of a Diary of the Weather; together with Draughts and Descriptions of Machines subservient thereunto; inscribed to the President and Fellows of the Royal Society', *Philosophical Transactions*, 1741, pp. 1–18.
38. Ibid., p. 1.
39. Ibid., pp. 3–4.
40. Ibid., pp. 4–5.
41. Mechanical explanations were not always viewed as antithetical to Hippocratic writings. Friedrich Hoffmann (1660–1742), for example, carefully documented mechanical explanations in the Hippocratic *Corpus*. See Lonie, 'Hippocrates the Iatromechanist' (n.6).
42. Theodore M. Brown, *The Mechanical Philosophy and the 'Animal Oeconomy': A Study in the Development of English Physiology in the Seventeenth and Early Eighteenth Centuries*, New York: Arno Press, 1981; Anita Guerrini, 'Isaac Newton, George Cheyne and the *Principia Medicinae*', in Roger French and Andrew Wear (eds), *The Medical Revolution of the Seventeenth Century*, Cambridge and New York: Cambridge University Press, 1989, pp. 222–45; Anita Guerrini, 'James Keill, George Cheyne and Newtonian Physiology 1690–1740', *Journal of the History of Biology*, **18**, 1985, pp. 246–66.
43. John Arbuthnot, *An Essay Concerning the Effects of Air on Human Bodies*, London, 1733, p. vii. For a discussion of this work, see Riley, *The Eighteenth-Century Campaign to Avoid Disease* (n. 3), pp. 20–26.
44. Arbuthnot, *An Essay Concerning the Effects of Air* (n. 43), p. vii.

45. Ibid., p. 152.
46. Ibid., pp. 50–51.
47. Stephen Hales, *Statical Essays: Containing Haemastaticks; or, an Account of some Hydraulick and Hydrostatical Experiments made on the Blood and Blood-Vessels of Animals*, London, 1733.
48. John Lining, 'Extracts of Two Letters from Dr. John Lining, Physician at Charles-Town in South Carolina, to James Jurin, M.D. F.R.S. giving an Account of Statical Experiments made several times in a Day upon himself, for one whole Year, accompanied with Meteorological Observations; to which are subjoined Six General Tables, deduced from the whole Year's course', *Philosophical Transactions*, **42**, 1743, pp. 493–509 at p. 492.
49. Ibid., p. 493.
50. John Lining, 'A Letter from Dr. John Lining, at Charles-Town in South Carolina, to James Jurin ... serving to accompany some Additions to his Statical Experiments printed in no. 470 of these Transactions', *Philosophical Transactions*, **43**, 1745, pp. 318–330 at p. 319.
51. John Huxham, *Observations on the Air and Epidemic Diseases from the Year MDCCXXVII to MDCCXXXVII inclusive; together with a Short Dissertation on Devonshire Colic, Translated from the Latin Original by his Son, John Corham Huxham*, London: J. Hinton, 1759. All citations from this work in this essay are to this edition. The original work is Huxham, *Observationes de aëre et morbis epidemicis ... 1727–1737, Plymuthi factae. Hic accedit opusculum de morbo colico Damnoniensi*, London: S. Austen, 1739.
52. Ibid., p. xii.
53. Aphorism XCVI, Arbuthnot, *An Essay Concerning the Effects of Air* (n. 43), p. 223.
54. Clifton, *The State of Physick* (n. 36), n.p.

Part III

Hippocratism in Eighteenth- and Nineteenth-century France and North America

CHAPTER EIGHT

Hippocrates and the Montpellier Vitalists in the French Medical Enlightenment

Elizabeth A. Williams

In 1801 a bust of Hippocrates was donated by the government of First Consul Napoleon Bonaparte to the newly renovated School of Medicine in Montpellier and installed in the school's quarters amid an elaborate ceremony.[1] Some three years later, for the first time in the long history of the Montpellier medical school, students who ascended to the *doctorat* formally swore the Hippocratic oath.[2] These two events – the first formal swearing of the Hippocratic oath and the installation of the bust of Hippocrates – are but two of many signs indicating the increased attention accorded in this period to the 'father of medicine' among the physicians of Montpellier, one of the most prestigious medical schools of continental Europe. Although Hippocrates had long been claimed as the source of many of Montpellier's best-known teachings on diagnostics, prognostics, pathology and therapeutics, the eighteenth century and early years of the nineteenth witnessed an intensification of this already pronounced interest in the physician of Cos. In the complex history of the declines and revivals of Hippocrates's reputation, this period must be regarded as one of the peaks in his prestige among European physicians – not least the physicians of Montpellier.

Medical historians have recently begun to show renewed interest in Hippocrates in his many guises, chiefly because interpretive and historiographical shifts of the last few decades have supplied new tools for exploring the diverse, sometimes directly conflicting, representations that have developed around enigmatic historical figures. This interest in representations of Hippocrates has tended to supplant an older historiography that, conceived in a confidently positivistic vein, usually sought to discover the 'true' Hippocrates and to gauge the genuineness of his disciples' claims to be carrying the Hippocratic banner.[3] Few scholars now seek to find the 'true' Hippocrates, or to sift the wheat from the chaff among his self-styled disciples. Instead, interest presently focuses on the ideological, professional and overtly political 'uses' of Hippocrates by physicians of earlier eras.[4]

This essay is situated within this historiographical frame. It examines the creation and manipulation of divergent images of Hippocrates to different ends at two moments in the unfolding of the medical Enlightenment by physicians of the Montpellier school. I will approach this matter by juxtaposing two texts, one written by Théophile de Bordeu and published in 1767, and another the oration delivered by Paul-Joseph Barthez to the audience that gathered in Montpellier in 1801 to install the bust of Hippocrates.[5] The question that I will ask is what view of disease, and more broadly of the medical art, the Montpellier physicians, – often characterised as the most important 'Hippocratists' in eighteenth-century France – intended to convey in assuming the label 'Hippocratic'.[6] As I hope to show, the content of this Hippocratism varied with the passage of time and the shifting personal and public commitments of the physicians who claimed Hippocrates's legacy. Bordeu used Hippocrates to argue for the simplicity of nature's works in both health and illness and for the availability of medical truth to the unlearned; Barthez used Hippocrates to insist on the complexity of disease and treatment and, concomitantly, on the indispensability of medical erudition and professional authority. As I will argue, these different constructions of Hippocrates reflected not only divergences in the training, ambitions and theoretical inclinations of these two important eighteenth-century physicians but also competing views of the medical practitioner's role, the character of the medical art and, most tellingly for broader medical history, the means by which the new medicine they represented – what would eventually be called 'Montpellier vitalism' – might establish a distinctive posture in a medical world transformed by powerful currents of reform and, finally, revolution.

As the Montpellier medical tradition has been relatively neglected in the historiography of French medicine (certainly in comparison to Paris), it may be worthwhile beginning with a brief introduction to the Montpellier school. Montpellier was the home of one of the oldest medical schools on the continent; it came into being some time in the eleventh century and received its first statutes in 1220. From the later Middle Ages onwards it occupied a prominent place in the European medical world as one of the chief Mediterranean centres of medicine.[7] In the seventeenth century Montpellier was principally known for its championing of medical chemistry against the neo-Galenism of the Paris faculty.[8] Then in the eighteenth century it became one of the most important sites for the development of medical vitalism, thanks largely to the efforts of the two figures considered here – Bordeu and Barthez.[9]

How and why did Montpellier come to be known as a centre of 'Hippocratic' medicine during the eighteenth century? The beginnings of the Hippocratic revival of this era in Montpellier are entangled with one of those mysteries in the history of medicine generated by antagonisms and jealousies dividing French and British chroniclers of medical tradition. In this case, the mystery involves the so-called 'English Hippocrates' – Thomas Sydenham. For a long time French medical historians have routinely recounted that, during his formative years as a practitioner, Sydenham studied in Montpellier and there imbibed his Hippocratism from Charles Barbeyrac, the physician generally credited in the literature on Montpellier as the instigator of the Hippocratic revival.[10] Indeed, Théophile de Bordeu was one of the physicians who, in recounting the history of medicine, claimed that Sydenham had taken 'all ... that was most valuable' in his work from Barbeyrac, to the point of calling him 'Sydenham ... of Montpellier'.[11] However, English-language historians of medicine generally do not accept this account.[12] Kenneth Dewhurst, in particular, has gone to some lengths to discredit this story, pointing out that Sydenham knew no French and that his good friend John Locke – who definitely did visit Montpellier in 1675–76 – made no reference to a visit by Sydenham to Montpellier in letters he wrote from France.[13] In this version of events Barbeyrac is supposed to have learned his Hippocratism from Sydenham (via his writings) rather than vice versa.[14]

Although there remains little doubt that the story of Sydenham in Montpellier is apocryphal, the relative importance of indigenous French sources of Hippocratism versus the influence of Sydenham in France still needs to be sorted out. What does seem clearly established is that a 'Hippocratic revival' began in France in the late seventeenth century, and that physicians in Montpellier were prominent in instigating and perpetuating it.[15] It is, at any rate, indisputable that from the late seventeenth century onwards Montpellier physicians regularly – though with varying degrees of conviction and to diverse ends – claimed Hippocrates as their master.

To establish the setting for the particular constructions of Hippocrates developed by Bordeu and Barthez, it should first be emphasised that Hippocrates was invoked in eighteenth-century Montpellier, as he was throughout Europe, principally as the founder of observational medicine. In this respect, Hippocrates was used by Montpellier physicians as by physicians everywhere else to contrast the virtues of 'observation' to all the errors – the tendency towards system-building, the reliance on dogma and authority, the recourse to philosophy or theology – ritually laid at the door of unenlightened medicine.[16] However, in Montpellier, Hippocrates was used more specifically as a tool in the struggle that the architects of medical vitalism waged against iatrochemistry and iatromechanism. The Montpellier physicians used Hippocrates particularly to contest the prestige of Hermann Boerhaave, the great Leiden teacher and practitioner, and his version of mechanist medicine – although, ironically, Boerhaave was also praised by his contemporaries and later medical historians alike as one of the chief revivers of Hippocrates.[17] Nonetheless the vitalist physicians of Montpellier argued that iatromechanists betrayed the heritage of Hippocrates in neglecting the individual patient in favour of purported mechanist universals; in focusing on the search for spurious causes of disease rather than on cures; in investigating malfunctions of hypothetical body parts rather than keeping in view the sick person, and so on.[18] One able spokesman for vitalism, Jean-Joseph Ménuret de Chambaud, wrote of Boerhaave, for example, that 'nothing was less Hippocratic, less in conformity with the free and varied march of nature than the metaphysical divisions and subdivisions' that formed the basis of Boerhaave's theories.[19] The vitalist physicians claimed that, in contrast to these system-builders, they recognised, with Hippocrates, that there were no diseases as such, but rather an infinity of fleeting, variable, endlessly transformable pathological states.[20]

Such sentiments were expressed in texts published during the 1730s, when François Boissier de Sauvages first launched an assault on iatromechanism from his lectern in Montpellier to and, indeed beyond, the dawn of the era of clinical medicine in France – the period at which this essay concludes. Embedded within these generalities of the vitalist–mechanist struggle, however, were important differences of thinking and approach that illuminate some of the key features of Enlightenment medicine and its transformation in the charged circumstances of the medical revolution of the 1790s.

Bordeu and the truth of nature

Paradoxically, Théophile de Bordeu is perhaps most famous for a text that he did not write and, indeed, was not published for decades after his death and that of its true author. This text was Denis Diderot's *Rêve de d'Alembert*. There Bordeu figured as d'Alembert's learned interlocutor in a dialogue about the fundamentals of cosmology, and he was made to espouse a pantheist doctrine of a universal life principle animating all matter. Bordeu, in fact, espoused no such view, limiting his inquiry regarding the life principle to problems of physiology and pathology – the nature of sensitivity, the character of glandular function, and the signs and symptoms of chronic maladies such as scrofula and *colique de Poitou*. He wrote nothing on cosmology and seldom referred in his writings to matters outside the sphere of medicine.[21]

Powerful affinities of thought and temper drew Diderot and Bordeu together, but if Diderot had chosen Bordeu for this fictional role purely because he sought a notorious figure his choice would have made sense in view of Bordeu's fame as a practitioner in Paris. A native of Béarn, Bordeu studied at the University of Medicine in Montpellier from 1739 to 1743, practised for a time in his native region, and then moved to Paris in the late 1740s. After another brief stint in the south at the end of the decade, he settled definitively in Paris in 1751. His success there was impressive. From the publication of his first major treatise, a study of glandular function, Bordeu built a reputation both as a theorist and as a practitioner in exalted social circles. He was one of the consultants called to the deathbed of Louis XV, and it was long expected in Paris that he would be appointed First Physician of the realm. His disappointment in this ambition was attributed to the profound enmity shown towards Bordeu by members of the Paris Faculty of Medicine, many of whom he had offended in a long career of iconoclastic medical writing that often used revered Parisian figures as targets.[22]

Bordeu's text of 1767, *Recherches sur le tissu muqueux, ou l'organe cellulaire, et sur quelques maladies de la poitrine*, was one of a number of treatises Bordeu composed on problems of physiology, pathology and general medicine.[23] In it he set forth his understanding of the 'cellular tissue', the spongy, multiform matter that encased all the major organs and filled all the 'interstices' of the anatomical system.[24] This cellular tissue played a crucial role in Bordeu's physiological and pathological doctrine. In the language of eighteenth-century pathology Bordeu was often labelled a 'solidist' – that is, a theorist who believed the solids to be more important than the humours or fluids in bodily function, whether healthy or morbid.[25]

In fact Bordeu belonged in neither the solidist nor the humoralist camp; to him, the key element in both normal physiological function and in pathological conditions was neither solid nor fluid but what he called 'vital force'. While acknowledging that he could not define vital force, he nonetheless believed that, with its varying degrees of intensity and its protean manifestations, it was the essential element distinguishing life functions from the operations of brute matter.[26] Moreover, the cellular tissue played a crucial role in this framework in several respects. First, it provided a vehicle for concentrating on the whole vital system, as opposed to discrete anatomical parts. Vital force was distributed throughout the animal economy, although it was concentrated, Bordeu believed, in three 'centres' – the head, the diaphragm and the abdomen. Similarly, the cellular tissue was found throughout the body, providing what Bordeu called a 'pocket' (*poche*) for the individual organs and abetting (or subverting) their actions at all times. Second, the cellular tissue was, along with the circulatory system proper, one of the primary pathways for movement of the humours; indeed, an essential component of health was the easy permeability of the cellular tissue. (One of Bordeu's most serious complaints against the mechanists was that they confined humoral movement to circulatory pathways that, in his estimation, were often wholly imaginary.) Third, and perhaps most important, the cellular tissue exhibited, for whatever reason, varying degrees of vital force and therefore functioned as a kind of anatomical substratum for the manifold powers of life itself, chief among them nervous sensitivity. Nevertheless, closely linked as the cellular tissue was to the nervous system, it was not its direct corollary and it did not depend for its functions on the movement of nervous impulses. Thus the cellular tissue could explain a multitude of phenomena that had no observable relation to the topography of either the circulatory or the nervous pathways.[27]

Bordeu used a variety of strategies to convince his readers that his theory of the *tissu muqueux* was valid, but none was more elaborate or impassioned than his invocation of the father of medicine in support of his thinking. He decried what he perceived as the general neglect of Hippocrates: who now, he asked, reads or understands Hippocrates? Bordeu attributed this unhappy state of affairs to the pernicious influence of the system-builders who, in their arrogance and devotion to the thinking of the moderns, ignored Hippocrates's genuine medical observations and insights. Although Bordeu mentioned iatrochemistry in passing, his real target here was medical mechanism which, he believed, had made William Harvey, the 'author of the circulation', into an all-powerful authority and had come to ascribe all physiological phenomena of any importance to the circulatory system. The wrongheaded pathology of the mechanists was, moreover, matched by their therapeutics. Mechanists had nothing to offer patients but copious, often murderous, bleeding; all other features of medical art had been lost.[28]

Bordeu continued his attack on the mechanists by arguing that, since they were captive to the circulatory model, they could not appreciate the insights of Hippocrates, who had neither known nor used it. Mechanists besmirched the reputation of Hippocrates, he argued, by claiming that phenomena he had faithfully described were anatomically impossible and his teaching therefore outmoded. In reaction against such claims, Bordeu was stepping in, as he put it, 'to save the honor of Cos'.[29] Quoting liberally from the *Coan Prognostics*, the *Aphorisms*, and the *Epidemics*, he argued that some of Hippocrates's most telling observations – phenomena that any honest physician must admit encountering in bedside practice – found a clear explanation within his own framework of the cellular tissue.

The focus of Bordeu's discussion was on illnesses of the chest, although he made passing reference to a host of ills afflicting the stomach, the head and other body regions. One example may suffice to illustrate his use of Hippocrates to demonstrate the cellular tissue theory and vice versa. Bordeu's characteristic procedure was to quote, sometimes at great length, an excerpt from Hippocrates and then show how his own cellular tissue theory could elucidate Hippocrates's observations in a way that 'modern theory' could not. One such excerpt, drawn from the *Coan Prognostics*, read as follows:

> One can expect [to encounter] an enlarged parotid in a sick person who has laboured breathing along with tension in the hypochondrium, acute fever, and some shivering. ... Such patients, if bilious, are also subject to abscesses around the ears.[30]

Bordeu recognised that some of these symptoms might be interrupted if remedies were applied, but he insisted that 'if the malady were left to itself the prognosis of Cos would take place [as] ... such a course of events follows the dictates of nature'. Indeed, Bordeu concluded, 'The phenomenon could not be otherwise: it is wholly necessary given the position and mechanism of the cellular substance of the chest'. In Bordeu's opinion, knowledge of cellular tissue illuminated all the events described by Hippocrates, such as the swelling of the parotid, which resulted from the fact that it 'is located precisely at the point ... where the cellular tissue of the chest joins with that ... of the neck'. It was to this 'depot' that the 'partially cooked [cuite] ... almost purulent' matter associated with the malady was carried by the cellular tissue.[31]

Bordeu anticipated a spirited objection to this account from theorists who explained all pathological phenomena by reference to the circulation: 'But, someone will say, this language overthrows the modern theory, which is founded on incontestable principles [that] ... demonstrate that all maladies are situated in the vessels.' He further imagined his detractor 'trampl[ing] on this jargon of the ancients, which is nothing more than the tacit admission ... of ignorance of the circulation'. It was such incomprehension of Hippocrates's observations, Bordeu argued, that had caused them first to 'fall under suspicion and then to be forgotten and scorned'.[32] Moreover, this posture of the moderns had not only caused Hippocratic wisdom to be lost but had dictated 'methods of treatment that appeared to be the necessary corollaries' of the modern approach.[33]

Bordeu presented scores of such observations from Hippocrates, all of which, he argued, would appear meaningless if viewed from the 'accepted point of view' but which were perfectly comprehended and, indeed, revealed in all their brilliance when seen in light of the cellular tissue theory. Having demonstrated his case with particulars, he then speculated on how and why it could be that Hippocrates was so consistently right and the 'moderns' so thoroughly wrong. And it was here that Bordeu linked his Hippocratism to one of the most powerful themes in Enlightenment discourse. In emotive phrases, Bordeu recalled that he and his fellow students in Montpellier had been led astray by professors who talked endlessly of blood globules and fibres of all shapes and sizes;[34] it was only when he went out among the people that he heard another language – the true language of life and vitality, sickness and healing. The people spoke to me, Bordeu wrote,

> ... of serosities that from the head fell to the chest; of these same serosities that moved from the back of the head and were evacuated by the nose, by the eyes, by the ears; of excesses of sun and damp that carried aqueous, cold, [and] heavy humours into the throat, the nose, and the gums.[35]

This was the language of Hippocrates – a language that the learned professors had concealed from Bordeu and his fellow students, but one that *the people spoke*. How could this be? How could the people know what erudite physicians did not? This seeming paradox was, in fact, easy to explain: Hippocrates and the people of the countryside round Montpellier both spoke the 'language of nature'.[36] Retrieving and learning to speak this language was the only means of undermining the influence of abstractions and false systems.

Similarly, Bordeu counselled a therapeutics based on nature; repeatedly in this treatise, after surveying the physiological details of a given condition using the Hippocratic symptoms as his starting point and then the cellular tissue theory as the pathological explanation, he concluded that the violent therapeutics of the moderns, the upholders of the circulation theory, were murderous. Excessive bleeding had carried off many a patient who should have been left to the healing powers of nature; the violent purgatives often coupled with such bleeding finished off others. He lamented that he himself had once killed a patient in this way – a physician who had insisted on violent treatment and whose counsel Bordeu had been too inexperienced to resist. But he had learned, subsequently, by carefully reading and reflecting on the words of the father of medicine, and now his own practice was in conformity with both Hippocrates and nature.[37]

This text of Bordeu's is one of many produced by Montpellier physicians of this era in which they claimed for their tradition a distinctive understanding of the virtues and power of nature. No term carried greater weight, of course, in Enlightenment discourse, and it would be impossible to sort out here the many meanings attached to it in medical contexts, let alone in broader philosophical and scientific contexts.[38] Even in Bordeu's own use of the Hippocrates/nature equivalency, moreover, there were tensions and complexities, some of which emerge clearly if this work of 1767 is compared to another text, Bordeu's article, 'Crise' published in the *Encyclopédie* in 1754. This famous piece is one of the great masterpieces of Enlightenment medical writing. Learned, ironic, sceptical, it perfectly embodies the critical mode for which the encyclopaedic project was both hailed and pilloried. The specific issue Bordeu addressed in the entry was the validity of the 'critical days', those days on which, according to Hippocratic–Galenic orthodoxy, a malady achieved 'crisis' and began its 'march' towards resolution. Of this seemingly modest topic Bordeu made a vehicle for meditation on medical tradition and the fundamental character of disease. In this text Hippocrates played a rather different role from that of the pure translator of nature Bordeu assigned him in the treatise on the cellular tissue. Indeed, in this instance, Hippocrates exemplified what Bordeu saw as a lamentable pattern in the history of medicine, the readiness of physicians to subordinate their own observations to the explanatory power of 'systems'. Bordeu culled from the *Aphorisms*, the *Epidemics* and the *Coan Prognostics* what he regarded as Hippocrates's general teaching on the critical days and then discussed in detail the additions to, and developments of, the doctrine made by Galen, other ancients and the Arabic physicians. Although Bordeu acknowledged that Hippocrates contradicted himself on details, and that Galen had imputed to Hippocrates 'serious errors' on the subject, he argued that there was nonetheless a coherent Hippocratic doctrine of the critical days that had alternately inspired admiration and scorn among 'Moderns' who sought guidance from it in devising practical therapeutics. Hippocrates's contradictions troubled Bordeu, but his principal objection to the very enterprise of counting the days of an illness stemmed from his hostility to the view that nature's works could be thought to exhibit mathematical regularity: 'Nature has its laws, but one can neither count nor classify them.'[39] To explain this aberration of Hippocrates – his resort to the authority of number – Bordeu took his lead from Celsus who had written that, in this instance, the great master, led astray by his admiration for the Pythagoreans, had adopted their teachings despite the violence done thereby to his own observations.

In this text, then, Hippocrates represented physicians who allowed 'dogmas' and 'systems' to blind them to the unsullied truths available to observation, a host of whom figured in the historical commentary that followed Bordeu's exposition of the critical days doctrine. Prominent among these system-builders were the physicians who were to become the standard targets of vitalist criticism: Galen himself (with his 'vivid imagination, his genius incapable of supporting doubt'); Boerhaave and Friedrich Hoffmann; and, crucial to Bordeu in this phase of his campaign against mechanism, the Montpellier professor and one-time First Physician Pierre Chirac and his own teachers in Montpellier who had embraced '*Chiracisme*'.[40] This doctrine, which Bordeu likened to 'Cartesianism in physics', overthrew the ancients, treated Hippocrates and Galen as 'mere empirics', and devised a curative method that disregarded the crises of nature. Here, in the cool tones of the medical philosophe, Bordeu described the therapeutic measures to which *Chiracisme* had given rise – endless bleeding and purging tied in no way to the 'time' of the malady – measures on which, in private, he heaped scorn.[41]

Thus, as Bordeu moved through his analysis, he shifted gradually from the errors of the original critical days doctrine to those of physicians who, in rejecting it, abandoned the broader Hippocratic understanding of the natural march of disease. By the end of the piece Hippocrates had subtly re-emerged as the bearer of the truth of nature, all the more to be revered for having survived the rigours of philosophical criticism. Bordeu made no final declaration on behalf of the doctrine of the critical days, nor did he retreat from the view that even the great Hippocrates had, in this case, been 'seduced' by the spirit of system. Yet in excoriating contemporary adversaries Bordeu made clear that any doctrine that neglected the 'march of nature' – whether out of admiration for a false clarity or a yearning for the prestige of philosophy or mathematics, undermined true medicine. Just what phenomena constituted the march of nature, he concluded, would be understood fully only when a multitude of observations was amassed by physicians prepared to heed its signs. This task could not be the work of the physician who taught medicine 'in the schools' and was 'obliged to attach [himself] to a system' (the 'misfortune of the professor's condition'). Nor could it be undertaken by the 'ordinary, popular physician' who had no time to reflect and sought only 'determined rules' of practice. Such work could be performed only by the 'legislator of the art, the philosophical doctor who began as witness [and] who from practitioner becomes a great observer'.[42]

This piece, written early in Bordeu's career, gives only a few hints of where, ultimately, his own efforts to discern the march of nature would lead him. One sign appeared in his reference to the Chiracians as physicians who viewed disease as a direct attack on 'the vital principle', rather than, as Bordeu argued, the natural effort of the vital principle to restore the body to health. Another indication of his future course was the section he devoted to James Nihell's *Observations nouvelles et extraordinaires sur la prédiction du crises par le pouls* (first French edition 1748), a work that set Bordeu on what was to be a 20-year quest to replace Hippocrates's uncertain doctrine of the critical days with a sure prognostic device – the reading of the pulse.[43] It was to be this work on the pulse that fulfilled the promise Bordeu displayed with such virtuosity in the *Encyclopédie* and that made of him a 'legislator of the art'.[44] With it, wrote one reviewer, Bordeu added 'new luster to ... Hippocratic medicine' by providing 'an ingenious and coherent system of practice' that guided practitioners round the perils attendant on interrupting the work of nature.[45]

It might seem that the unambiguous Hippocrates/nature dyad of Bordeu's 1767 text is irretrievably lost amid his more complex utterances on Hippocrates, disease and the medical art made in the studies of the critical days and of the pulse. And, indeed, no purpose would be served in obscuring the tensions in Bordeu's uses of Hippocrates and corresponding constructions of the nature of disease and the ends of medicine. Yet there is a crucial level at which these various representations of Hippocrates reinforce one another, and that lies in Bordeu's construal of the accessibility of the truths of nature. Who, in Bordeu's reading, was empowered to read nature, and why? The answer to this question was ambiguous: Hippocrates could read nature, when he acted as master–observer and avoided the seductions of system-building; the 'legislator of the art' could because his vision was not clouded by the ambition and vanity of the abstract theorist; the people could because they saw with the eyes of the nature of which they themselves were part.

It was to become an increasingly important element of Montpellier's self-promotion that the vitalist medicine taught there was built on this style of observation, and that such observation was the legacy of Hippocrates – the master whom only Montpellier continued to heed. The theme of Montpellier's unique appreciation for Hippocrates was developed with great ingenuity and style by the physician who, in the late 1760s, emerged as Bordeu's most forceful champion – Ménuret de Chambaud. Ménuret was the first of the Montpellier vitalists to argue that genuine observation of nature, and therefore the preservation of the Hippocratic heritage, were properly the work of men of the provinces, who understood the infinite variety of the countryside and the folly of resorting to false universals to explain the vitality or feebleness of its products or inhabitants.[46] In the early nineteenth century Montpellier's promoters would develop this refrain into an elaborate equivalency between Montpellier and Cos.[47] But before Ménuret's inspired theme could be developed, a discordant note was sounded by the next master theorist of Montpellier vitalism, Paul-Joseph Barthez.

Barthez and the complexity of the medical art

I turn now from Bordeu's text of 1767 to a very different one, Barthez's oration in honour of Hippocrates delivered in 1801. Barthez was born in 1734, a decade after Bordeu, and was perhaps just sufficiently different in age to render him immune to Bordeu's style of Enlightenment reverie about the transparent truths of nature. Unlike Bordeu, he came from the immediate Montpellier region; his father was an important landowner, one of his brothers was a magistrate for Montpellier's most important court and another was a successful, if minor, *homme de lettres*. By origin, then, Barthez was much more urban than Bordeu, who hailed from the Béarnais countryside. Like Bordeu, Barthez studied and took his medical degree in Montpellier and then tried his fortunes elsewhere. In the early 1750s he lived briefly in Paris, where he attended the salon of Baron d'Holbach. After a stint as a military physician, he joined the Montpellier professoriate in 1760. In subsequent decades Barthez devoted his energies principally to teaching and to work on his *chef d'oeuvre*, *Nouveaux élémens de la science de l'homme*, published in 1778. In the 1780s he divided his time between Montpellier and Paris, where he pressed relentlessly for official preferment over his colleagues in Montpellier on a range of issues, both significant and petty. When the Revolution broke out, Barthez published a pamphlet denouncing the radical excesses of the Revolution and then went into seclusion in Narbonne, where he remained throughout the upheavals of the revolutionary years. When the Montpellier school of medicine was reopened in the mid-1790s Barthez was initially passed over for reappointment to the faculty, but he had powerful friends (including Jean-Antoine Chaptal and the soon to be Archchancellor of the Empire, J.-J.-R. Cambacérès) who used their influence to have him nominated once more. Although Barthez was widely resented and mistrusted in Montpellier, his reappointment as professor was of great benefit to the faculty, which was now engaged in a struggle for its existence against claims made in the capital that Paris should be the country's sole centre of medical teaching. By the 1790s Barthez enjoyed a great reputation. His *Nouveaux élémens de la science de l'homme* was widely seen as the essential vitalist text and Barthez himself as the chief prophet of the new sect.[48] More important in the turbulent political environment that Montpellier's defenders now had to negotiate were Barthez's ties to powerful people in both medical and larger political circles.[49]

If Barthez's medical reputation and his political connections are taken into account, it is perhaps obvious why it was Barthez who – despite the hostility towards him in Montpellier and, more germane to this essay, his idiosyncratic thinking on Hippocrates, disease and the medical art – was chosen to deliver the public oration that was the centrepiece of the ceremony staged to install the bust of Hippocrates in 1801. In any event, this ceremony was, as indicated at the beginning of this essay, a clear sign of the growing devotion to Hippocrates in Montpellier. And Barthez's oration ought, if the history of Montpellier's 'Hippocratism' were as neat as local accounts have often had it, to have fitted into a framework similar to that just examined for Bordeu: Hippocrates as the father of observational medicine; Hippocrates as the faithful listener at the bedside of the sick; and Hippocrates as the voice of Nature itself.[50]

But, in fact, this was one of those points where history fails to offer a neat picture. For the Hippocrates evoked by Barthez differed from Bordeu's Hippocrates in crucial respects. Hippocrates was still, in Barthez's fashioning, the father of observational medicine: in his oration Barthez duly delivered the required encomium to observation over sterile system-building. But, in other ways, Barthez's Hippocrates was very different from that conjured by his heralded vitalist predecessor. First, Hippocrates – in this address supposedly devoted to his 'genius' – was not really the focus of Barthez's words at all. The 'genius' whose spirit actually inspired the meeting was Napoleon Bonaparte, the 'first magistrate of the republic, this extraordinary man who ... after attaining the highest degree of military glory proved himself jealous of [the further glory] of protecting and encouraging the sciences and the literary arts'.[51] In such endeavours, said Barthez, Bonaparte stood with Alexander and Caesar, and it was alongside these great ancients that Hippocrates stood.

Barthez's listeners must have known, on hearing this opener, that they were a long way from Bordeu's Hippocrates, who shared with sick peasants a natural language of health and healing. Indeed Barthez made it clear that a view of the people very different from that conveyed by Bordeu was one of the insights to be gained from studying the works of Hippocrates. According to Barthez, Hippocrates had joined with the 'ancient legislators of Greece' in insisting that the people must not be left to follow the 'natural progress of their degeneration' but must be guided by the state and by religion. Singling out for praise not the *Aphorisms* or *Prognostics* that Bordeu had emphasised but rather Hippocrates's great anthropological treatise *Airs, Waters, Places*, Barthez represented this as a work whose principal virtue was to illuminate the links between morality and politics, climate and government. If the physician integrated such counsel into his work in 'practical medicine', Barthez concluded, he could fashion himself as 'a god for other men'.[52]

This matter was something of a side-issue, however; the central theme sounded in Barthez's oration on Hippocrates – and here he broke sharply with Bordeu – concerned Hippocrates as master-creator of the medical art. Barthez lamented that physicians had for so long portrayed Hippocrates as counselling nothing but recourse to the 'healing power of nature'.[53] He acknowledged that nature could effect cures but only, so his experience taught, of the simplest maladies. For 'grave and complicated' illnesses, nothing could replace the physician's skill.⁵⁴ Barthez reminded his listeners of what he himself had taught, throughout his years as professor of 'practical medicine', about medical art and method. Resisting the unwonted recourse to nature, he had always held that the 'natural' method must be supplemented by the 'empirical' and the 'analytical', the former based on the physician's past practice and including, when necessary, 'brusque' interruptions of nature's course, the latter aiming to resolve the malady into discrete 'elements' and devising treatments accordingly.⁵⁵ Thus, far from endorsing Bordeu's view that learned professors could lead the student of medicine astray while the people could guide him to the truths of nature itself, Barthez emphasised the importance of medical erudition. Of all the characteristics required of the good physician, Barthez held, none was more important than good education and training. Hippocrates himself had defended medicine, Barthez claimed, against detractors who criticised the art while 'lacking utterly the knowledge required [to understand] what constitutes, in essence, medical science'.⁵⁶

Now it might be observed that this text of Barthez's functioned principally as an exercise in flattery of the political luminaries who, in donating the bust of Hippocrates to the Montpellier school, made a welcome show of support for the institution. And, if so, the question might arise of whether it is really very illuminating to juxtapose two texts so different in format, audience and apparent intention as Bordeu's learned treatise of 1767 and Barthez's bombastic oration of 1801. Bordeu's text presented an innovative theory in physiology and pathology and hued closely to the minute particulars of cases of illness and treatment. Barthez's piece, by contrast, was essentially a piece of propaganda on behalf of a practitioner (himself), an institution (the Montpellier medical school), and a set of political and ideological loyalties (Bonapartist conservatism).

Yet, if Barthez's remarks on Hippocrates are culled from his other works, treatises as theoretically serious as Bordeu's work on the cellular tissue, it becomes clear that this oration of 1801 – though chiefly focused on the public and political uses to be made of Hippocratism rather than on specific pathological or therapeutic guidance physicians might take from it – nonetheless reflects Barthez's long-held and often-stated convictions about the father of medicine, the character of health and disease, and, most important, the necessity of the medical art. Barthez's emphasis on the complexity of disease, and the absolute necessity of a medical art cultivated by men who were laboriously trained, was a theme that ran straight through his teaching and writing. To him, the proposition that understanding and curing disease was a simple matter of listening reverently to a nature whose voice could also be heard by humble folk was anathema: diseases were complex and so were treatments. Yet, interestingly, Barthez used precisely this view of the complexities of disease to support the vitalist framework Bordeu had supported by invoking the simplicity and genuineness of the language of nature. To Barthez, the character and workings of the vital principle were the most complicated and difficult matters physicians had to face. Indeed, it was the complexity of the actions of the vital principle that rendered foolish the mechanists' search for immutable 'laws' of pathology and of therapeutic practice. Arguing in this vein, Barthez held that Hippocrates was great not for recognising virtually self-evident truths of health and illness, as Bordeu had urged, but for demonstrating with his minutely observed bedside cases a view of disease as infinitely variable and individual in character. Physicians, he insisted, 'never saw two illnesses of the same species'. Indeed, properly speaking, there were no diseases but rather 'infinite variations in different individuals' of pathological phenomena and, generally, of the workings of the vital principle.[57]

Yet even this mild affirmation of Hippocrates was lacking in Barthez's discussions of Hippocratic therapeutics. In his *Cours de thérapeutique*, Barthez made only a few references to Hippocrates and these were, for the most part, either neutral or openly critical, dismissing various recommendations of Hippocrates as suitable only to 'the art in its infancy'.[58] Barthez's neglect of Hippocrates in this regard contrasts markedly with his favourable references to various 'moderns', a roster that even included many of his avowed mechanist adversaries.[59] Happy as he was, then, to unfurl the banner of Hippocrates in defence of 'the art' generally and of Montpellier tradition in particular, Barthez brushed the master aside when he obscured knowledge of the complexities of disease and treatment laboriously compiled by medical *érudits* since the days of Cos.

Conclusion

Where does the comparison of these texts leave us? As my general references to vitalism should indicate, I do see Bordeu and Barthez as serving, in some respects, the same gods. Both took the mechanist system-builders as their target and proselytised on behalf of vitalist conceptions that, at the level of physiological explanation at least, shared a good deal in common. To these ends both physicians mobilised Hippocrates, who taught, as they saw it, a view of illness that emphasised its systemic, variable and ultimately indefinable nature.

Yet, in other respects, these constructions of Hippocrates worked to very different effect. Of primary importance in the transition from Bordeu to Barthez is the eclipse of the view of nature as offering up, to any who would listen, ancient and unassailable truths, and its replacement with the view that 'art' alone could discern these truths – in this case, a medical art painstakingly constructed out of the materials gathered by the 'erudite'.

Why this shift took place, and where its significance lies, can be interpreted in a number of different lights. To some extent, a biographical analysis is fruitful: Bordeu and Barthez cultivated very different loyalties of place and memory. In all his writing, including his sometimes painfully honest letters to his family, Bordeu expressed a nostalgic longing for the rude simplicity of his native Béarn.[60] By contrast, Barthez never let anyone forget his status as a sophisticated member of the provincial elite. Institutionally and professionally, the value of shifting away from a view of nature and disease that saw medical truths as readily accessible to any would listen, and towards a view that emphasised the essential role of the highly trained physician and the expertly organised school, was something Barthez apparently took for granted. And this pattern fits well with the particulars of the careers of these two physicians: Bordeu, despite his well-documented complaints about the financial uncertainty of the high-society physician and the sufferings inflicted on him by unscrupulous professional rivals, accepted as given the fundamental organisation of medicine and expressed no need to defend the structures within which he operated.[61] Barthez, by contrast, witnessed first-hand, in the later years of the ancien régime and from his exile in Narbonne through the revolutionary era, the threats that faced the provincial medical school and medical elite amid the transformations worked by the French medical revolution. Ultimately, of course, it was Barthez's vision that, generally speaking, won out – if not in Montpellier, then certainly in most centres of nineteenth-century medicine. As has often been remarked, the dominant trope of nineteenth-century medicine would be not the nature that spoke directly about disease and affliction but the nature whose secrets were forced by the ever more sophisticated instruments of medical art.

Yet, as events would prove, Barthez's peculiar version of what Paul Starr calls the 'legitimate complexity' defence of medical authority was itself doomed to obsolescence.[62] Barthez saw the ideal physician as a figure who blended bookish erudition and analytical acumen with intuitive power in observation. In company with Bordeu and other vitalists, he had scant regard for the weapons of emergent localist medicine – microscopes, laboratory tests, statistical charts – a medicine that, for its part, would seldom waver in asserting that nature was to be actively manipulated rather than passively regarded. Yet for Montpellier medicine the inutility of Barthez's quirky construction of medical complexity – and of Hippocrates as master-inventor of an esoteric medical art – ultimately made little difference. His 1801 oration proved to be a momentary fillip along the otherwise resolute course by which Montpellier's defenders promoted a construction of Montpellier medicine – its traditions and its future – that they serenely called 'Hippocratic' and indiscriminately attributed to the founding fathers of Montpellier vitalism, Bordeu and Barthez. The differences that had, in fact, divided the acclaimed founders of Montpellier 'Hippocratism' over what constituted genuine Hippocratic teaching on the nature of disease and the medical art were brushed aside by Montpellier's nineteenth-century standard-bearers as incidental. That Hippocrates was made to stand for all these views – of Bordeu and Barthez, but also of those who in subsequent years blithely synthesised their competing constructs – suggests perhaps the clearest conclusion to be drawn from this material: that it is precisely the enigmatic legacy that best serves the ends of rhetorical struggle and most readily survives transformations of vision and of historical circumstance.

Notes

1. The ceremony installing the bust of Hippocrates was held on 4 messidor, an IX (1801). In the adoption of Hippocratic symbolism, the government of the First Consul was anticipated by the Convention: in the year III the Committee of Public Instruction had decreed that the seal of the newly founded Ecoles de Santé would carry a 'head of Hippocrates engraved after the [fashion of] antiquity': Archives de la Faculté de Médecine de Montpellier [hereafter AFMM], Register S107, p. 65.
2. The taking of the Hippocratic oath was decreed by the Ecole de Médecine on 17 messidor, an XII; a text of the oath was transcribed in the faculty registers in both Latin and French. See Louis Dulieu, *La médecine à Montpellier*, 4 vols, Avignon: Les presses universelles, 1975–1990, Vol. 4, p. 134.
3. See, for example, the distinctions drawn between genuine and purported Hippocratism in Erwin H. Ackerknecht, *A Short History of Medicine*, rev. edn, Baltimore: Johns Hopkins University Press, 1968: 'In spite of his frequent declarations of reverence for Hippocrates, Galen was no Hippocratist' (p. 74); 'Hippocrates, the empiricist, was to him [Paracelsus] the only respectable medical authority of the past. ... But thoroughly un-Hippocratic was his medieval belief that God was a direct source of medical revelation and knowledge' (p. 106). Similarly, F.N.L. Poynter refers to Thomas Sydenham as 'the *first* among the moderns to lead medicine back to the true road, to the Hippocratic method of observation and experience' and also to Sydenham's work on epidemic constitutions as 'being truly Hippocratic'; see Poynter, 'Sydenham's influence abroad', *Medical History*, 17, 1973, pp. 223–34 at p. 224. In another instance, G.A. Lindeboom distinguishes between the 'real Hippocratic medicine' of Boerhaave, based as it was on natural science, and that of Sydenham, 'who did not appreciate the usefulness of natural science'; Lindeboom, *Herman Boerhaave: The Man and his Work*, London: Methuen, 1968, pp. 55–56.
4. The inaugural text in this vein in English-language scholarship is Wesley D. Smith, *The Hippocratic Tradition*, Ithaca, NY: Cornell University Press, 1979.
5. Théophile de Bordeu, 'Recherches sur le tissu muqueux, ou l'organe cellulaire, et sur quelques maladies de la poitrine', in *Oeuvres complètes de Théophile de Bordeu*, 2 vols, ed. A.-B. Richerand, Paris: Caille et Ravier, 1818, Vol. 2, pp. 735–96; Paul-Joseph Barthez, *Discours sur le génie d'Hippocrate*, Montpellier: Tournel, an IX [1801].
6. This assessment of the Montpellier tradition has been vigorously promoted by physicians and historians in Montpellier itself since the eighteenth century. See, for example, Jacques Lordat, *Exposition de la doctrine médicale de P.-J. Barthez, et mémoires sur la vie de ce médecin*, Paris: Gabon, 1818; Frédéric Bérard, *Doctrine médicale de l'Ecole de Montpellier, et comparaison de ses principes à*

ceux des autres écoles d'Europe, Montpellier: Jean Martel, 1819; Léon Delarbre, *Etude sur Sauvages, ses oeuvres et sa doctrine*, Montpellier: Imprimerie centrale du Midi, 1880; François Granel, 'Charles Barbeyrac (1629–1699), rénovateur de l'hippocratisme', *Monspeliensis Hippocrates*, 1, 1958, pp. 6–15. Modern historians who have endorsed this judgement include Jacques Roger, *Les sciences de la vie dans la pensée française du XVIIIe siècle*, rev. edn, Paris: Albin Michel, 1993, p. 620; Sergio Moravia, 'Philosophie et médecine en France à la fin du XVIIIe siècle', *Studies on Voltaire and the Eighteenth Century*, **89**, 1972, pp. 1089–1151; Russell Maulitz, *Morbid Appearances: The Anatomy of Pathology in the Early Nineteenth Century*, New York: Cambridge University Press, 1987, pp. 13–14. The argument made here develops further the discussion of Hippocratism in Montpellier offered in my *The Physical and the Moral: Anthropology, Physiology, and Philosophical Medicine in France, 1750–1850*, New York: Cambridge University Press, 1994.

7. Montpellier's early history is treated in Sonoma Cooper, 'The Medical School of Montpellier in the Fourteenth Century', *Annals of Medical History*, ns, **2**, 1930, pp. 164–95; Joseph Calmette, 'Introduction', *Cartulaire de l'Université de Montpellier publié sous les auspices du Conseil de l'Université de Montpellier*, Montpellier: Maison Lauriol, 1912; see also Dulieu, *La médecine à Montpellier*, Vol. 1 (n. 2); C. C. Gillispie, *Science and Polity in France at the End of the Old Regime*, Princeton, NJ: Princeton University Press, 1980, pp. 217–18.

8. Allan Debus, *The French Paracelsians: The Chemical Challenge to Medical and Scientific Tradition in Early Modern France*, New York: Cambridge University Press, 1991; Howard Solomon, *Public Welfare, Science, and Propaganda in Seventeenth Century France: The Innovations of Théophraste Renaudot*, Princeton, NJ: Princeton University Press, 1972.

9. The vitalist tradition in Montpellier is treated in Elizabeth Haigh, 'The vital principle of Paul Joseph Barthez: the clash between monism and dualism', *Medical History*, **21**, 1977, pp. 1–14; idem, 'Vitalism, the soul and sensibility: the physiology of Théophile de Bordeu', *Journal of the History of Medicine and Allied Arts*, **31**, 1976, pp. 30–41; François Duchesneau, *La physiologie des Lumières: Empirisme, modèles et théories*, The Hague: Martinus Nijhoff, 1982, pp. 361–404; Williams, *The Physical and the Moral* (n. 6), esp. chapter 1.

10. Granel, 'Charles Barbeyrac' (n. 6). Granel attributes this tradition to a physician named Vires; Kenneth Dewhurst traces it to P. Desault, *Dissertation sur les maladies vénériennes*, Paris, 1733. See his *Dr. Thomas Sydenham (1624–1689)*, Berkeley: University of California Press, 1966, pp. 27–28.

11. Théophile de Bordeu, 'Crise', *Encyclopédie ou dictionnaire des sciences, des arts et des métiers*, Paris: Briasson, 1751–65, Vol. 4, pp. 471–89 at p. 477.

12. It does show up in some older English-language textbooks of medical history; Fielding H. Garrison, for example, wrote that 'no less than Sydenham was a pupil of Charles Barbeirac in Montpellier' in his *An Introduction to the History of Medicine*, 4th edn, Philadelphia: W.B. Saunders, 1929, p. 282.

13. Dewhurst, *Sydenham*, (n. 10), pp. 27–28.

14. See also Poynter, 'Sydenham's influence abroad', (n. 3).

15. Historians date this revival somewhat differently. Henry Guerlac dates 'a revived interest' in *Airs, Waters and Places* to the period 'shortly before Montesquieu's time' and takes as a benchmark the space allotted to Hippocrates in Daniel Leclerc's *History of Medicine* (which Guerlac dates at 1699); see Guerlac, 'Humanism in Science', in *Essays and Papers in the History of Modern Science*, Baltimore: Johns Hopkins University Press, 1977, p. 14, n. 17; Wesley Smith also

singles out Leclerc's work (whose first edition he dates at 1696) among French commentators on Hippocrates in the era from Bacon to the nineteenth century; see Smith, *The Hippocratic Tradition* (n. 4), pp. 21–23. Sergio Moravia traces French Hippocratism to Barbeyrac's work 'just on the eve of the century of Enlightenment'; see Moravia, 'Philosophie et médecine' (n. 6). Jacques Roger points out that all through the seventeenth century Hippocratic paraphernalia formed part of the 'culte exigeant' of French medicine but that the works of Hippocrates, like those of Galen, were known principally through compendia and manuals; see Roger, *Sciences de la vie* (n. 6), p. 14, n. 17.

16. In the late seventeenth and early eighteenth centuries, Montpellier physicians who espoused otherwise conflicting doctrinal positions invoked Hippocrates as the genuine teacher of 'observation'. The First Physician Pierre Chirac, who shifted at mid-career from iatrochemical to iatromechanist principles, used Hippocrates to argue for observational medicine; see Julian Martin, 'Sauvages's nosology: medical enlightenment in Montpellier', in Andrew Cunningham and Roger French (eds), *The Medical Enlightenment of the Eighteenth Century*, Cambridge: Cambridge University Press, 1990, pp. 111–37 at p. 114. From the period when François Boissier de Sauvages began teaching in Montpellier in the 1730s, the Hippocratic mantle began to be claimed with special fervour by the Montpellier physicians identified first with animism (Sauvages and a few little-known disciples) and then with vitalism. References among the latter physicians to Hippocrates as the source of genuine methods of observation include Sauvages, *Nosologie méthodique, dans laquelle les maladies sont rangées par classes, suivant le système de Sydenham, & l'ordre des Botanistes*, Paris: Hérissant, 1771, Vol. 1, pp. 11–13; Louis de Lacaze, *Idée de l'homme physique et moral*, Paris: H.L. Guérin and L.F. Delatour, 1755, pp. 4–5, 57–68; Paul-Joseph Barthez, *Nouveaux élémens de la science de l'homme*, 2 vols, 2nd edn, Paris: Goujon, 1806, Vol. 1, p. 28; Vol. 2, p. 87. See also Charles-Louis Dumas, *Principes de physiologie ou Introduction à la science expérimentale, philosophique et médicale de l'homme vivant*, 4 vols, Paris: Crapelet, 1800–03, who contrasted the methods of Hippocrates to those of the 'philosophers' who came after him in the 'science of man' (p. 96).

17. Poynter, 'Sydenham's influence abroad' (n. 3), pp. 226–27; Lindeboom, *Herman Boerhaave*, (n. 3), pp. 8, 42, 55. On the use made of Hippocrates by another celebrated eighteenth-century 'mechanist', Friedrich Hoffmann, see Iain M. Lonie, 'Hippocrates the iatromechanist', *Medical History*, **25**, 1981, pp. 113–50. Iatrochemists in Montpellier occasionally invoked Hippocrates, but they were just as often critical of him and did not construct a full-blown 'chemical Hippocrates'; see the reference to Chirac in n. 16 and the discussion in Bordeu, 'Crise' (n. 11) where he quotes Chirac as designating Hippocrates and Galen as 'mere empirics' (p. 480).

18. These animadversions extended also to Albrecht von Haller, of whom Bordeu wrote that 'when it is a matter of a small muscle [or] an anatomical shape ... M. Haller spares himself nothing; he cites authors with an abundance that does honor to his erudition, he undertakes painful researches ... [yet] when it is a matter of pathology, he has nothing to say, nothing to cite': Bordeu, 'Crise' (n. 11), p. 479.

19. Jean-Joseph Ménuret de Chambaud, *Eloge historique de M. Venel*, Grenoble: J.J. Cuchet, 1777, p. 62. Ménuret charged that since the time of Harvey's 'vain and false discoveries' mechanist physicians had been interested only in 'pieces and fragments, without links, without relations, and without liaisons' (p. 21)

20. Sauvages's rejection of mechanism in favour of what he saw as the Hippocratic

conception of 'nature' inaugurated this line of argument; see Sauvages, *Nosologie méthodique* (n. 16), Vol. 1, p. 62, where he argues in favour of the 'Hippocratic' definition of illness as 'le concours des symptômes ... mutuellement liés ensemble'; see also pp. 13–14, 17, 24, 25 (against the search for causes), 67–68 (on 'nature'), 118–19 (the view that 'strictly speaking, all maladies are *individual beings*'). See also Bordeu, 'Recherches sur les maladies chroniques', in *Oeuvres complètes* (n. 5), pp. 797–800.
21. Denis Diderot, *Le Rêve de d'Alembert*, ed. Jean Varloot, Paris: Editions sociales, 1962. On the place of this work in the evolution of Diderot's thinking about life, see Roger, *Les sciences de la vie* (n. 6), pp. 585–682.
22. Biographical sources on Bordeu include A.-B. Richerand, 'Notice sur la vie et les ouvrages de Bordeu', in *Oeuvres complètes de Bordeu* (n. 5), pp. i–xxiv; 'Notice de M. Lefeuve sur Bordeu', in Théophile de Bordeu, *Recherches sur l'histoire de la médecine* [1764], rev. edn, Paris: Auguste Ghio, 1882, pp. 7–80; 'Bordeu', *Dictionaire des sciences médicales: Biographie médicale*, Vol. 2, pp. 387–402; Louis Dulieu, 'Théophile de Bordeu', *Dictionary of Scientific Biography*, Vol. 2, pp. 301–2; Bordeu's conflicts with Parisian physicians are detailed in the editor's notes to his correspondence; see Théophile de Bordeu, *Correspondance*, ed. Martha Fletcher, Montpellier: Centre national de la recherche scientifique, Université Paul Valéry, nd, esp. Vol. 2, pp. 222–26.
23. Although first published in 1767, this work was apparently largely composed in the late 1740s. In publishing a serialised version of the work, Augustin Roux remarked that it had been in the hands of the censor Bruhier in 1749; [Roux], *Journal de médecine, chirurgie et pharmacie*, **26**, March 1767, pp. 195–96. All references here are to the text found in Bordeu, *Oeuvres complètes* (n. 5), pp. 735–97.
24. Bordeu defined cellular tissue as 'un composé d'atômes ou de petits corps collés les uns sur les autres ... la substance gluante, plus ou moins tenace, qui est la vraie substance cellulaire': 'Tissu muqueux' (n. 5), pp. 735–36.
25. Barthez, *Science de l'homme*, (n. 16), Vol. 1, pp. 25–30.
26. Williams, *The Physical and the Moral* (n. 6), pp. 32–41.
27. Bordeu, 'Tissu muqueux' (n. 5), pp. 735–36, 738, 752–53, 755; on Bordeu's place in the development of tissue theory, see John M. Forrester, 'The homoeomerous parts and their replacement by Bichat's tissues', *Medical History*, **38**, 1994, pp. 444–58.
28. Bordeu, 'Tissu muqueux' (n. 5), pp. 760, 763–64, 777.
29. Ibid., p. 768.
30. Ibid., pp. 761–62. Bordeu's citations to Hippocrates for these passages were given as follows: 'Coac., no. cvii' and 'Coac., no. cxxvi' (pp. 761–62). I have not checked these citations against editions of the Hippocratic writings in use in the period. On editions of Hippocrates frequently used in eighteenth-century France, see Roselyne Rey, 'Anamorphoses d'Hippocrate au XVIIIe siècle', in Danielle Gourevitch (ed). *Maladie et maladies, Histoire et conceptualisation: Mélanges en l'honneur de Mirko Grmek*, Geneva: Droz, 1992, pp. 257–76.
31. Bordeu, 'Tissu muqueux' (n.5), 762.
32. Ibid., p. 763.
33. Ibid., pp. 763–64.
34. Ibid., p. 777. A similar observation had been made by Sauvages about his teacher Antoine Deidier, who held the chemistry chair at the University of Medicine from 1697 to 1732; according to Sauvages, Deidier viewed 'troubled circulation' as the 'principle of all maladies'; Sauvages, *Nosologie methodique* (n. 16), Vol. 1, p. 4.

35. Bordeu, 'Tissu muqueux' (n. 5), p. 777.
36. Ibid., pp. 777–78.
37. Ibid., p. 777.
38. D.G. Charlton, *New Images of the Natural in France: A Study in European Cultural History, 1750–1800*, Cambridge: Cambridge University Press, 1984; an excellent bibliographic survey appears on pp. 221–22.
39. Bordeu, 'Crise' (n. 11), p. 488
40. Ibid., pp. 474, 478, 480–82.
41. Bordeu cited his teacher Antoine Fizes (professor of chemistry at Montpellier from 1732 to 1765) as a typical practitioner of *Chiracisme*. In his correspondence he called Fizes 'un sot, un butor et voilà tout!'; Bordeu, *Correspondance* (n. 22), Vol. 2, p. 188.
42. Bordeu, 'Crise' (n. 11), p. 489.
43. Nihell's work was first published in English in 1741.
44. Théophile de Bordeu, *Recherches sur le pouls*, Paris, 1756.
45. [Augustin Roux], 'Suite des recherches sur le pouls par rapport aux crises', *Journal de médecine, chirurgie et pharmacie*, 8, April 1758, pp. 291–305. Roux, a native of Bordeaux, edited the *Journal de Médecine* from 1762 to 1776. A habitué of the *coterie holbachique*, he was closely associated with Diderot and was one of the strongest defenders in Paris circles of Bordeu and the new Montpellier-based approach to medicine that would come to be known as vitalism. On his Paris career, see Alan Charles Kors, *D'Holbach's Coterie: An Enlightenment in Paris*, Princeton, NJ: Princeton University Press, 1976, esp. pp. 185–88.
46. See, for example, Ménuret, *Eloge historique* (n. 19), pp. 48–53. This crucial theme in vitalist polemics is explored in my forthcoming study of Montpellier vitalism in the eighteenth century.
47. Frédéric Bérard, *Doctrine médicale de l'Ecole de Montpellier, et comparaison de ses principes à ceux des autres écoles d'Europe*, Montpellier: Jean Martel, 1819, pp. 24–32, 270–98.
48. The introductory essay to a new publication of the Société médicale d'émulation referred to 'the illustrious professor Barthez, the glory and pride of the old school of Montpellier'; see 'Discours préliminaire', *Mémoires de la Société médicale d'émulation*, 1, an VI/1797, pp. i–xiii.
49. Barthez's many honours and awards were capped in 1806 (shortly before his death) with his appointment to the medical entourage of Napoleon Bonaparte. Biographical sources on Barthez include 'Paul-Joseph Barthez', *Dictionaire des sciences médicales: Biographie médicale*, Vol. 1, pp. 572–88; Ruth Schwartz Cowan, 'Paul-Joseph Barthez', *Dictionary of Scientific Biography*, Vol. 1, pp. 478–79; Louis Dulieu, 'Paul-Joseph Barthez', *Revue d'histoire des sciences*, **24**, 1971, pp. 149–76; Alisa Reich, 'Paul Joseph Barthez and the Impact of Vitalism on Medicine and Psychology', PhD dissertation, University of California at Los Angeles, 1995.
50. See the sources cited in note 6 above.
51. Barthez, *Génie d'Hippocrate*, p. 4; all references in the text are to the edition cited in note 5 above.
52. Ibid., p. 39.
53. Ibid., p. 8.
54. Ibid., p. 25.
55. For these particulars about his classification of healing methods, Barthez referred his listeners to his *Nova doctrina de fonctionibus naturae humanae*, Montpellier, 1774 and to his courses. See also L. Rouzet's introduction to Charles-Louis

Dumas, *Doctrine générale des maladies chroniques*, 2nd edn, Paris: Gabon, 1824, p. xii.
56. Barthez, *Génie d'Hippocrate* (n. 5), pp. 30, 52.
57. Paul-Joseph Barthez, 'Cours de thérapeutique', Ms. 256, Bibliothèque de la Ville de Montpellier, p. 23.
58. Ibid., p. 165.
59. References to Hippocrates in this text are found at pp. 162, 165, 177, 189, 200, 205, 250, 300 and to various 'mechanists' at pp. 2, 4, 7, 17–18, 19, 21, 23, 58–59, 65, 71, 75, 76, 184, 250: ibid.
60. In May 1754, for example, Bordeu wrote that he thought of Barèges (the site of the mineral waters his father superintended) as his 'retreat, exile, place of repose, place to hide away my troubles'; Bordeu, *Correspondance* (n. 22), Vol. 2, p. 113; see also other relevant comments at Vol. 1, pp. 107, 113, 158; Vol. 2, p. 26. Yet it should be noted that Bordeu also sometimes rejoiced at the excitement of life in Paris. In light of such comments, his public yearning for the simplicity of the Midi might be interpreted simply as a self-promoting pose. If so, however, it was a pose he could have thought rewarding only if he expected his sophisticated readers to enjoy, and perhaps share, in it.
61. Bordeu, *Correspondance* (n. 22), Vol. 2, pp. 6, 115–17; Vol. 3, pp. 75, 100; on his sufferings at the hands of Paris rivals, see the sources cited in note 22.
62. Paul Starr, *The Social Transformation of American Medicine*, New York: Basic Books, 1982, p. 19.

CHAPTER NINE

The Rhetoric of Hippocrates at the Paris School

Ann F. La Berge

> ... each has the right to hippocratise to his delight and to transform ad libitum the old sage into a solidist, a humoralist, a vitalist, an organicist, an animist, a iatrochemist ... .[1]

So wrote Louis Peisse, the medical journalist, frequent contributor to the *Gazette médicale de Paris*, and member of the Academy of Medicine, in his 1857 book, *La médecine et les médecins*, while discussing the recent debate in the Academy over organicism and vitalism.[2] Peisse compared the Hippocratic writings to the Bible, claiming that all the medical sects used Hippocratic texts as freely as religious sects used the Bible. He went on to say that, since in medicine there was no superior authority to interpret the texts and fix the dogmas, each could use Hippocrates to his own advantage. For Peisse, Parisian physicians used Hippocrates to justify any position whatsoever.

Until recently such uses of Hippocrates would have been as troubling to historians as they were to Peisse. The dominant historiographical tendency was to measure the various portrayals of Hippocrates and his medicine against some notionally real Hippocratic medicine, and to categorise as truly Hippocratic only those that matched such medicine.[3] The trend today, however, is to take a more agnostic position on the veracity of portrayals of Hippocrates and his medicine. Instead, what Peisse described as 'hippocratising' is now taken as an opportunity for historians to explore the cultural worlds of the 'hippocratisers'. Put simply, the various uses and portrayals of Hippocrates can tell us much more about those who produce them than that they failed to measure up to a particular image of Hippocrates and of his medicine.

Focusing on early nineteenth-century Paris medicine, this essay explores the different ways in which French physicians employed Hippocrates polemically to fashion their own reputations and careers. As such, there were as many 'Hippocrateses' as there were physicians striving to make a living, all reflecting the particular interests and agendas of those who invoked his name. Yet if Hippocrates had different meanings for French physicians, they all agreed that the roots of French medicine lay in ancient Greece. Thus the invocation of his name also implied recognition of a foundational myth which provided an image of strength and unity in the face of diversity and external challenges.

Hippocratic rhetoric thus served a double function. It served, on the one hand, to promote individual careers and reputations and, on the other hand, to provide a special identity for Paris medicine as a whole.

The birth of the clinic: Hippocrates at the early Paris School

When eighteenth-century physicians invoked Hippocratic medicine, they typically referred to a meteorological and environmental medicine, derived in part from *Airs, Waters, and Places*.[4] Yet, as Roselyne Rey notes, such a model of medicine began to disappear with the introduction of quantification and pathological anatomy, which made the Hippocratic concept of idiosyncrasy untenable and undermined humoral medicine. Attention increasingly came to focus on Hippocrates as the founder of the observational method. Hippocratic medicine, Paris physicians agreed, was a pristine, innocent time – similar to the state of nature for political and social theorists[5] – before physicians perverted it with their systems. 'La médecine rendu à son unité primitive.'[6] But, if Paris physicians agreed on the need for a return to the principles of Hippocratic medicine, they disagreed on what these principles were, or the extent to which modern medicine should go beyond them. Hippocrates was variously portrayed as a *médecin-philosophe*, an empiricist, a sceptic of Enlightenment values and a pathological anatomist. The point can be demonstrated by exploring the different images of Hippocrates of four of its major figures – Cabanis, Pinel, Corvisart and Laennec.

Cabanis: Hippocrates as médecin-philosophe

Pierre-Jean-Georges Cabanis' (1757–1808) portrayal of Hippocrates reflected his involvement in the construction of Enlightenment medicine and the revolutionary fervour of the new Paris School, established in 1794: he was both a member of the faculty from 1796 to 1804 and a legislator, representing the School on the Council of 500. To Cabanis, Hippocrates provided the proper starting point for the Enlightenment physician defending medicine and medical reform. As a faculty member, he prepared lectures on texts from Hippocrates in which he stressed the significance of Hippocrates for modern clinical medicine. An Ideologue who subscribed to the sensualist philosophy of Condillac, Cabanis believed that Hippocrates had been the first empiricist, had liberated medicine from philosophical systems and had applied the true method of observation. Yet this Hippocrates was no enemy of philosophy. On the contrary medicine and philosophy were inseparable in his practice. He was the archetypal *médecin-philosophe*.

Cabanis' views on Hippocratic medicine are well set out in the first of 12 memoirs that would become *On the Relations between the Physical and Moral Aspects of Man*,[7] and presented to the National Institute for the Sciences and Arts in 1796. With a wonderful boldness and arrogance, combined with a seemingly unbounded optimism about the progress of the human spirit, in this work Cabanis epitomises the age of Enlightenment and Revolution in France. His reverence for the ancients is clear, and when he speaks of the ancients and of Greece, the reader is reminded of Cabanis' France:

> Greece was not only the mother of the arts and of liberty; that philosophy whose universal lessons alone are capable of perfecting man and all his institutions was born here. ... What more beautiful spectacle is there than that of an entire class of men unceasingly occupied in seeking the means to improve human destiny, to tear peoples from oppression, to fortify the social relations, to bring to the public morals that energy and elegance that have never since anywhere been united to the same degree.[8]

Cabanis lists the principal 'benefactors of the human race' as Pythagoras, Democritus, Hippocrates, Aristotle and Epicurus. As he explains:

> Although Hippocrates is more especially celebrated for his work and his success in the theory, practice, and teaching of his medical art, I include him here because he related, as he himself said, PHILOSOPHY TO MEDICINE, AND MEDICINE TO PHILOSOPHY.[9]

Thus Cabanis portrayed Hippocrates as the original *médecin-philosophe*:

> As the doctor and the philosopher, combined in his writings, are absolutely inseparable there, one cannot separate that which regards the one when speaking of the other.[10]

Central to his portrayal of Hippocrates as the original *médecin-philosophe*, was Cabanis' perception of him as the founder of observational medicine.[11] This Hippocrates was not, however, a *radical* empiricist. Instead, he had arrived at a felicitous combination of the empirical and the rational to produce what Cabanis considered the original and true observational method:

> I repeat, medicine is identified in his writings with the rules or the practice of his method, they cannot be separated. ... But I am speaking to men who know too well that in the proper methods is found, as it were, all the rational philosophy of each century and of each writer.[12]

Continuing his discussion of the methodological contributions of Hippocrates, he referred to Hippocrates as

> ... a man for whom the art of putting truths in logical sequence was no less familiar than was that of discovering them. He was equally suspicious both of those precipitate views that generalize on insufficient data, and of that impotence of the spirit that, not knowing how to perceive relations, harps eternally on individualities, without result. Who better than he was ever able to apply to the different parts of his art these general rules of reasoning, this superior metaphysics that embraces all the arts and all the sciences?[13]

For Rey, Cabanis' portrayal of Hippocrates as *médecin-philosophe* was crucial to what she regards as the impoverishment of the Hippocratic *Corpus* and the reduction of philosophy to epistemology and methodology. Cabanis, she claims, reinforced a tendency since the beginning of the eighteenth century to progressively strip 'Hippocrates of everything that had been attributed to him in the past'.[14] The result, Rey argues, was that what was held to be important, again, was the 'spirit' of Hippocrates – to use Cabanis' term – an art of method, rather than the doctrine. As the subsequent discussion makes clear, this portrayal fails to capture fully the complex ways in which Hippocrates was portrayed in nineteenth-century French medicine.

Pinel: the empiricist Hippocratist

If Cabanis saw Hippocrates as a *médecin-philosophe*, the nosologist and protopsychiatrist, Philippe Pinel (1745–1826) tended to see him as an empiricist. Pinel was a proponent of the medical science of man, or anthropological medicine: an approach that had flourished among the Ideologues in Paris as well as in Montpellier where Pinel had studied under Barthez. Like Cabanis, Pinel subscribed to the reciprocity of the physical and moral, and he and Cabanis shared similar theories of illness and approaches to therapy. Both emphasised observation and the study of man as ways to reform social, political and moral life. Both also appealed to the ancients, especially Hippocrates, as a guide to medical reform.[15] But Pinel was also an Anglophile, heavily influenced by the British empirical approach to the sciences, exemplified most of all by Bacon. Indeed, he considered Bacon and Sydenham as the true successors of Hippocrates.

A representative Pinelian text, *The Clinical Training of Doctors: An Essay of 1793*, provides a good general idea of Pinel's Hippocratism.[16] Pinel favoured a return to what he regarded as the simplicity of Hippocratic medicine which he claimed had existed before the construction of systems and complicated therapies. With Hippocrates as guide, therapeutics within the clinic could be streamlined, and one could 'dispense with the profusion of treatises on pharmacy and materia medica produced since the days of Galen'.[17] Instead, physicians should recognise that 'dietetics was the first, the chief, and often the only part of medicine used by Hippocrates for the care of illness'.[18] For Pinel, Hippocrates meant simplicity, and the simple was the natural, and the simple and natural were true. Thus he emphasised the importance of 'reducing therapy to its simplest elements and showing clearly how nature proceeds when man does not interfere'[19] – the *vis medicatrix naturae*.

Pinel's Hippocrates was more than a resource for scientific therapeutics. He was also a sure guide for a proper method. Whatever progress had been made since Hippocrates, 'one need only imitate the Father of Medicine and his method of observation, description of diseases, and respect for nature in his therapy'.[20] Hippocrates headed the list of 'the true observers of all ages'.[21] As a general guide, 'the physician must not deviate from the high road of observation and experience ... .'[22] Following Sydenham's emphasis on *Airs, Waters, and Places*, Pinel also argued that to understand the true history of diseases it would be necessary to analyse the 'influence of the seasons and of each year's medical constitution';[23] to 'assess the topography, meteorology, and medical constitution of various years, the detailed circumstances of the patient's history, etc.'.[24] Thus, while Pinel acknowledged that 'meteorological observations were imperfect in Hippocrates's time',[25] he illustrates the importance that eighteenth- and early nineteenth-century French physicians placed on the role of meteorology and topography in understanding disease, especially epidemic disease.[26] He opined:

> An exact topography can be singularly revealing about the special characteristics and treatment of illnesses usually prevalent on teaching wards. It indicates the productions of the soil, the way of life that the inhabitants lead, their customary exercise or physical labor, the food they eat, and whatever may have a marked influence on the animal economy and later its functions. Whoever, says Hippocrates, will have scrupulously studied these facts, will better know the constitution of each season and each year, the prevalent illnesses in summer and winter, and all the dangers that changes in living habits and nourishment may entail.[27]

Pinel condemned physicians who failed to take what he considered a Hippocratic approach, while castigating those, such as the Dutch physician Anton de Haen (1704–1776), of abandoning the fundamentals of Hippocratism: 'But it is wrong to proclaim, as De Haen does (*Rat. med.* part 8, cap. I) that one follows the Hippocratic method scrupulously, and then proscribe it by totally neglecting its principles.'[28] Merely paying lip service to Hippocrates would not do. Pinel harshly criticised physicians who neglected 'all true [Hippocratic] principles',[29] 'the high road of observation and experience'.[30]

Corvisart: the sceptical Hippocratist

If Cabanis' and Pinel's Hippocratisms were informed by Enlightenment optimism, that of Jean-Nicolas Corvisart (1755–1821) represented a more sceptical vision of (especially humoral) medicine.[31] Corvisart, who succeeded Desbois de Rochefort at the Charité hospital in 1788, became professor of clinical medicine at the new Ecole de Santé in 1794. Three years later he was appointed professor at the Collège de France. Finally, in 1804, he gave up this post to become personal physician to Napoleon. He was the teacher of both Bayle and Laennec. Corvisart took a radically different approach to Hippocrates from that of Cabanis and Pinel, venerating the divine old man but emphasising the dark side of nature; for him, the pathological was normal, to be expected. Nature was not beneficent; nor did it exhibit healing powers. Birth was merely a prelude to the long downhill struggle of life that led to death.[32] Thus, Corvisart's Hippocrates departed from the more optimistic Enlightenment outlook towards mastery over disease and asserted that the 'inevitable death to a vast number of beings ... is a melancholy and incontrovertible truth'.[33]

Not only did Corvisart challenge the widely accepted notion of the beneficence of nature, attributed by other physicians to Hippocrates, but he also denied the idea of the uniformity of the natural world and the moral goal of moderation.[34] For example, Corvisart said of the heart: 'how far its action is from being uniform and moderate!'[35] Like Hippocrates, he emphasised the influence of politics and political unrest on health: the heart's 'organic lesions were more frequent in the horrible times of the revolution, than in the usual calm of social life'.[36] Corvisart did not believe that cures were possible in the case of diseases of the heart and circulatory system – the prognosis was death. Nor was prevention possible, for he asserted that it was impossible to prevent either the moral or the physical causes of such diseases.

Corvisart, like Pinel, highlighted inequalities in health and hygiene. Thus he commented that a few people, practising the rules of hygiene and with good fortune on their side, might escape disease, but the poor were damned to bad health and early death and there was very little that practitioners could do to challenge such inequalities.[37] Agreeing with Cabanis, Corvisart argued that philosophy and medicine should be united, 'an alliance so expressly enjoined by Hippocrates'.[38] The real physician for Corvisart was the one 'who is capable of pronouncing and keeping the oath of Hippocrates'; he ventured that, 'philosophy will never be separated from medicine'.[39]

And yet this avowedly Hippocratic physician denied the notion of equilibrium, of natural perfection, of a self-correcting organism:

> This ideal temperament is remote from the effective temperament. No one is born with organic perfection. Every one of us comes into this world more or less imperfect, whence arises a certain defect of equilibrium in the functions.[40]

Nor did he believe in the healing power of nature: nature could not cure; nor could the physician. Yet, for Corvisart, this did not mean that the physician had no important role to perform. After all, Corvisart had never assumed that the physician's main goal was curative, or that the healing power of nature would allow all patients to be cured.[41] Ever the realist, he recognised limits: 'in proportion to the species of organization bestowed by nature, the consequence even of life, after having produced the organic diseases, is the cause of death.'[42]

Hippocrates as pathological anatomist: Laennec's Hippocrates[43]

Yet another vision of Hippocrates is evident in the work of René-Théophile Laennec (1781–1836), pathological anatomist and inventor of the stethoscope. Laennec saw Hippocrates as a critic of Pinelian nosology, an advocate of pathological anatomy, who subscribed to the notion that an exploration of the human voice by means of auscultation could be a way to diagnose diseases of the chest. All these ideas appeared in Laennec's 1804 MD thesis, which had as its epigraph a quote from 'On Ancient Medicine':

> Medicine is not a new science. ... But anyone who, casting aside and rejecting all these means, attempts to conduct research in any other way or after another fashion, and asserts that he has found out anything, is and has been the victim of deception.[44]

Writing his thesis in haste, Laennec argued that, whereas most physicians claimed to understand and to adhere to the Hippocratic method, few understood the Hippocratic doctrine – the 'systematic' ideas about diseases, including symptoms and concepts used to enable the physician to make sense of the facts. In a challenge to Pinel's nosological categories, Laennec explained that the Hippocratic doctrine made a fundamental distinction between specific symptoms and common, non-specific symptoms: Hippocrates wanted to distinguish diseases on the basis of organic lesions, a pathological–anatomical approach to disease limited only by his practical training and education. In an effort to explain Hippocrates's ignorance of internal organic diseases, Laennec claimed that Hippocrates had just not opened enough bodies. Laennec and his Hippocrates did point out, however, that some diseases left no traces or lesions.

Laennec's thesis on Hippocrates served to establish his own reputation within the highly competitive Paris School, but it was only partly successful. Jacalyn Duffin suggests that Laennec may have seen himself as the successor of Michel-Auguste Thouret, who at the time held the chair of Hippocratic medicine and rare diseases, which had been established in 1794. His hopes came to nothing when the faculty abolished the chair of Hippocratic medicine and rare diseases in 1811, but his interest in Hippocrates and ancient medicine persisted and, in 1821, he published an essay entitled 'Fevers according to the doctrine of Hippocrates and the findings of pathological anatomy'. According to Duffin, Laennec had to find a way of explaining what he saw as the very real limitations of pathological anatomy and the importance of physiology in disease. He did this, she claimed, by seeking 'to inform his own research in the fundamental question of nosology with ancient clinical experience, re-examined in the light of pathological anatomy'.[45]

Not only did Laennec invent a Hippocrates to suit his doctrinal needs, he also sought to fashion himself as the Hippocrates of Paris medicine, finding a direct link between Hippocrates and himself on auscultation. Thus, in his *Treatise on the Diseases of the Chest*, Laennec describes Hippocratic succussion:

> There exists still another means of ascertaining the existence, during life, of the pneumo-thorax complicated with purulent effusion, which I have also several times alluded to in the first part of this work – I mean by exciting the sound of fluctuation by the succussion of the chest. This method was practiced by Hippocrates, or his disciples, and is described by the author of the treatise De *Morbis* ... .[46]

Although most historians have accepted Laennec's own account of how he came to invent mediate auscultation, questions remain about how the idea came to him. In a later version of his work he gave credit for direct auscultation both to his friend Gaspard-Laurent Bayle, who had died in 1816 and to Hippocrates.[47] There were clear advantages in attributing claims of priority to deceased predecessors, especially if one of them was Hippocrates. Such a tactic lent a certain prestige to Laennec's discovery, while opening up a professional space which did not have to be shared with any contemporaries, notably Corvisart. (Although Laennec had studied with Corvisart, he denied that the latter had used direct auscultation, while acknowledging that Corvisart had listened to patients' hearts by placing his ear close to their chests.) While George Weisz has made us aware of the changing fate of Laennec's reputation after his death and how he came to be canonised by later generations, the work of Duffin and Mirko Grmek shows how he fashioned himself as a hero during his own lifetime.[48]

Broussais and the Hippocratic discourse: revolution and reinvention

If Cabanis, Pinel, Corvisart and Laennec sought to portray Paris medicine as a return to Hippocratic values, François Broussais (1772–1838), wanted to take it in quite a different direction. A pathological anatomist known primarily for his system of 'physiological medicine', Broussais hoped to return to a simpler, more straightforward medicine, like the self-proclaimed Hippocratists. But unlike the latter, he wanted to erase 2000 years of medicine and start anew. Broussais found Pinelian medicine complicated and ineffective, and wanted to eliminate in one stroke Hippocrates, Galen and all the great physicians and to topple Pinel's domination of Paris medicine. In such a way, he fashioned himself as the saviour of Paris medicine, standing for the simple, the modern and the effective – all in opposition to Pinel's version of Hippocratic medicine.

Because of his pathological–anatomical orientation, Ackerknecht regarded Broussais as a 'gravedigger' of Hippocratism.[49] Broussais, whose reputation plummeted at the hands of nineteenth-century positivists, was rediscovered by Ackerknecht and, since then, has received considerable historical attention.[50] While acknowledging the importance of these recent works, for my discussion

I want to turn to two nineteenth-century commentators, both of whom have served as important primary sources for twentieth-century accounts: Louis Peisse and Jean-Baptiste Bouillaud.⁵¹ Both Peisse and Bouillaud challenge Ackerknecht's account of Broussais as a gravedigger of Hippocrates.

Writing about Broussais in 1827, medical journalist Louis Peisse confidently declared: 'M. Broussais is unquestionably the most remarkable medical writer of the present age.' He continued: 'He has wrought a medical revolution in France, favorable in many respects, unfavorable in others, but in every way worthy of attention.'⁵² Peisse inclined favourably toward Broussais and thought he had been 'wrongly judged, not through ignorance, but through the spirit of party'.⁵³ Peisse considered Broussais an innovator because he had singlehandedly broken the hold of the ancients.⁵⁴ Although Broussais' first book, *The History of Chronic Inflammations*, was a 'work of pure observation, abounding in just and discriminating views of pathological anatomy', it was his *Examination of Systems of Nosology*, published in 1816, that effected the medical revolution, containing a totally new medical system that 'destroyed the reigning opinions and cried down the labors of his predecessors and contemporaries'.⁵⁵

With this work Broussais mounted what Peisse considered to be a brutal attack on the Pinelian approach. Peisse commented on Broussais' manner: 'It was important, above all things, that his attack should be made roughly, resolutely, and with unerring directness.'⁵⁶ Yet

> ... he was cautious how he borrowed from or made concessions to Pinel, whom he supplanted; – he sought no countenance nor support in ancient and foreign doctrines. He presented himself from the first as alone with his opinions, declaring of no avail the past and the present. To indicate plainly the extent of his mission, he went back to all the epochs in the history of medicine. He questioned the correctness of Hippocrates, venerated and guarded so long, – he attacked Galen and Boer[r]have, always illustrious in fame, but long since nullities in science. ... Arrived at the end of the last century, he combated Barthez and the school of Montpellier, and finally, placing himself in the midst of his contemporaries, he put forth all his efforts to overthrow the Pinelism of France. ...⁵⁷

The result of Broussais' strategy, according to Peisse, was to do 'for medicine what Descartes did for all the other sciences. ... He has shown us the medical edifice elevated by so many centuries, such as it was in reality – only a vast scaffolding with no solid or enduring support'.⁵⁸ But Broussais' abandonment of Hippocrates was not so complete as it initially might seem, for he effected this revolution by using Hippocratic principles to demolish Hippocratic medicine:

> With a great power of logical examination, he has exhibited the absurdity of its [Hippocratic medicine's] principal dogmas, time-hallowed though they were; the radical defects of medical language, and the innumerable errors which these defects had produced and perpetuated. ... M. Broussais,

with that characteristic hardihood of spirit which distinguishes him, has dared to attack, not only the systems, but the observations which sustain them. Experience, always and everywhere appealed to, appears to him to have been the most frequently fallacious, as it had already appeared to Hippocrates.[59]

The result of this attempted Broussaissian demolition of Hippocratic–Pinelian medicine, as every student of the Paris School knows, was that for about 15 years, from 1816 until the early 1830s, medical Paris was polarised. Writing in 1827, Peisse commented:

> This revolution has not, however, been effected without opposition; from its origin, on the contrary, it stirred up a controversy which still continues. The medical journals were divided in the debate, and became the theatre of a warm and animated contest.[60]

Both Rey and Ackerknecht point out that physicians with a predominantly pathological anatomical orientation, such as Laennec and Broussais, brought about the demise of the more holistic version of Hippocratism, the medical science of man tradition, characterised by Pinel.[61] Peisse explained that physiological medicine reduced medical practice to two indications, and offered leeches and abstinence as a kind of universal remedy: 'it has many charms for those young doctors who find it exceedingly convenient to learn their whole materia medica in fifteen minutes, and the science of diagnosis in a week.'[62] But its success was due to more than ease and simplicity.

> Its prodigious success is owing, less to the positive knowledge which it has brought into the science of medicine, than to the auspicious direction which it has given to pathology and therapeutics. It has strongly insisted on the necessity of associating disease with the organs; of referring symptoms to their true causes; it has introduced into the language of science, a precision hitherto unknown;[63]

Yet, even though he was sure that Broussais had provided the death-knell for Pinel's Hippocratic medicine, Peisse believed Broussais' physiological doctrine would not endure: 'Already do new innovators find it insufficient.'[64]

If, in 1827, Peisse portrayed Broussais as the death-knell of Hippocratism, his 1838 necrology of Broussais provided quite a different message. Had Broussais really been all that revolutionary, he queried, and how enduring was this revolution from the vantage point of 1838? Was Hippocratic medicine really dead? According to Peisse, Broussais' 'scientific life had been over for a long time, and death struck only the man'.[65] Yet during his scientific career, Peisse argued that he had 'tried to dominate more than to convince, and in his campaign against ancient medicine, he seemed less to want to reform science than to turn the [Paris] school upside down'. For Peisse, Broussais used Hippocrates as a foil by which he could elevate himself to the position of power he wanted and so effect a revolution in Paris medicine. 'In general Broussais established nothing except by opposition.' Peisse suggested, 'The author [Broussais] presented [his doctrine] as a protest of the modern spirit against the ancient spirit.'[66] Referring to Broussais' use of Hippocratic rhetoric, Peisse commented, '... its value as a critical instrument was great, and its inventor wielded this instrument with an unequaled vigour.'[67] What was, then, the fate of Hippocratic medicine? Did Broussais really demolish it? Peisse takes a moderate position: 'The ancient medicine was reconstituted, but not the ancient medical spirit.'[68]

If Peisse questioned the extent of Broussais's break with Hippocrates, Jean-Baptiste Bouillaud began to reconstruct Broussais as the true heir of the father of medicine. Bouillaud was a leading disciple of Broussais, a philosopher of science and medicine and a physician trained at the Paris School, and he constructed what became the received view of Paris medicine. Thus we can turn to him to investigate the role of Hippocrates and Hippocratic medicine in his story about the Paris School. The first part of his *Essai sur la philosophie médicale* (1836) was a history of medicine, up to and including the Paris School. His account became a principal source for Ackerknecht, when he wrote his *Medicine at the Paris Hospital*.[69]

Although Bouillaud claimed adherence to several Hippocratic doctrines, he did not consider himself a Hippocratist. He referred to the Hippocratic physicians as 'they', and declared himself to be an eclectic. However, Bouillaud used Hippocrates to establish Paris medicine as the best and most advanced in the world. First, he confirmed the myth of Hippocrates as the true creator of medicine, arguing that 'it is to the Paris Faculty of Medicine that belongs the honour of the definitive restoration of Greek medicine'.[70] Second, he also sought to establish a link between Hippocrates and specific leaders of the Paris school, such as Laennec:

> As for the first idea of auscultation, it goes back, as we have seen here, to Hippocrates himself. Laennec was the first to call attention to the passage, generally forgotten, in which the oracle of Cos spoke of this method.[71]

Using Pinel to support his point of view, Bouillaud contended that one could pay homage to Hippocrates without claiming too much. Specifically, one could not assert that Hippocrates had observed all, that his wisdom was for all times. Yet if Paris medicine had rediscovered lost Hippocratic methods, it had also gone beyond Hippocrates. Much had escaped Hippocrates's observations, and important medical advances had occurred in the intervening years. He found Pinel's ideas noteworthy and saw them as a reply to 'those modern hippocratists for whom progress consists in marching backwards, and who would like to take medicine back twenty centuries.'[72]

Thus, for Bouillaud, the Paris School was a vast improvement over ancient medicine: 'the time is long gone when all the sentences of Hippocrates could be considered as so many oracles.'[73] Since he had neither positive anatomical and physiological nor precise physical and chemical knowledge, Hippocrates could only rely on observations of exterior phenomena. Bouillaud noted that Hippocrates had not opened cadavers, and hence was at a disadvantage in his observations. Ancient medicine was good as far as it went; it just didn't go far enough. Paris medicine, whose physicians could take advantage of new techniques and new knowledge, was far superior.

Bouillaud, like Peisse, argued that Broussais had effected a medical revolution – the 'medical revolution of 1816', he called it. Since both history and science were progressive, Bouillaud argued that the Pinelian–Hippocratic system was destined to perish, like any system: 'All was prepared for a new medical revolution: all that was missing was the coming of a medical messiah who would accomplish this regeneration. This messiah finally appeared, under the name of M. Broussais.'[74] For Bouillaud, Broussais was the death-knell of Hippocratic medicine in its Pinelian incarnation. Broussais struck the 'mortal blow to the *most generally adopted doctrine* by the publication of this famous *Examination*, which appeared in 1816'.[75] Bouillaud commented that the repercussions were still being felt after 20 years.

Although a great blood-letter in the spirit of his master, Bouillaud allied himself with the eclectics, those moderates who claimed to be partisans of both past and present. Thus, while Bouillaud was an ardent admirer of Broussais, he also saw important medical wisdom in the teachings of Pinel and the Hippocratists. Furthermore, Bouillaud was favourable towards Laennec, supposedly, Broussais' arch-enemy, 'one of the men whose name honors medical France the most'.[76] Indeed, after Broussais, Laennec was 'the greatest medical illustration of his epoch'. Like Broussais, Laennec took the pathological–anatomical approach to disease, and for Bouillaud pathological anatomy was 'the only basis of positive knowledge in medicine'.[77]

The first rupture with Hippocratic medicine for Bouillaud, as later for Foucault, came with Xavier Bichat. Bichat moved Paris medicine in the direction of normal and pathological anatomy and physiology, but it was Broussais, Bichat's student, who realised the full revolution that Bichat had started. Broussais' fundamental principle was that, like Bichat, he believed that medicine ought to be based on anatomy and physiology. But unlike Bichat, who eschewed causes, Broussais wanted to ask why. The institutional basis of Paris medicine provided the framework for both Bichat and Broussais. Thus Bouillaud emphasised the centrality of the clinical institutions. The hospitals were the *sine qua non* of Paris medicine. Here was the principal difference between the original Hippocratic medicine and Paris medicine. Hippocrates lacked the institutional basis to practise a true clinical medicine that had finally come to fruition in Paris.[78]

One of Bouillaud's major concerns was the defence of systems. Broussais was justified in his system of physiological medicine, Bouillaud argued, for facts alone did not constitute science or knowledge. He argued against Gaspard-Laurent Bayle who maintained that empiricism was the methodological heart of the Hippocratic tradition. Bouillaud's Hippocrates was no radical empiricist. Instead, Bouillaud asserted that Hippocrates and his followers recognised the importance of reasoning and theory in order to make sense of observations:

> No, never, no matter what Bayle and all those of his school say, the Hippocrates, the Sydenhams, the Morgagnis did not teach the heresy that one attributes to them. Doubtless, they accorded observation all the worth due it in medicine; but they never could have thought that it suffices to have eyes and patience to be a complete observer.[79]

The great observers, Bouillaud maintained, needed theories and systems. This need was exemplified by their use of aphorisms – generalising statements that made sense of observations and provided guidance and direction for physicians. Hippocrates himself was thus the original and great systematiser.

In such a way, Bouillaud portrayed Broussais, the physician who supposedly demolished Hippocratism, as one who recaptured the true Hippocrates. He agreed with Corvisart that it was the changes of systems that make great men, and it was the latter who invariably determine the epochs of medical revolutions. Thus, in Bouillaud's account, Broussais was the man of the epoch, the great man of Paris medicine, the Hippocrates of Paris medicine, in the same way that Hippocrates was the great man of ancient medicine.[80] Laennec may have thought he was the Hippocrates of Paris medicine, but Bouillaud gave the honours to Broussais.

Montpellier defends its Hippocratic heritage

As Bouillaud constructed Paris medicine as the heir of Hippocrates, Montpellier physicians became concerned that their claims to the Hippocratic heritage were being challenged. In April 1837 Risueño d'Amador, professor of general pathology and therapeutics at the medical faculty of Montpellier and a corresponding member of the Academy of Medicine, came to Paris to read an essay to the Academy on the calculus of probability applied to medicine.[81] Risueño D'Amador's main argument was that the calculus of probability was an inappropriate tool for the natural and medical sciences, where variation was the norm and the variables were too numerous to be controlled. He also raised many other objections which, taken together, constituted a spirited defence of Montpellier Hippocratism against what Risueño d'Amador perceived to be the extremes of Paris medicine. Just as Bouillaud had claimed Hippocrates for Paris medicine, Risueño d'Amador claimed Hippocrates for Montpellier medicine. The general message was that Parisian physicians – in this case, the numerists – had subverted and distorted Hippocratic medicine, while he and his fellow Montpellier physicians practised and preached true Hippocratism.

Risueño d'Amador defended what he regarded as the Hippocratic method of inductivism against critics who accused it of sterility and impotence. He claimed that these critics, the numerists, wanted to introduce a new instrument, 'the calculus, that is what they call the numerical method'.[82] Whereas the numerists saw medical statistics as an extension of, and an improvement on, the inductive method, the Montpellier physician argued that, in fact, the numerical method was just another system, destructive of the 'true inductive method,' by which he meant the great and historical inductive method of Hippocrates, Aristotle, Sydenham and so on. He contrasted the methods with which 'the great observers drew their portraits of disease' with the 'puerile procedure, exact and necessarily unfaithful, of which the numerists have given several examples'.[83]

For Risueño d'Amador the 'true inductive method' was the ancient method of induction: 'and by induction I mean this *natural* and *simple* method that Hippocrates used, 2,000 years ago with a success which inspired both the admiration and despair of modern science, formulated into rules three centuries ago by Bacon ... .'[84] Like Pinel, for d'Amador the key words were *natural* and *simple*. Hippocratism was a method 'as natural to the spirit as the action of seeing and looking is to the eye'.[85] It was part of the essence of humanity; it was the way humans worked. He argued that, since physicians already possessed the one true method, they should innovate by making discoveries but *not* by developing new methods. There was no need to alter the spirit of science or art. Hence, Risueño d'Amador echoed a conservative message: the 'old way' – the way of Montpellier medicine – was the true and best way.

Risueño d'Amador's defence hinged on agreement on the correct means of observing. The science of numbers could not replace the art of medicine and portraiture: 'To count and note everything which presents itself to the senses is not to observe properly; it is only a mechanical operation ... .'[86] The great observers did not proceed this way. They painted portraits of disease. Just as in art, techniques and mechanical processes could not replace the 'careful hand of a good artist', so in medicine medical statistics could not replace the careful observations of a good – that is, Hippocratic – physician. Arithmetical combinations could not replace the physiognomic descriptions that physicians admired in Hippocrates and all the other great masters. 'What a mistake you are making!' he confidently proclaimed to the numerists.[87] Put another way, the numerical method, 'destroys true art and true observation, substituting for action of the [true, that is, Hippocratic] spirit, and the individual genius of the practitioner, a uniform, blind, and mechanical routine.'[88]

Not to be outdone by Risueño d'Amador, Bouillaud called on the same Hippocratic tradition to defend the numerical method. The numerical method was, he argued, part of the Hippocratic method of observation and was not in opposition with any of the elements of which the 'great experimental and rational method' is composed. His use of Hippocrates was no less firm for being tacit: everyone knew that the 'great experimental and rational method' referred to Hippocrates.[89] Other participants in the debate also called on

Hippocrates to defend their position. So, for example, eclectic and proto-urologist Pierre Rayer cited the first Hippocratic aphorism to show how fallacious experience and observation could be and had been over the centuries. The calculus of probability and the numerical method were both ways of improving upon the method of observation, but they were not, as Risueño d'Amador had argued, in opposition to Hippocrates's great method. Rather, they were a way to perfect it.[90]

Rayer went one step further, highlighting the underlying motives of the whole debate: that Montpellier physicians felt threatened by Paris medicine and turned to Hippocrates to defend their medicine.[91] Thus Rayer mounted a great defence of the Paris School. An eclectic like Bouillaud, he defended the contributions of the ancients while subscribing to the progress of the moderns. And what medicine best exemplified the best of ancient and modern medicine? Paris medicine, of course.[92]

From the experimental to the vitalist Hippocrates

Broussais may have tried to banish Hippocratic medicine from the Paris School but, for different reasons, physicians kept appropriating and reinventing Hippocrates. One of these was Gabriel Andral (1797–1876), known as the father of haematology, who credited Hippocrates as the real founder of Paris medicine. Thus in his 1843 essay on pathological haematology, Andral saw him as the origin of 'the three great points of view, which, now abandoned, and now again adapted, have produced the three systems of solidism, humoralism, and vitalism'.[93] As Andral put it:

> One of the characteristics, and I venture to say one of the glories of the present medical epoch, is to have understood what incomplete and necessarily erroneous results these minute subdivisions of the science [of medicine] conduces ... .[94]

Andral favoured an integrative, or eclectic, approach and urged adopting a variety of methods and orientations to further knowledge of disease and therapeutics. Hippocrates had had a 'beautiful ensemble' worked out, Andral claimed, but lamented that 'few physicians remained faithful to these principles'.[95]

Andral's goal in publishing *Pathological Hematology* was to justify his study of the blood. First, he used Hippocrates to support his neo-vitalism, arguing that a solidist, organic approach would not suffice: the old Hippocratic humours, or fluids, of the body might be the seat of disease as well. Second, he used Hippocrates to support his methods of studying the blood, implying that had Hippocrates lived in nineteenth-century Paris, he would have used medical chemistry and microscopy.[96] The Hippocratic emphasis on observation included all possible means of observing. Andral's Hippocrates ruled out mere speculation, or reasoning by deduction. Ancient physicians sought the origin of disease in elementary principles – in this case, the constituent humours. Reacting to those physicians who proposed that the physical sciences could serve as a model for medicine, Andral propounded a notion of medical humanism, a rediscovery of ancient texts by modern observers. Whereas those who favoured the physical sciences had denied that the blood could, by its alterations, play a part in the production of disease,[97] now it was time to restore a humoral approach.

Andral noted the 'absolute contempt' of physicians of Bichat's generation for the application of chemistry to physiology and pathology. But Bichat was an exception, accepting the validity of a humoral approach. His contemporaries ignored Bichat's vindication of humoralism, Andral argued. Not only did many in the Paris School reject the use of chemistry to study the blood; they also rejected microscopy.[98] For Andral, this earlier epoch was to be distinguished from his own, for whereas in the late eighteenth and early nineteenth century, the early era of Paris medicine, physicians rejected chemistry and microscopy, by the early 1840s, 'the glory of returning to the experimental method, to the microscope, as it has done to the chemical study of the blood, was reserved for our epoch'.[99] Just as Laennec's Hippocrates had been a pathological anatomist, Andral's Hippocrates was an experimentalist. The inheritors of the Hippocratic tradition were his heroes of the Paris School, Bichat and Magendie.

In the 1850s overt references to Hippocrates seemed to wane in debates over the Paris School. Thus he had little place in the debate over microscopy which took place at the Academy of Medicine (October 1854 to January 1855), despite the threat that this technique posed to older clinical ideals.[100] We might have expected Parisian clinicians to call on Hippocrates to defend their clinical ideals. But they did not. Hippocrates did not emerge as a would-be microscopist. Instead, what we find is an observational, clinical ideal – which could have been called Hippocratic – but was now simply called Paris medicine.

Yet this should not be taken to mean, as Ackerknecht asserts, that Hippocratism was a dead letter.[101] A month after the microscopy debate ended, Hippocrates was vigorously invoked in support of vitalism during a debate between Parisian and Montpellier physicians on medical nomenclature.[102] Were diseases to be based on pathological anatomy, the name of the afflicted organ – the so-called organicist approach associated with Pierre-Adolphe Piorry? Or would the traditional terms suffice? Piorry, defending organicism, claimed that he and the other leading Parisian physicians stood for modern, progressive, evolutionary medicine and that new discoveries necessitated a new language. Those who defended the older medical language he called Hellenists or Hippocratists. We need not be detained by the details of the debate over vitalism and organicism, or the renewed rivalry between Montpellier and

Paris that it spawned. The main point is that, again, proponents of all the various vitalist positions – three according to Bouillaud [103]– called on Hippocrates to defend their turf. Each group claimed to be the heir of the true Hippocratic tradition. It was within this context that Peisse made his statement about hippocratising that appears at the beginning of this essay.

Other evidence also supports a renewal of Parisian interest in Hippocrates in the 1850s. For example, Charles Daremberg notes that Andral gave a series of lectures on Greek medicine between 1852 and 1854. The course was intended to be on general pathology, and Andral was going to give a historical overview, but Daremberg comments that it began and ended with Greek medicine.[104] A number of works on vitalism were also published, such as Auber's *Traité de la science médicale* (1853) and Jaccoud's *De l'humorisme ancien et moderne* (1859). Williams reports that the third edition of Barthez's *Nouveaux éléments de la science de l'homme*, edited by Barthez's nephew, was published in 1858, prompted by the general debate on vitalism at the Academy of Medicine.[105]

I began with Peisse and it is worth ending with him, for he illustrates the ways in which Hippocratism was invented and reinvented in early nineteenth-century Paris medicine:

> The Hippocratic doctrine which has been cited in all ages, and always with admiration, is difficult to define, or rather it is, like many others, a consecrated name, but which has not and cannot have any precise signification. Hippocratic medicine has also been called the medicine of observation, but all doctrines have claimed for themselves the same foundation. Hippocrates, like all other physicians, observed, and true it is that no one ever observed more faithfully, and then he theorized on his observations. It has been erroneously pretended, that he had no system, but his physiological and pathological principles governed his practice. This doctrine, it is true, did not consist in those physiological phantasies [sic], which men of the present day, called Hippocratic physicians, pretend to be governed by. As to his practice, it was no other than the expectant method, wise, judicious and proper, when there were no good reasons for more energetic procedures. For my own part, I conceive that this system has, in all times, excited the admiration of good practitioners, because other modes of treatment, resulting from their contemporary systems of doctrine, were all more or less murderous.[106]

Peisse suggested that Broussais had identified the problems of Hippocratism:

> M. Broussais has, in effect, clearly shown that this Hippocratic doctrine, of which it is pretended that a school even exists in the present age, is only a collection of traditional opinions, inconsistent in themselves, with no common bond of connexion, and altogether in arrear of the actual condition of science.[107]

His comments can also serve as a conclusion, for it was these very inconsistencies that made Hippocrates so appealing to Paris physicians. Hippocrates could stand for virtually any position within Paris medicine, and was used in inconsistent and contradictory ways. It is these inconsistencies and contradictions that make Hippocrates so appealing to historians as a valuable means of exploring the divisions within Paris medicine during this period.

Notes

1. Louis Peisse, *La médecine et les médecins*, 2 vols, Paris: Baillière, 1857, Vol. 1, pp. 236–37.
2. *Bulletin de l'Académie de Médecine*, 20, 1856, pp. 549–906. Cited in ibid., Vol. 1, p. 226.
3. Roselyne Rey, 'Anamorphoses d'Hippocrate au XVIIIe siècle', in Danielle Gourevitch (ed.), *Maladie et maladies: histoire et conceptualisation: Mélanges en l'honneur de Mirko Grmek*, Geneva: Droz, 1992, p. 275; Erwin Ackerknecht, *Medicine at the Paris Hospital, 1794–1848*, Baltimore: Johns Hopkins University Press, 1967, p. 57.
4. Rey, 'Anamorphoses' (n. 3) and Ackerknecht, *Paris Hospital* (n. 3). This was true of European medicine in general. See also William F. Bynum, *Science and the Practice of Medicine in the Nineteenth Century*, New York: Cambridge University Press, 1994, p. 3.
5. Roselyne Rey, 'Anamorphoses' (n. 3) pp. 257–76; Michel Foucault, *The Birth of the Clinic*, New York: Vintage, 1973, chapter 4.
6. Ackerknecht, *Paris Hospital* (n. 3) p. 37. This was the caption on a bronze medal struck in 1797 at the creation of the dissection school in Paris. On the medal the portraits of Fernel and Paré were united, symbolising the union of medicine and surgery during the French Revolution. On this topic see also Toby Gelfand, *Professionalizing Modern Medicine: Paris Surgeons and Medical Science and Institutions in the 18th Century*, Westport, CT: Greenwood Press, 1980; I use this expression to refer to the notion of a primitive unity, a halcyon time before there were medical divisions – a medical state of nature identified with Hippocrates.
7. P.J.-G. Cabanis, *On the Relations between the Physical and Moral Aspects of Man*, ed. George Mora, with introductions by Sergio Moravia and George Mora, 2 vols, Baltimore: Johns Hopkins University Press, 1981, p. xi. This translation and edition is based on the 2nd edition of Cabanis, *Rapports du physique et du moral de l'homme*, published in two volumes in Paris in 1805. On Cabanis, see also Martin S. Staum, *Cabanis: Enlightenment and Medical Philosophy in the French Revolution*, Princeton, NJ: Princeton University Press, 1980; Sergio Moravia, 'Cabanis and his Contemporaries', in *Relations between the Physical and Moral*, (above) ed. George Mora, pp. vii–xliv; also, Ackerknecht, *Paris Hospital* (n. 3), pp. 3–8. On Cabanis, the ideologues and the medical science of man, see also Elizabeth Williams, *The Physical and the Moral: Anthropology, Physiology, and Philosophical Medicine in France, 1750–1850*, New York: Cambridge University Press, 1994.
8. Cabanis, *Relations between the Physical and Moral* (n. 7), pp. 36–37. Cabanis exemplifies a broader cultural interest in classical Greece in the eighteenth and nineteenth centuries. This is, of course, well known in art and architecture, literature and politics and this general interest no doubt contributed to the renewed interest in Hippocrates. Just as Cabanis, while writing about Greece, seems to be writing about France, so Olga Augustinos notes that many travel accounts, while purportedly about Greece, were really about France. See, on this topic, Olga

Augustinos, *French Odysseys: Greece in French Travel Literature from the Renaissance to the Romantic Era*, Baltimore: Johns Hopkins University Press, 1994.
9. Cabanis, *Relations between the Physical and Moral*, (n. 7) p. 37 (emphasis in original).
10. Ibid., p. 41.
11. Ibid., p. 42.
12. Ibid., p. 43.
13. Ibid., p. 45.
14. Rey, 'Anamorphoses', (n. 3), p. 264.
15. Dora B. Weiner, 'Introduction', *The Clinical Training of Doctors: An Essay of 1793*, ed. and with an introduction by Dora B. Weiner, Baltimore: Johns Hopkins University Press, 1980; and Williams, *The Physical and the Moral* (n. 7), chapter 2.
16. Pinel, *Clinical Training*, (n. 15).
17. Ibid., p. 83.
18. Ibid., p. 81.
19. Ibid., p. 83.
20. Ibid., pp. 85–86.
21. Ibid., p. 94.
22. Ibid., pp. 85–86.
23. Ibid., p. 67.
24. Ibid., p. 68.
25. Ibid., p. 69.
26. This preoccupation was embodied institutionally in the work of the eighteenth-century Royal Society of Medicine and the nineteenth-century Paris Academy of Medicine. Both institutions had epidemic commissions that gathered meteorological and topographical information from provincial medical correspondents with the aim of uncovering laws of epidemic disease. On the Royal Society of Medicine, see Caroline Hannaway, 'The Société de Médecine and Epidemics in the Ancien Régime', *Bulletin of the History of Medicine*, **46**, 1972, pp. 257–73; on the epidemic commission of the Paris Academy of Medicine and its role in public health see George Weisz, *The Medical Mandarins: The Paris Academy of Medicine in the Nineteenth and Early Twentieth Centuries*, New York: Oxford University Press, 1995, chapter 4; and Ann F. La Berge, *Mission and Method: the Early Nineteenth-Century French Public Health Movement*, New York: Cambridge University Press, 1992, chapter 3.
27. Pinel, *Clinical Training*, (n. 15), p. 72.
28. Ibid., p. 86. Weiner comments, however, that when de Haen followed van Swieten from the Netherlands to Vienna, he routinely performed autopsies before his medical students. See ibid, p. 96, n. 2. However, Pinel may have made an unjust accusation. Erna Lesky suggests that physicians like de Haen were rooted in the Hippocratic foundations of Viennese empirical medicine. On this, see Erna Lesky, *The Vienna Medical School of the 19th Century*, Baltimore: Johns Hopkins University Press, 1976, pp. 26, 75–76.
29. Pinel, *Clinical Training*, (n. 15), p. 87.
30. Ibid.
31. Ackerknecht, *Paris Hospital*, (n. 3), p. 84.
32. On Corvisart's dark view of nature, see Randall Albury, 'Heart of darkness: J.N. Corvisart and the medicalization of Life', *Historical Reflections/Réflexions Historiques*, **9**, 1982, pp. 17–31. See also Randall Albury, 'Corvisart and

Broussais: Human Individuality and Medical Dominance', in Caroline Hannaway and Ann La Berge (eds), *Constructing Paris Medicine*, Amsterdam, Atlanta: Rodopi, 1998, pp. 221–50.
33. Jean-Nicolas Corvisart, *Essay on the Organic Diseases and Lesions of the Heart and Great Vessels*, trans. Jacob Gates, New York: Hafner, 1962, p. 25. Reprint of 1812 edition and translation by Gates. First published in French in Paris in 1806.
34. An excellent source remains Clarence Glacken, *Traces on the Rhodian Shore: Nature and Culture in Western Thought from Ancient Times to the End of the Eighteenth Century*, Los Angeles: University of California Press, 1967.
35. Corvisart, *Diseases of the Heart*, (n. 33), p. 28.
36. Ibid., p. 30.
37. On this elitist point of view, that of private hygiene, see William Coleman, 'Health and hygiene in the *Encyclopédie*: a medical doctrine for the bourgeoisie', *Journal of the History of Medicine and Allied Sciences*, 29, 1974, pp. 399–421.
38. Corvisart, *Diseases of the Heart*, (n. 33), p. 33.
39. Ibid., pp. 33–34.
40. Ibid., pp. 268–69.
41. Ibid., p. 271.
42. Ibid., p. 274.
43. This material on Laennec relies almost exclusively on Jacalyn Duffin, *To See with a Better Eye: A Life of R.T.H. Laennec*, Princeton, NJ: Princeton University Press, 1997. See also Ackerknecht, *Paris Hospital*, (n. 3), pp. 88–97.
44. Cited in Duffin, *Laennec*, (n. 43), p. 52.
45. Ibid., p. 75.
46. R.T.H. Laennec, *A Treatise on the Diseases of the Chest*, trans. and with a preface and notes by John Forbes, New York: Hafner, 1962, pp. 346–47. Originally published in London in 1821 by T. and C. Underwood.
47. Duffin notes that the Montpellier-trained physician François Double had recommended immediate auscultation in 1817, and suggested that Laennec may have been inspired by Double's suggestion. Curiously, as Duffin points out, Laennec did not mention Buisson's 1802 thesis, which she claims led Laennec to contemplate the meaning of auscultation and the exploration of the human voice.
48. Part of this discussion relies on Duffin, *Laennec*, (n. 43), chapter 6. The Grmek reference, cited by Duffin, is Mirko Grmek, 'L'invention de l'auscultation médiate: retouches à un cliché historique', *Revue du Palais de la Découverte*, 22, 1981, pp. 107–16, esp. p. 110. See also George Weisz, 'Creating the Posthumous Laennec', *Bulletin of the History of Medicine*, 61, 1987, pp. 541–62; and Louis Peisse, *Sketches of the Character and Writings of Eminent Living Surgeons and Physicians of Paris*, trans. Elisha Bartlett, Boston: Carter, Hendee and Babcock, 1831, p. 79. Originally published in Paris as *Les médecins français contemporains* in 1827–28. Peisse's example was Nicolas Desgenettes.
49. Ackerknecht, *Paris Hospital*, (n. 3), p. 96.
50. Erwin Ackerknecht, 'Broussais, or a Forgotten Medical Revolution', *Bulletin of the History of Medicine*, 27, 1953, pp. 320–43; Weisz, 'Creating the Posthumous Laennec', (n. 45); Jean-François Braunstein, *Broussais et le matérialisme: médecine et philosophie au XIXe siècle*, Paris: Méridiens-Klincksieck, 1986; Michel Valentin, *François Broussais, Empereur de la Médecine*, Dinard: Association des Amis du Musée du Pays de Dinard, 1988; Jacalyn Duffin, 'Laennec and Broussais: the "Sympathetic" Duel', in Hannaway and La Berge (eds), *Constructing Paris Medicine* (n. 32), pp. 251–74; Williams, *The Physical and*

the Moral (n. 7), pp. 166–75; and Georges Canguilhem, *The Normal and the Pathological*, New York: Zone Books, 1991, esp. pp. 47–64.
51. Jean-Baptiste Bouillaud, *Essai sur la philosophie médicale et sur les généralités de la clinique médicale*, Paris: Rouvier et le Bouvier, 1836; Peisse, *Sketches* (n. 48); and Louis Peisse, 'Broussais' obituary published in the *Gazette médicale*, 24 November 1838, reprinted in Louis Peisse, *La médecine et les médecins* (n. 1), Vol. 2, pp. 389–404.
52. Peisse, *Sketches* (n. 48), p. 22, for both quotations.
53. Ibid., pp. 22–23.
54. Ibid., p. 23.
55. Ibid., p.26.
56. Ibid., p. 27.
57. Ibid., pp. 27–28.
58. Ibid., pp. 37–38.
59. Ibid., p. 38.
60. Ibid., p. 40. On the Laennec–Broussais struggle, see Duffin, 'Laennec and Broussais',(n. 50).
61. Rey, 'Anamorphoses' (n. 3); Ackerknecht, *Paris Hospital*, (n. 3), p. 96. On the medical science of man tradition, see Williams, *The Physical and the Moral* (n. 7).
62. Peisse, *Sketches*, (n. 48), p. 51.
63. Ibid., p. 52.
64. Ibid., p. 69.
65. Peisse, *La médecine et les médecins* (n. 1), Vol. 2, p. 390.
66. Ibid., Vol. 2, pp. 392–93.
67. Ibid., Vol. 2, p. 394.
68. Ibid., Vol. 2, p. 403.
69. For a fuller account of Bouillaud's construction of Paris medicine, see Ann La Berge and Caroline Hannaway, 'Paris medicine: past and present perspectives', in Hannaway and La Berge (eds), *Constructing Paris Medicine* (n. 32), pp. 1–69.
70. Bouillaud, *Essai sur la philosophie médicale*, (n. 51), pp. 8–9.
71. Ibid., p. 85, n. 2.
72. Ibid., p. 5.
73. Ibid., p. 4.
74. Ibid., p. 85.
75. Ibid., p. 72 (emphasis in original). François Broussais, *Examen de la doctrine médicale généralement adoptée*, Paris: Méquignon-Marvis, 1816.
76. Bouillaud, *Essai sur la philosophie médicale* (n. 51), p. 85.
77. Ibid., p. 88.
78. Ibid., pp. 101–12.
79. Ibid., pp. 161–65. Quote, p. 165. For a good discussion of the meaning of observation, indeed the whole rhetoric of observation, see Weisz, *Medical Mandarins* (n. 26), p. 163. See also Williams, *The Physical and the Moral*, (n. 7), p. 94.
80. Bouillaud, *Essai sur la philosophie médicale* (n. 51), pp. 171–75.
81. *Bulletin de l'Académie Royale de Médecine*, 1, 1836–37, pp. 622–806. Hereafter referred to as 'Statistics debate', followed by the page number. On the debate over the numerical method and the introduction of medical statistics into Paris medicine, see Terence Murphy, 'Medical knowledge and statistical methods in early nineteenth-century France', *Medical History*, **25**, 1981, pp. 301–19. See also John Rosser Matthews, *Quantification and the Quest for Medical Certainty*, Princeton, NJ: Princeton University Press, 1995, chapter 2; Theodore M. Porter,

The Rise of Statistical Thinking, 1820–1900, Princeton, NJ: Princeton University Press, 1986, pp. 151–62.
82. 'Statistics debate' (n. 81), p. 645.
83. Ibid., pp. 645–47. Quotation, p. 647.
84. Ibid., p. 654 (my emphasis).
85. Ibid.
86. Ibid., p. 663.
87. Ibid., p. 664.
88. Ibid., pp. 678–79.
89. Ibid., p. 700.
90. Ibid., p. 780.
91. On the use of the rhetoric of Hippocrates by Montpellier physicians, see Williams, *The Physical and the Moral* (n. 7), pp. 63–66. For a general historical account of the uses of Hippocrates, see Wesley D. Smith, *The Hippocratic Tradition*, Ithaca, NY: Cornell University Press, 1979.
92. 'Statistics debate' (n. 81), pp. 780–88.
93. Gabriel Andral, *Pathological Hematology. An Essay on the Blood in Disease*, trans. J.F. Meigs and Alfred Stillé, Philadelphia: Lea and Blanchard, 1844, p. 15. This work was first published in French in Paris in 1843.
94. Ibid., p. 6.
95. Ibid., p. 5.
96. This was a recognisable appropriation. Galileo used the same tactic in 'Letters on Sunspots' to claim that had Aristotle lived in seventeenth-century Italy, he would have looked through a telescope. See Galileo, 'Letters on Sunspots', in Stillman Drake (ed.), *Discoveries and Opinions of Galileo*, New York: Doubleday/Anchor, 1957, p. 118.
97. Andral, *Pathological Hematology* (n.93), p. 25.
98. Ibid., p. 26.
99. Ibid., p. 27.
100. *Bulletin de l'Académie Impériale de Médecine* (1854–55), 3 October–16 January, pp. 7–447. On the microscopy debate, see Ann La Berge, 'Dichotomy or integration? Medical microscopy and the Paris clinical tradition', in Hannaway and La Berge, *Constructing Paris Medicine*, (n. 32).
101. Ackerknecht, *Paris Hospital* (n. 3), p. 99. Ackerknecht dates this from the 1830s.
102. See note 2. Hereafter referred to as 'Vitalism–organicism debate', followed by the page number.
103. 'Vitalism–organicism debate', (n. 102) pp. 694–95.
104. Charles Daremberg, *Histoire des sciences médicales*, Paris: Baillière, 1870, p. ix. These lectures were published, according to Daremberg, in *l'Union médicale* from 1852 to 1854.
105. Williams, *The Physical and the Moral* (n. 7), p. 47, n. 7.
106. Peisse, *Sketches* (n. 51), pp. 28–29.
107. Ibid.

CHAPTER TEN

Making History in American Medical Culture: The Antebellum Competition for Hippocrates

John Harley Warner

During the past decade, historians have paid increasingly close attention to the ways in which individual historical figures are remembered, represented and commemorated, and especially to how their images change over time, being refashioned to serve particular social, political and intellectual agendas. In part, this reflects a wider historical preoccupation with appropriation, representation and storytelling as important cultural practices. At the same time, it reflects a growing historical awareness that, in the process of constructing cultural heroes, nations, social movements and professions alike create models that embody their aspirations, validate their endeavours and reaffirm their perceptions of self. Recent studies in the history of medicine on John Hunter, René Laennec, Louis Pasteur and Walter Reed have shown that, as one historian lucidly put it, 'the way in which the idol is conceived is affected by the interests of those who claim to be his acolytes'.[1] Collectively, such studies have gone beyond the banal observation that medical and scientific heroes are appropriated and reconfigured to serve the contingent, and sometimes divergent, agendas of their commemorators: they begin to show how selective depictions of medical heroes and anti-heroes give the historian a revealing window into the cultures that produced particular representations.

The American celebration of Hippocrates displays the constitutive role that historical storytelling has played in medical culture. During the antebellum era, the most pervasive depiction of Hippocrates was as archetypal empiricist, as avatar of a particular epistemological stance that resonated powerfully with larger social, intellectual, and political currents in ways that encouraged physicians to see it as a powerful instrument in promoting bids for authority and programmes for professional uplift. A diverse array of medical Americans deployed his image as empiricist hero, the central focus of this essay, in recounting stories about medical history that called for revolt while invoking the theme of return, playing on the authentic 'firstness' of Hippocrates. This making of medical history reveals deeply rooted assumptions about how professional authority and public esteem were best to be won and maintained in a culture that relied on tradition to preserve order while looking optimistically to the selective overthrow of established authority as an avenue to radical social change.

The portrayal of Hippocrates as 'the father of medicine' was commonplace in antebellum America – that is, the United States between the 1820s and the end of the 1850s, the decades that preceded the Civil War. A professor at the Vermont Academy of Medicine was typical in opening his first lecture of 1820 by telling the class that, as one student wrote in his notebook: 'Hypocrates existed about four hundred years before the Birth of Christ. He was of the Esclepian Family. This illustrious character is called the Father of Medicine.'[2] In commemorative oratory, such as introductory addresses delivered at medical schools and presidential addresses presented at medical society meetings, Hippocrates was routinely brought forward as an indispensable actor in the story of medical history that was told and retold as a central ritual of professional culture. Anti-orthodox physicians – such as homoeopaths and hydropaths – frequently shared in this convention, as did a student at the homoeopathic Hahnemann Medical College in Philadelphia when he wrote in his 1856 MD thesis that 'one of the most sagacious observers & industrious men that ever lived was Hippocrates, Coan Sage, entitled the Father of Medicine'.[3]

Some physicians recognised that, often, Hippocrates was cited by medical practitioners who knew nothing about the Hippocratic writings; they were merely making a facile allusion to a professional founders myth. The conservative Philadelphia medical professor John Redman Coxe, prefacing his own 1846 translation of a collection of Hippocratic treatises from Latin into English, complained that 'our teachers refer to them ex cathedra; our books continually quote them; and yet, not one in a hundred of the Profession, at least in America, have ever seen them, and if interrogated, could not inform us of what they treat'.[4] Worse still, Coxe charged two decades earlier, were physicians 'who may deem the writings of Hippocrates to be useless, or even unworthy of perusal, whilst yet they join in senseless acclamations to his worth, and in tributes of respect to his memory'.[5]

What gave the invocation of his name by physicians more than merely ornamental value, however, was the important professional place occupied by history in antebellum American medicine. At least through the first two-thirds of the nineteenth century, much of the professional definition and authority that later physicians would derive from science came instead from history. It was medical history and the values it displayed that validated the orthodox practitioner's standing and soundness as a 'regular' physician, confirming participation in a learned tradition and identity as a professional. History placed physicians in a continuing lineage and affirmed the links with the past that gave them legitimacy. At a time when a multitude of irregular healers were competing successfully for recognition and clients, recounting an historical story that displayed two millennia of enduring tradition was a tool that orthodox physicians could use to set themselves apart.⁶

Much professional argument, moreover, was cast as historical polemic. But it is critical to see that this form of history-making was not simply a culturally enhancing, but detachable, framework for presenting medical ideas, as it would become in most twentieth-century texts; rather, it *was* medicine. Engagement with classical texts was not merely a leisure activity for the cultivated physician but, rather, an engagement with a living medical tradition – not an antiquarian pursuit but a medical one. History was a prominent part of both transmitting and defending a medical position, whether it was a matter of conveying the established canon to students in a classroom or introducing a new idea to colleagues at a medical society meeting. Accordingly, it was both to second and to validate the particular argument he sought to promote that a medical student in Nashville, Tennessee asserted in his 1857 MD thesis that 'it is due to the immortal Father of Medicine to say, that the ordeal of twenty three hundred and seventeen years [*sic*] experience, has undiminished the lustre of many of his teachings, nor lessened the value of his practice'.⁷

Certainly, the Hippocrates deployed in these accounts was highly malleable, just as his authority could be pressed into service by not only divergent, but sometimes warring, medical camps – orthodox doctors and homoeopathic physicians, for example. And his teachings (or putative teachings) were not always viewed uncritically. 'Though Hippocrates discovered the true path in medicine,' one admiring orthodox physician told members of the St Louis Medical and Surgical Society in 1845, 'he did not always adhere to it.'⁸ The following year, another physician proposed that 'Hippocrates laid down the principles of a sound philosophy but forgot them when he began to speculate concerning disease'. He concurred that Hippocrates deserved to be designated 'the *"Father of Medicine,"*' but judged that 'when he leaves the region of fact and approaches the borders of theory, he betrays a weakness common to men – his speculations are flimsy, and oftentimes most absurd'.⁹

Other physicians defended the doctrines of Hippocrates, not on the grounds that they were correct but on the grounds that medicine was a progressive science and improvements in knowledge were to be expected. At the turn of the nineteenth century the Philadelphia medical professor Benjamin Rush had criticised Hippocrates for 'his *ignorance* in anatomy' in general and his confusion of arteries with veins in particular, an assault that Rush redoubled in lectures to students published in 1811.¹⁰ Coxe, a former student of Rush, later launched a public rebuttal when in 1829 he delivered 'An Introductory Lecture in Vindication of Hippocrates' to medical students at the University of Pennsylvania. 'Surely, if our medical ancestors of only two centuries past are not blameable for their ignorance in respect to the circulation,' Coxe argued, 'it can scarcely be deemed just to asperse the character of a man who lived twenty centuries ago, for a deficiency in the same particular.'¹¹ As Coxe insisted, 'The truth is, the views of Hippocrates, even if absurd; are those of a great, a vigorous, and a master mind; unaided by any very extensive means of previous inquirers; yet unshackled by the past, or contemporary authority!'[12] Real error, other defenders charged, rested with physicians who adhered unthinkingly to the scriptural teachings of Hippocrates rather than to the spirit and methods he espoused – those who 'pinned their faith upon Hippocrates' in ways that left them 'constantly praising learning at the expense of knowledge'.[13]

Most regular physicians who spelt out the shortcomings in Hippocratic theory tempered their criticisms by suggesting that Hippocrates – practising in a different age, in a different era, and on different peoples – might well have been correct in his therapeutic tack, even if the same treatments might be inappropriate for the constitutions, environments and civilisation encountered in the nineteenth-century United States. 'Whatever might have been the advantage, in Greece, of this truly Hippocratic *expectation*,' the Philadelphia physician René La Roche commented in 1829 on the therapeutic plan that relied on the healing power of nature, 'it does not require much experience in the diseases of this country, to discover that it is not so well calculated to ensure success here as a more energetic mode.'[14] 'You all know that the climate of Greece is equable & serene & that the people of that country in the time of Hippocrates still cherished the simplicity of their Republican habits,' John Eberle told Jefferson Medical College students in his 1827 class on the theory and practice of medicine, using this as a springboard for his assertion that treatment suiting the ills of modern Americans had to be more boldly interventionist than what had been appropriate for the sick looked after by Hippocrates.[15]

What is striking, though, is that most depictions of Hippocrates in antebellum American medicine were not only positive but also remarkably consistent in the characteristic of 'the father of medicine' they made most prominent – namely, direct empirical observation of nature. There was not one Hippocrates but many; yet, by and large, representations made him stand above all else for empiricism and against rationalism, for an allegiance to simple, unadorned truth and against the rationalistic indulgence that fostered artificial embellishment and the mystification of medical knowledge. 'Hippocrates', one physician asserted in language that was typical, 'separated medicine from phylosophy [*sic*]; he showed that observation is the only true guide to those truths, which nature permits the human mind to reach. A just appreciator of systems, he abandoned them to others, who gave themselves to the guidance of imagination.'[16] It was the achievement of Hippocrates, an Albany, New York student wrote in his 1840 MD thesis, to initiate the extrication of medicine from 'the labyrinthian morass of speculation and hypothesis'.[17] Hippocrates provided a venerable touchstone of empiricism, and it was this epistemological stance that antebellum American physicians most vividly made him represent.

My focus in this essay is not so much on a discourse about Hippocrates as on how this predominant image of Hippocrates was deployed in a wider discourse about the state of American medicine and programmes for reform. My leading aim, in turn, is to explore and explain what it was about this particular construction of Hippocrates as avatar of empiricism that held such powerful resonances in antebellum American culture. It is not difficult to comprehend how American physicians were able to plausibly present Hippocrates as a symbol of direct empirical observation of nature, for their concern was not so much a quest after the historical Hippocrates than to represent a figure endowed with those attributes they esteemed. Thus, what chiefly needs to be explained is why some Americans so stridently depicted Hippocrates as a radical empiricist and why they so ardently celebrated this particular depiction as an important instrument in explaining the past, giving meaning to the present and offering a plan for the future.

Hippocrates at the barricades: promoting the French Revolution in American medicine

While the depiction of Hippocrates as an empiricist hero was common across a wide range of physicians in antebellum America, those who as a group most energetically displayed and proselytised this image were those who had studied in France and who, in the process, had come to see themselves as disciples of the Paris Clinical School. After Waterloo and peace, Paris had become a Mecca for foreign medical students and practitioners, including at least 1000 Americans who made the journey across the Atlantic for medical study during the antebellum decades. As these Americans returned home, promoting the lessons of the Paris School (as they interpreted them) became a task central both to defining their own identity and to establishing a plan for the cognitive and social reformation of American medicine.[18]

Underlying the way in which Americans who became disciples of the Paris School tended to think about French medicine was the tacit assumption that it represented something fundamentally new, that it marked a critical departure from the medicine of the past. As Americans who studied in France were drawn into professional interactions after their return home, their claims for the importance and newness of the Paris School became increasingly systematic and stylised, and nowhere more so than in their presentation of history. Glossing over all subtleties, their account of medical history was this: since the collapse of the classical Greco-Roman world, Western medicine with only a few notable exceptions – Vesalius, Sydenham, Morgagni and Hunter – was dominated by rationalism and speculation, and this was exacerbated in the Enlightenment by the reigning spirit of system. The Paris School that emerged in the wake of the French Revolution marked a break, a valiant revolt against the dogma and speculative embellishment of ancien régime medicine. But it marked a break only with the medical errors of the past rather than with medical tradition itself, for it involved a return to Hippocratic observation of nature. With liberation from the spirit of system in sight, and with the empiricist pathway to truth revealed, it was now up to the acolytes of the Paris School to carry on the good fight and establish a new medical order.

Indeed, of all the messages American physicians transmitted home from Paris, the one that most distinctly characterised their programme for American medicine was the animus against speculation and for the empirical pursuit of facts, against rationalistic systems and for knowledge rooted in the collection of observed facts. They could have presented this cluster of commitments as Baconian, for in fields ranging from natural science to religion American appeals to Baconianism were pervasive.[19] The representation by American physicians of the medical empiricism they encountered in Paris as something distinctly French, however, grew from the way they viewed and wished to portray medical history. They depicted the Paris School as a revolt against nearly two millennia of epistemological delusion, but one that at the same time could be framed as a return to a much earlier, more authentic Hippocratic empiricism. Both the Frenchness and newness of the Paris School helped make it a distinctive banner under which the Americans could mount their own campaign. Presenting their epistemological position as a radically new French empiricism, rather than as yet another expression of Baconianism, therefore was essential to an historical narrative on which they relied both to define the meaning of the Paris School and to clarify their role as its emissaries. Telling an historical story that situated the Paris School at an abrupt disruption in the course of medical thought helped validate the importance of the programme to which they had consecrated themselves while it underscored the promise of the newly mounted battle against medical systems. Even though most American physicians did not take up their account of history intact, and often neglected to stress the role of the Paris School that its disciples so celebrated, the campaign against the spirit of system that this account of history was designed to propel became perhaps the most powerful intellectual impulse in antebellum American medicine.

In private writings this version of history was tacit knowledge that there was no need to spell out. In public rhetoric, however, it was a story they told again and again. Professional rituals such as introductory and commencement addresses at medical schools particularly offered occasions to present this historical narrative. But because recounting history was such an in-built part of ordinary professional argument and persuasion, it often appeared in didactic lectures to students, in textbooks and in technical contributions to medical journals as well. Already common in the 1820s and 1830s, as the number of committed disciples of French medicine grew this account of history became commonplace during the 1840s and 1850s. Told initially to persuade students and colleagues – an act of proselytism designed to convince others to embrace

French ways – over time it increasingly functioned as a form of righteous action, an affirmation of a shared creed recounted less to convert the unenlightened than to reassure the faithful.

The French revolution in medicine, as these Americans told the story, represented a fresh start in reconstructing medical knowledge. 'A BICHAT, a BECLARD, a BROUSSAIS, have been given to the world; ignorance and error are now trembling, tottering, falling!' one physician told members of a local medical society in South Carolina in 1837. 'The flimsy theories and unphilosophical writings of many from the time of HIPPOCRATES, to the present, are now being exploded and consigned to the depository of the antiquary.'[20] Echoing this view, a Boston physician asserted flatly in 1836 that 'disease has never, until quite recently, been investigated'. Direct empirical observation was just beginning to expose the 'incomprehensible mysticism and absurd speculations of the closet dogmatists upon the nature of disease'.[21]

Often made early in the antebellum period to assert the newness and importance of what was just appearing from Paris, by the mid-century such historical claims generally were more reflective but no less intent on identifying the Paris School as a new departure. In 1848, for example, the French-experienced Philadelphia physician Alfred Stillé used the preface to his *Elements of General Pathology*, which he titled 'Medical Truth', as a forum for reaffirming his Parisian faith as the foundation for a new medical order. 'The theories which ruled the world successively, have disappeared one after another, like succeeding fashions in equipage and dress, while many of the *facts* recorded two centuries before the Christian era, recur in the daily walks of our profession, precisely as the Father of Medicine inscribed them on his tablets,' he began.[22] But the great observers, Hippocrates 'as well as all his successors, until very recently, preferred to communicate the general results, rather than the elements of their experience, in the form of aphorisms, or short, pithy maxims, which were easily remembered by their pupils'. A more rigorous use of observation as a basis for medicine was required, Stillé insisted, and:

> ... it became necessary, therefore, that the moderns should apply themselves to the *natural* history of disease, and build up the science anew, from its very foundations, by slow and gradual labour. Thus it is, that nearly the whole domain of pathology, such as we now possess it, is of very recent acquisition.[23]

Stillé nodded approvingly to Bacon, but denied that his method had instigated a new departure in medicine:

> It is somewhat remarkable, that although these precepts were promulgated more than two hundred years ago, and many physicians since that time have professed to guide their inquiries by the Baconian philosophy, yet not until within twenty or thirty years has any one carried them into literal execution.[24]

The Paris clinician Pierre Louis, Stillé continued, was the first to develop this method in medicine and to put it to productive use, not only asserting, but acting on, the conviction 'that the science of medicine is founded *alone* upon the observation of facts, to the *entire exclusion* of all hypothetical reasoning'. Stillé noted that 'from the beginning of time to the present day, the same material phenomena have been presented to the senses, but in medicine, with comparatively little profit, until a recent date'; it was the Paris School that had revealed a new pathway to lasting change.[25]

What such disciples of French medicine as Stillé sought to convey by presenting history in this way, and what others took away from their words, were not necessarily the same thing. It was fully possible to take up the call to battle against speculation without embracing the proposition that the Paris School marked the critical turning point between the old medicine and the new, and many American physicians followed this course. The programme for reassessing established knowledge, after all, comported very well with broader movements in American thought. Not only professionals, but educated Americans in general, spoke much about the error of blind allegiance to the teachings of authority and the importance of making independent judgements on the basis of free observation. This became even more widely pronounced with the Jacksonian era calls for each American man and woman to exercise their democratic duty by making up their own minds about all that concerned the social, political and natural worlds. In the medical profession, as elsewhere in American society, rhetorical allegiance to independent thinking was routine. 'Blind devotion to authority is an obstacle to the acquisition of knowledge', a medical professor in Kentucky told a new class of students in 1825, echoing preceptors throughout the country, Paris-experienced or not.[26] Even calls within medicine for empirically determined fact were expressed in rhetorical conventions that, as the next section will explore, had much wider social and political resonances.

The wider dissemination of the empiricist campaign against speculative systems of pathology and therapeutics is especially evident in antebellum MD theses, in which students, reproducing the depiction of medical history they had been taught, presented the battle against systems as the leading intellectual campaign of their era. In the anti-system orthodox MD theses that proliferated, ordinarily the first task was to display the longstanding oppression of medicine by systems, persisting through the present. 'System-making is a characteristic of the times,' one medical student at Transylvania began his thesis in 1841. 'The marks of this fondness for theorizing are nowhere more plainly perceptible than in the history and progress of Medical Science. Scarcely does one fair fabric of hypothesis and conjecture crumble into dust, ere another superstructure, composed of the same flimsy materials, rises upon its ruins.'[27] The following year, another student at the same school wrote:

> In looking back over the history of medical science; we observe nothing that has exerted a more baneful influence upon the curative art, or therapeutic application of medicines; than the many systems that have been established.[28]

Each student then went on to catalogue the dire consequences of system-building, chief among them ineffective practice and a block to progress. The evils of unorthodox medicine were likewise attributed to system-building, for not only Cullenism, Brownianism and Cookeism, but equally Thomsonianism, hydropathy and homoeopathy were brought forward as examples of the absurd systems of practice to which unchecked speculation could lead. Even in confronting only the systems of orthodox physicians, another thesis writer complained, the medical student could well feel overwhelmed by what he called 'the gush of speculation'.[29] Identifying evil, and loudly deploring it, provided a vehicle to reform, a plea for physicians to recognise that the spirit of system was dangerous, however seductive, and that facts rather than speculations provided the only sturdy foundation for the medicine of the future.

The putative newness of the Paris School and the epistemological break with tradition it was made to stand for had a singularly powerful appeal for physicians self-conscious of the newness and cultural potential of their own nation, liberated, as many saw it, not only from the Old World but from the burden of the past. The radical empiricism of the French revolution in medicine offered a basis for creating a new medical tradition, and its newness enhanced its symbolic value. Citizens of the New Republic persistently contrasted the intellectual despotism of the Old World with the freedom of thought of the New. Thus an American physician wrote from London in 1839:

> Here improvement is checked and cramped by old forms and old customs, that they cannot shake off. – With us we have no such thing, we look at things without prejudice, – try all things reject the worthless or useless and improve upon the good.[30]

Perceptions such as this encouraged the conclusion that Americans, of all peoples, were suited to embracing the new departure represented by the Paris School and bringing it to fruition, and Americans often returned from Paris with proud confidence in American destiny. One Alabama medical student could optimistically claim in his 1857 thesis that 'the day of personal authority and universal sway in our science has passed and the great American principles of free thought and free speech, prevails'.[31] History – medical and civil – combined in giving American physicians a special mission. As the physician Austin Flint, writing from Paris in 1854, asserted, 'It rests with ourselves to take a national position, as regards the science of medicine, in keeping with the political importance of our republic.'[32]

In the account of history that the American disciples of French medicine urged, then, there were wide-ranging professional and cultural reasons to stress the newness of the Paris School. Without contradiction, however, they used history to reveal continuities between the features of Parisian medicine they admired and a thread of truth that extended backward in time. The crusade against the spirit of system, according to this depiction of it, was in some respects a return to Western medicine's classical roots; and for the American disciples of Parisian medicine, as for some among their French medical heroes such as Pierre-J-G. Cabanis, Philippe Pinel and René-T-H. Laennec (explored in the contribution to this volume by Ann F. La Berge), Hippocrates especially represented a useable past.

Hippocrates was to be admired for freeing himself from the speculation prevalent in his time and for providing a model of empirical observation of fact that distinguished him from the centuries of speculative theorists that ensued, from Galen onwards. As one student at the Albany Medical College wrote in his 1840 thesis:

> Although the science at his day was in its infancy, and himself entangled in the labyrinthian maze of speculation and hypothesis, yet notwithstanding this he deemed all our knowledge in medicine, to consist in the observance of actual phenomena and their generalization.[33]

'Hippocrates has left us a masterpiece which excites our surprise and admiration, when we remember the remote age in which it was written,' one medical professor asserted in 1845, proposing that, to understand the reasons for such lasting success his students need only recognise 'with what care that great man avoided the delusive guide of imagination'.[34] So, too, did another physician, critical of occasions in which Hippocrates 'philosophizes concerning disease', as in discussions of humoral pathology, hold up his writings on epidemics as a model of the empirical revelation of enduring truths: 'He is here the historian of nature, and his descriptions will continue true to the end of time.'[35] That the products of empirical observation had survived intact testified to the durability of fact, contrasted with the frailty and ultimate transience of speculations.

Invoking the example of Hippocrates was a way of blunting the potentially unsettling radicalness of the claim that medical science was in its infancy. But it also provided one way of proclaiming a new departure in medicine without denying a longer lineage that was an important source of the profession's identity and confidence. It retained what was good from the past – 'those glorious principles handed down to us from Hypocrates and other Fathers', as one medical student put it[36] – while positing a revolution that not only overthrew past errors but continued full circle to restore something important that had been lost – that is, Hippocratic observation of nature. Hippocrates was portrayed as standing stalwart with the American disciples of the Paris School at what Pierre Louis told one of his Boston pupils it was their duty to defend – namely, a '[b]arrière contre l'esprit du système'.[37]

This theme of return, like assertions of the newness of the Paris School and its epistemology, was rooted not only in a particular understanding of the medical past but also in broader conventions in American thought and rhetoric. Indeed, it has been suggested that the theme of return was the one unifying motif that recurred in all the diverse movements for social change during the Jacksonian era.[38] Just as political and social reformers demanded change not only in the name of progress but also by calling for a return to a more authentic, simpler, ancestral American past, so medical reformers seeking to dispel the spirit of system sought to both break with the past and simultaneously return to an older, purer, ancestral past represented by the most revered of the medical fathers, Hippocrates.

Hippocrates, the 'true physician', and the cultural meaning of empiricism

These coexisting themes of revolt and return are clearly exemplified in the thought of the American disciple of the Paris School, Elisha Bartlett. In his empiricist manifesto *A Philosophy of Medical Science* (1844), Bartlett gave the fullest account offered by any American of the philosophy of the Paris School and its place in the wider history of medical epistemology and medical knowledge. Erwin Ackerknecht, indeed, regarded the book as 'the only systematic formulation of the philosophical approach of the great Paris clinical school', and by merit of this claimed for Bartlett the title 'the philosopher of the Paris clinical school'.[39] In Bartlett's text, as in his lectures to students, he assailed rationalism and urged in its place close, empirical observation of fact after the Paris model.[40]

Medical hypotheses and theories, Bartlett argued:

> ... have only rendered more obscure and difficult what was sufficiently so before their intervention; and they have ever impeded the progress of the science which they professes to promote. Not only so, but they have almost always acted injuriously upon the practical applications of the science of medicine.[41]

He insisted that:

> ... so far as medical science has any just title to the appellation; and so far as medical art possesses any rules, sufficiently positive to be worth anything, it is owing, exclusively, to the diligent, unprejudiced, and conscientious study of the phenomena and relationships of disease. The sole tendency of every departure from this study, – the sole tendency of every attempt to refer these phenomena to certain unknown and assumed conditions, for the purpose of rendering them *rational*, has been to hinder the progress and improvement of the science and the art. So has it ever been, so will it ever be.[42]

He catalogued in detail the systems that had reigned, each in its turn, and underscored excessive reliance on rationalism as the fundamental flaw that characterised all of them, denouncing Cullenism, Brownism, Rushism, Broussaisism 'and all the host of other so called rational *isms*'.⁴³ Pathological systems were '*a priori* abstractions, under the misnomer of laws, or principles', and it was not merely deluded but dangerous to deduce therapeutics from them. Bartlett concluded:

> I hope that the true character of all these pretended medical doctrines is now sufficiently obvious to the reader. I hope he is prepared to judge them according to their deserts, and to assign them their appropriate position *without* the pale of legitimate science.⁴⁴

In the place of such system-building he proposed 'a pure philosophical empiricism'.⁴⁵

Bartlett's critics and admirers alike agreed that his was a radical book, one that held up the banner of the Paris School as the standard under which the medical profession would, once and for all time, revolt against the spirit of system. Critics denounced him for slighting Bacon and accused him of being 'blinded by his ardor to demolish speculative theories'.⁴⁶ On the other hand, supporters, many among them physicians who had spent time in Paris, applauded his singleminded zeal. The Paris-experienced Alabama physician Josiah Clark Nott, for example, reviewed it as 'the most remarkable medical book yet written in this country'. By undermining the 'hypothetical explanations' and 'baseless visions' of rationalistic systems, Bartlett had shown that 'Galenism, Cullenism, Brownism, Rushism, Broussaism, like Cookeism and Thompsonism now stand only as monuments of the fallacy and madness of human reason; because they are hypothetical explanations of facts, and not legitimate deductions from them'.⁴⁷ Stillé made a similar appraisal of the book, privately in a letter to the Boston pupil of the Paris School George C. Shattuck jr, recognising in Bartlett's arguments 'those of my own medical creed, & of yours, & of all of us who have been brought up in the school of that "Prince of medical logicians" Louis'. He continued:

> [Bartlett] has settled the question whether a priori reasoning can discover new truths in medicine. His work should be considered a sufficient answer to hypothesis-mongers of all sorts whether within or without the medical profession. Its style is clear, correct, and logical; it shows a thorough mastery of his subjects, a love of truth for its own sake, and a certain dignified inflexibility becoming one who has undertaken to call to account the worshippers of idols.⁴⁸

Yet, like other American physicians who shared his Parisian faith, however much Bartlett celebrated the radical newness of Parisian epistemology, he also pointed back towards Hippocrates. Accordingly, despite Bartlett's energetic advocacy of the numerical method of Louis (to whom he dedicated his *Philosophy of Medical Science*), Bartlett explained in a footnote:

I have devoted no separate chapter to a formal exposition of what has been called the 'numerical' method of observation. The reason of this omission must be obvious to every reader of my book.

As he continued:

This method is no new thing. Its elements are as old as Hippocrates: and there is hardly an individual writer on practical medicine, of any authority or importance, from his period to our own – including those who have been most unsparing in their abuse of the method – who has not used it.[49]

His aim was not to diminish the credit owing to Louis, but to insist that all lasting contributions to medical knowledge had been the product of empirical observation. Laennec, Andral and Louis, Bartlett explained, like the first of such true observers, Hippocrates, 'imbued with the same spirit, guided by the same principles, and steadfast in their allegiance to the same doctrines, have resisted the influences of a fascinating but false philosophy, and have worked faithfully and diligently in their only true vocation, – *the study and analysis of phenomena and their relationships*'.[50]

Bartlett's celebration of Hippocrates as progenitor of the empiricist programme was especially clear in an introductory address he delivered in 1852 at the College of Physicians and Surgeons in New York, later published as *A Discourse on the Times, Character and Writings of Hippocrates*. His address opened with inventive and richly detailed scenes of the Greek physician at the bedside, tableaux calculated to evoke a distant time and place as much as to convey information. But Bartlett soon turned the attention of his listeners to Hippocrates or, rather, to what Bartlett imagined Hippocrates would have said had he been invited to speak at such an occasion: 'the Valedictory Address to the graduating class of the school of Cos, at the term of the first year of the 95th Olympiad.' He would have begun 'by warning his hearers against the subtle and dangerous errors of superstition' and perhaps of 'the system of his Cnidian neighbors,' Bartlett suggested. 'He would speak of the great revolution that had so recently taken place in the Greek mind, even then only partially accomplished.' Then, Bartlett continued, 'he would have warned his hearers against the seductive but dangerous influences of the philosophers', those whose systems were based on 'empty hypothesis and idle speculation' rather than 'observation and experience', and 'he would have shown that they had accomplished nothing, and that in the very nature of things they could accomplish nothing, for the real advancement of knowledge'. Hippocrates, in other words, was unmistakably cast as the first sensual empiricist, and was made to look as distinctly Parisian as possible. Indeed, in speaking by proxy for Hippocrates, Bartlett used language remarkably similar to that he used in his own *Philosophy of Medical Science*.[51]

But lest the slower members of his audience might fail to draw the connection between past and present, Bartlett went on to spell it out. Hippocrates, in the first volume of Littré's translation, *Ancient Medicine*, had exposed the errors of the 'speculative philosophers', those whose 'system ... consisted in vague, shadowy, hypothetical, *à priori* speculations and conjectures'. As Bartlett put it:

> The true character of medical science, and of these *à priori* hypothetical systems, could hardly be more clearly and succinctly stated, more logically argued, or more happily and forcibly illustrated, than it is in this Essay. And this is the very question that still divides medical opinion – that is unsettled to-day, as it was when this Essay was written; dogmatic rationalism, on one side – simple, philosophical empiricism, on the other.

Framed this way, the French empiricist revolt against system appeared no less a revolution, but a revolution that could claim a return to reassuringly antiquated and venerable beginnings.[52]

The programme for reforming American medicine launched under the banner of empiricism, which was proselytised most vigorously by the disciples of French medicine but taken up by others as well, was far from monolithic. But three leading objectives to the reform brief nonetheless can be identified. First, by escaping the reign of rationalistic systems, the regular profession would shed those features of its knowledge and practice that had come most under attack, depriving anti-orthodox critics of their targets. Second, by cultivating empirical observation of nature, regular physicians would improve the character of their knowledge and practice, with the expectation that such betterment would duly win public favour. And, third, having undermined the attack on orthodox medicine, regular reformers would go on to use the ideals of empiricism and anti-rationalism to discredit their irregular competitors, thereby affirming the superiority of regular medicine in ways consonant with American values.

What remains a little puzzling about the programme to use empiricism as a platform for uplifting the regular profession – a programme in which Hippocrates was depicted as primal prophet of the empiricist faith – is its sheer durability in the face of a discouraging paucity of social change. The antebellum decades did witness a substantial transformation in orthodox medical thought and practice – most especially a self-conscious move away from reliance on expansive systems of pathology and therapeutics. But signs that the regular profession's standing was significantly elevated as a consequence – the aim reformers so routinely and confidently proclaimed – were few. Only in the final third of the century would the extraordinary rise in public esteem for the medical profession that became so pronounced in the twentieth century commence, and, perhaps ironically, when this change did come it was linked to both a different programme for medical epistemology and a new relationship between epistemology and authority in American society. Yet, by and large, antebellum reformers did not conclude that the problem was intractable or that its potential was exhausted, and continued with undiminished vigour to proselytise sensual empiricism and anti-rationalism as engines of social uplift.

Indeed, the epistemological programme that Paris-returned physicians had begun to urge by the 1820s intensified during the 1830s, 1840s and 1850s.

However, the persistence of regular doctors in their campaign to bring professional uplift through epistemological change cannot be fully understood in terms of an operational account of a reform agenda that went largely unfulfilled. As I have argued elsewhere, the appeal of an ideal of empiricism must be partly ascribed to the social status of this epistemological position in America.[53] During the first half of the nineteenth century a shift from rationalism towards empiricism was evident in varying degrees throughout Western medicine; but the peculiar socioeconomic, political, and intellectual milieu of the antebellum United States redoubled the meaning that this epistemological stance held for the American physicians who returned from Paris and for other regular medical reformers who took it up. The ideal of empirical truth had particularly powerful resonances in the wider culture of antebellum America and represented a tool for unmasking fraud and imposture both within the ranks of the orthodox profession and among its rivals.

Antebellum society was beset by a fear of deception, and was paranoid about being taken in and exploited. On the one hand, an American fascination with trickery and masquerade made possible the success of P.T. Barnum and his self-admitted cultivation of the art of humbug. On the other hand, anxiety about deception and its social consequences in daily life was deeply rooted in American culture. Karen Halttunen has neatly captured these anxieties by pointing to the looming images of the painted woman and the confidence man as two archetypal counterfeits – representations of imposture and hypocrisy that threatened American society and were duly assailed. What these two imagined characters shared was a disregard for truth and a power to deceive through false appearances. The painted woman, more often a woman of fashion than a prostitute, seduced through the guises of extravagant embellishment and false etiquette not the authentic charms of natural simplicity. The confidence man also pretended honesty – a calculated forthrightness that was merely deceit – as the lure to draw in his victims. Especially after 1830, advice manuals warned boys and girls to guard against such disguises, but the greater fear was that American youth might themselves be transformed into practitioners of deception. What matters here is not the particular types of imposture this rhetoric warned against – Jacksonian political oratory, for example, was cast in much the same mould and portrayed its own roster of malefactors – but rather the wider preoccupation it represents: dishonesty, artificial adornment and calculated deception – all betrayals of Republican virtue – were threatening to undermine American society.[54]

This preoccupation with deception and its social consequences, pervasive in antebellum American rhetoric, was a central theme in the oratory and writing of physicians. 'Our age is one of imposture and unbounded credulity,' a student at an orthodox Kentucky medical school observed in his 1850 MD thesis, voicing a commonplace perception, 'deception & craftiness is the order of the day, and public sentiment and belief very unsteady'.[55] If quacks were dismissed as deceivers by their very nature, more disturbing were regular physicians suborned by the arts of deception. Overcrowding in the medical profession was identified as one source of the problem for, as orthodox leaders complained, it compounded the in-built trickery of quacks with a resort to trickery by well-educated, regular-bred physicians desperate to win a competitive edge. Orthodox medical schools, locked in competition, also succumbed to this malaise. As Stillé wrote from Philadelphia to Shattuck in 1848:

> The tricks, the falsehoods, the quibbles & equivocations, the downright frauds & moral felonies practiced by some of the medical schools of this city are enough to disgust an honest physician with his profession, and make him tear the diploma which confers upon him a title borne by so many whose proper place would be at the plough-soil or behind the counter.[56]

Indeed, as Stillé reiterated a decade later, he believed that, not just among doctors but among lawyers and clergy members as well, authentic professional knowledge and skill had grown less important than the power to charm by false appearances. As he pointed out to Shattuck, 'Learning, & science, & skill are but so many hindrances to professional success, unless their possessors combine them with the cunning & the impudence of the charlatan.'[57]

For many regular physicians the lament about dishonesty and deception in medicine was part of a wider lament about the condition of American society and its values. Politics, in particular, reflected the ills that plagued medicine. Complaining in 1840 about a country 'where commerce is synonymous with swindling', Stillé protested against 'the contempt for virtue and uprightness' that he believed to pervade popular politics.[58] Speaking before an entering class of medical students in Philadelphia in 1854, Stillé denounced the quack, the medical system-builder and the political pretender alike. 'The shallow politician, the trickster of popular favor, the great man's familiar spirit, the creature of accident, may sometimes glide into place and power,' he told the students, cautioning them that in medicine 'the way is not smoother than in the political arena, nor the rivalry freer from shocks and strategems'. He warned that:

> ... the smooth and plausible deceiver, the crafty panderer to the sins and follies of patients, the cringing sycophant of doctors of renown, the oracular expounder of solemn nonsense, – or even the insolent denouncer of all science, the dealer in shameless imposture, the trader in nostrums, the brazen-browed quack, in fine, – may plate his sins with gold, and be worshipped by the people, as was the golden calf of ancient times.[59]

As a Tennessee medical student stated pointedly in 1857, 'Most Physicians must have their hocus pocus upon which to ride into Practice as does the Politician into office.'[60]

Epistemological issues, then, were routinely expressed in an emotionally resonant idiom that spoke to anxieties deeply rooted in both medical and the broader culture. As Stillé put it in his *Elements of General Pathology* (1848), a textbook he prefaced with an essay entitled 'Medical Truth', this ideal of truth was a bulwark against 'metaphysical subtlety, the dreams of genius, or the frauds of charlatanism'. Its lesson was 'to abandon every hypothesis ... [and] to lay aside the pride of reason'.[61] His own aim was to avoid the false allurements of speculation and the false promises of reason, to avoid the temptation 'to speculate on fanciful analogies, rather than to extract truth from facts'.[62] In the rhetorical forms that became commonplace among regular physicians, epistemological positions became distinctly value-laden, with empiricism and rationalism linked not only to divergent ways of knowing but more profoundly to integrity and dishonesty respectively. On the one hand, empirically determined medical fact was rhetorically identified with sincerity, honesty, authenticity and, above all, simple, unadorned truth. On the other, rationalism was identified with deception, trickery, hypocrisy and fraud, while its fruits were framed as seductive, alluring and captivating, but ultimately false.

And, yet, everybody who practised medicine claimed experience as a sanction for their ideas and practices. Even those whom Paris-returned physicians denounced as the rankest speculators – be they a professionally eminent system-builder such as Benjamin Rush or a proudly unlettered anti-professional such as Samuel Thomson – confidently asserted that their medical explanations and interventions grew out of experience and were validated by success in practice. As one New Hampshire physician wrote to Bartlett in 1847, 'Sometimes I long for the appearance of a good strong-headed, fearless exposition of the medical twaddle which under the name of Experience, flows in such streams from the press.'[63] How, then, did orthodox American physicians make *their* empiricism different from that of everyone else?

The image of an empiricist Hippocrates proved especially useful at this juncture. Just as the American disciples of the Paris School celebrated the newness of French empiricism while at the same time asserting its special legitimacy by linking it to a medical tradition extending back to Hippocrates, so orthodox physicians in general, by laying claim to the tradition of Hippocrates, could affirm that theirs was a professionally respectable, learned empiricism, methodologically and morally distinct from the ways of the mere *empiric* – a longstanding synonym for the charlatan. This was important partly because it framed French empiricism as a learned, cultured empiricism, something to be scrupulously distinguished from the empiricism of the host of upstart medical 'empirics' who claimed that experience was on their side. Some regular practitioners resorted to terms such as 'scientific empiricism' or 'rational empiricism' in an effort to distinguish professionally respectable empiricism from its more sordid alternatives: the modifier 'rational', however, in this case referred not to any epistemological position but was intended only to indicate that this empiricism was reliable and proper, rather than irrational. Even if 'rational empiricism' seemed an oxymoron that confused rather than clarified, its use pointed to the concerted effort by regular physicians to assert their allegiance to a professionally reputable empiricism somehow fundamentally different from the mere experience claimed by their competitors.[64]

The adherents of rationalistic systems, regular and irregular alike, came to be caricatured as medical deceivers, and the assault upon them by reformers consecrated to the professionally cultured empiricism represented by Hippocrates and by the Paris School gained in force by being cast in the language of deception and honesty, imposture and forthrightness, guile and character. Rationalistic systems and their mystification of medical knowledge were depicted as forms of trickery dangerous to the people's health and the social standing of the profession. 'Whether it stalks abroad bedecked with false advertisements, or lies more concealed and domesticated', a Philadelphia medical student urged, such deception and disguise 'must be considered as highly reprehensible and injurious to the physical well being of the community'.[65] Conversely, stripping away concealment was held up as an intrinsically noble professional pursuit. Thus, having just read Bartlett's *Essay on the Philosophy of Medical Science* in 1844, Stillé wrote to Shattuck saying, 'Dr. B. has done Science much good by showing her naked to the professed followers, many of whom venerate the Queen less than they admire her artificial trappings, her rich garments, & her glittering crown.' Stillé lamented that 'her unadorned perfections have little charm for them in whom the inventions of Art have taken precedence of Nature', but reaffirmed the commitment he shared with Bartlett and Shattuck to 'consult Nature honestly' in the pursuit of unembellished truth.[66]

Much the same language was used to decry sectarians as deceivers – as (in the words of one South Carolina medical student) 'impostors and vain pretenders'.[67] In the United States one American physician reflected in 1847, 'quacks and charlatans' – as he collectively denoted irregular practitioners – 'live in a state of piracy against the world, robbing and killing all, who come in their way, or are allured by a false flag.'[68] The success of Thomsonian and eclectic physicians in competing with regular practitioners was likewise attributed to their dishonest cultivation of the arts of deception. 'Thomsonian Doctors', a regular physician practising in a rural Louisiana parish wrote in his diary in 1837, 'have totally infested the Country ... & by decrying mineral medicines have cast doubts upon the regular medical faculty & have succeeded in fooling the people & killing thousands of the innocent dupes.'[69] The public, in his view, were beguiled by these 'Root Doctors', taken in, as they were, by other confidence men.

In a similar tone of despair, in 1855 a physician in Texas looking for a place to practice without being suborned to 'the practice of a cheat' also wrote despairingly to his brother about the success of homoeopathy, 'more especially when almost all of ones [sic] friends turn to those who will swindle them the deepest with their infinitesimal delusions and arrant nonsense'.[70] Particularly during the early years of homoeopathy in America, when many of its practitioners were German immigrants, physicians tended to frame homeopathy as 'nothing but German mysticism', redoubling its image as a speculative system by linking it to a widely held caricature of the German mind: homoeopathy, as one critic described it, was the 'result of habitual modes of thinking in Germany, – the result of a kind of unphilosophical dreaming among a people who often show themselves incapable of severe reasoning, as they are almost always transcendent in the observation of facts'.[71] Thus the author of *The Anatomy of a Humbug, of the Genus Germanicus, Species Homeopathia* (1837) tellingly urged that 'Germany is the land most congenial to ghosts, goblins and devils' and suggested that homoeopathy – 'baptized in the magic waters of that country' – was a throwback to 'the reign of magic and witchcraft'. He proceeded to represent homoeopaths as foreign confidence men 'duping and deceiving the credulous', as beguilers who 'consider the Yankees fair game and an easy prey'.[72]

By the 1830s, a counter-archetype to that of the medical deceiver had become prominent in regular medical rhetoric – the 'true physician' or, as often, the 'honest physician'. The attributes of the true physician were the antithesis of those of the deceiver: integrity, sincerity, and success won not by trickery but by honest dealings. 'True physicians', Stillé told his students, 'present an example of pure and noble aims, and of devotion to knowledge and benevolence, which bring their inseparable rewards, a clear conscience, the blessings of humanity, and a sufficiency of the world's goods.'[73] Above all, true physicians were precisely what they seemed to be: not only were their minds unfettered by devotion to a system but they also professed medical beliefs out of genuine conviction and an allegiance to medical truth rather than artful calculation.

Many regular physicians found singularly useable models of the true or honest physician in the same empiricist heroes they looked to in propelling the campaign against the spirit of system, and for much the same reasons. Viewed in this context, the language used in glorifying figures such as Hippocrates and Pierre Louis, formulaic and repetitive as it was, seems unmistakeably calculated to depict them as exemplars of an emerging American stereotype: the honest or true physician. For the disciples of the Paris School, moreover, the antiquity of the one model and the newness of the other attractively reaffirmed the dynamic of revolt and return that characterised the empiricist campaign.

Louis, as his Boston acolyte James Jackson jr, described him in 1832, was 'the most respectable and honest *truth-seekers* of the age', labouring 'to *learn* and not to *invent truth*'.[74] Bartlett, on revisiting Louis in Paris in 1846, two decades after he had first studied in France, eulogised the French clinician as one who spent his life 'not in barren speculation, but in ... a love for truth, which no temptation can alienate, which no passion or interest can corrupt, and which no obstacle can turn aside'. Louis, as Bartlett depicted him, was the antithesis of the confidence man, an embodiment of those characteristics that best represented the true physician:

> If honesty of purpose, straight-forward, unbending integrity; simplicity of character, and the highest and purest combination of personal and social qualities, can constitute legitimate titles to our veneration and love, no claims can be stronger than those of Louis.[75]

Hippocrates, no less than Louis, provided a sterling model of the true physician. More than this, and in a way no modern could, he also represented the prototype of the honest observer of nature unwilling to obfuscate simple medical truths through artificial embellishment, rationalistic indulgence or calculated guise. His example and his approach to attaining medical truth had stood the test of time, enhancing confidence in their authenticity – with all the resonances that concept carried with it in antebellum American culture. Hippocrates was held up as a model of medical virtue, integrity and ethics, an image sustained by the link between his name and the Hippocratic *Oath*, a fitting exemplar of the true physician's character.[76] Thus, a medical student attending lectures at Transylvania Medical College in Lexington, Kentucky wrote in 1821 to his brother, still serving his medical apprenticeship in nearby Frankfort, advising that as part of preparing for the profession, 'you should read the Life of Hippocrates'.[77] At the same time, as the first standard-bearer of professionally respectable empiricism, Hippocrates represented the direct, honest, undistorting observation of nature that was the true physician's ideal. Empirical observation 'creates nothing, it does not even invent anything, it only *sees things as they are*, and discovers truth in what it sees,' Stillé insisted. 'Such was the genius of Hippocrates,' he asserted, 'such *is* that of Andral, of Chomel, of Louis.'[78]

The characteristics shared by admiring depictions of Hippocrates and Louis – including, above all, honest allegiance to the simple, direct, empirical observation of nature – were core components in a professional ideal held up for emulation by American physicians. Thus, Samantha S. Nivision, in her 1855 MD thesis at the Female Medical College of Pennsylvania, urged that 'as when the vail of the Temple was rent assunder in the hour of the great sacrifice, opening the sanctuary to all worshipers, so the penenetralia [*sic*] of each mind are opened, for the true physician'.[79] Joseph P. Logan, speaking to the Atlanta Medical Society in 1855, denounced both 'the fondness for *mystery* in the medical profession' and the pervasive imposition of '*humbug*', and went on to suggest that professional degradation could partly be attributed to the failure of the public to discriminate between 'the unscrupulous pretender' who embraced these deceptions, on the one hand, and 'the true physician' on the other. 'Notwithstanding the number of parasites and scullions who are hanging on the outskirts of our army, and have ever been a clog upon our march and a blot upon our escutcheon,' he told the gathered members, 'there is a noble array of determined and true men, who constitute an invincible phalanx pressing on under the banner of truth and philanthropy.'[80]

In depicting the true physician as one marching 'under the banner of truth and philanthropy', Logan invoked ideals so lofty and vast that they might be dismissed as having little relation to the often self-serving world of medical reform. But the assembled physicians who heard his words would have understood them to convey a specific message and charge. It was their philanthropic duty – an obligation of their calling – to disclose deception both outside and inside the ranks of the regular medical profession. As a student of Bartlett at Transylvania University wrote in his 1844 MD thesis on 'The Moral Responsibilities and the Proper Qualifications of the Physician':

> It becomes the duty of the honest and philanthropic physician, not only to adhere, *himself*, to the strictest principles of moral rectitude, in the prosecution of his professional duties, but also to use all honorable means in his power, to expose and suppress professional intrigue and dishonesty, under whatsoever garbs they may present themselves, and by whomsoever practiced.

He continued:

> It is his duty, as a guardian to society, to expose popular humbugs that are often gotten up in the profession. All such deceptions are, as I conceive, *dishonest*, and in the highest degree degrading to the medical profession; and lasting odium and disgrace should be branded upon the character of all who are guilty of such high handed imposture.... to detect and expose that monster in the profession called *quackery*, in all its shapes and under all its clokes of disguise [*is*] the duty of the physician as a philanthropist.[81]

Disclosing deception, as his mentor Bartlett had done the same year in his *Essay on the Philosophy of Medical Science*, was framed as a philanthropic act.[82]

In the American context, then, divergent epistemological positions took on distinct moral valences. Those physicians who advocated the programme of epistemological reform they had witnessed in France, and others in America who took it up, systematically associated empiricism with truth and rationalism with falsehood, implicitly identifying these polar epistemological positions with good and evil respectively. The homiletic language they so often used in calling for change, and the way in which they depicted such models as Louis and Hippocrates, aptly reflected both how they understood the task at hand and the wider meaning they found in this crusade. It was their conviction that epistemological programmes bore moral meaning that gave their proselytism a sense of moral legitimacy, beneficence and philanthropic selflessness, as well as an underlying sense of mission that was more than merely metaphorical.

Counterhistories: contested filiation and the competition for Hippocrates

To the account of history that depicted Hippocrates both as empiricist hero and as precursor to the radical empiricists of the Paris School there were also counterhistories, including a story some orthodox doctors told, not to celebrate the Paris School but to expose its evils and to denounce the revolutionary changes claimed in its name. Challenging all that the disciples of French medicine held dear, some American physicians asserted that the Paris School represented nothing really new and charged that its programme to reform medical knowledge was misdirected and dangerous. To them, French medicine represented not a source of salvation for American medicine, but one of corruption.

The denigration of Louis but a simultaneous sturdy admiration for Hippocrates characteristic of this alternative account is revealing. In 1838, for example, Joshua Flint delivered an introductory address at the Louisville Medical Institute that accused Louis's programme of misdirecting practice and sought to strip it of all meaningful claims to newness. Having just returned from a brief visit to Europe, he used the occasion to discredit Paris as a place for Americans to study medicine, to denounce Parisian therapeutics as feeble and, above all, to disparage French medicine as dogmatic, noting that 'their systems are equally remarkable for their multiplicity and transitoriness'.[83] Flint began with an exposé of the rise and fall of Broussaisism, noting with satisfaction that François-J.-V. Broussais's tirade against all the speculative systems of the past had proved to be nothing more than ground-clearing for a new system of his own. He then turned to 'Laennec and his pupils', who maintained 'the exclusive precision of their own method with as much pertinacity as if Hyppocrates, Sydenham, and Morgagni had never lived'. He continued: 'And now we are in the midst of another "epoch," as they are fond of terming their successive dogmas – the "school of observation," par excellence, better known as the "numerical system."'[84] He affirmed that 'the method of observation is certainly good – indispensable; but it is a desperate push for originality to claim it, or its application to medical studies, as the invention of any modern master'.[85]

'Neither is this numerical system, as some claim for it, a return to the Hippocratic method of medical investigation', Flint insisted, having dismissed its novelty. 'The sage of Cos, indeed, employed observation, but always with a view to some specific conclusion, and not in the *omnium-gatherum*, irrelevant manner of our modern fact gatherers.'[86] He went on to reassert his 'reverence for the method of the Novum Organum', urging medical students in his audience who were contemplating study abroad to choose the less 'dazzling and seductive' lessons of British teachers over the French, and insisted that 'the *numerical system*' was 'hindering the progress of rational medicine'.[87] He concluded by noting that 'not long since, a large portion of the élite of our profession had realized a charm in *Broussaisism*', and warned that 'a similar infatuation has since doomed another body of ardent and promising young men, to the tread-mill of *Numericalism*'.[88] Instead of liberating medicine from rationalistic systems, in other words, the Paris School was denounced as the source of new ones. Flint told his students that he spoke to 'counteract this propensity for system-worship, and to overthrow the idols it has set up', insisting that far from being a modern Hippocrates, Louis was 'head of a sect'.[89]

Likewise, in 1840, the New York medical professor Martyn Paine published a two-volume work, *Medical and Physiological Commentaries*, which, in the appraisal of Louis's Boston pupil Henry Ingersoll Bowditch, had as its main object 'a violent attack' on the numerical method and on Louis in particular.[90] Paine, for his part, proudly affirmed that he undertook his denunciation of Louis 'in protecting my brethren, from Hippocrates to the present time, against his almost universal scorn and derision, – in demonstrating the fallacy of the assumption that "medicine is now in its infancy"'.[91] Accusations such as these led the advocates of French medicine not to rewrite their account of history but to reaffirm it more stridently than ever.

Anti-orthodox physicians, such as homoeopaths, also contested the account of history that the American disciples of the Paris School proselytised, and in turn urged a different story about the medical past that informed a different interpretation of its present and future. They too believed that, in the early nineteenth century, medicine had reached a crucial turning point, a moment of potential liberation from the long-entrenched reign of speculation, indulgent theorising and misplaced faith in the authority of elaborate, alluring and ultimately delusive rationalistic systems. Theirs was a different sensibility to the past, however, for their explicit goal was not reform but revolution in established allopathic tradition – the complete overturning of the old medical order. American homoeopaths who, like their orthodox competitors, believed that the New World held singular promise in the struggle for freedom from the corruption of the Old World and burdens of its history celebrated what they claimed as their special mission. As one homoeopathic editor asserted in 1851, in the inaugural issue of the *North American Homoeopathic Journal*, 'It is here that the battle is to be fought between the Goliath of the Old Medicine and the young David of the New'.[92]

Homeopathic physicians did not speak with a single voice, any more than did their orthodox counterparts. Yet regarded collectively, what is striking about homoeopathic narratives of medical history is the extent to which a pattern of revolt and return constituted a central motif. On the one hand, the teachings of Samuel Hahnemann represented a revolt against the past, the dawning of a homoeopathic era out of what one Philadelphia homoeopath called 'the thick darkness of Allopathic ages'.[93] As another homoeopathic practitioner, William H. Holcombe, later told of his own battle against 'Allopathic superstition' in his conversion narrative, 'I am about to portray the struggles of an ardent and inquiring mind, whilst emancipating itself from the bondage of authority, and emerging into the light and liberty of truth'.[94] But framing Hahnemann as the father of homoeopathy and instigator of a break with the past in no way demanded the dismissal of Hippocrates as the father of medicine: 'that his work contains many crude and erroneous notions [is] inseparable from the age in which he lived,' Joseph H. Pulte, a prominent homoeopath, wrote of Hippocrates in 1853.[95] 'Hippocrates stands high in the opinion of all medical men, who, however much they may differ on other points, are agreed as to that,' Joseph Laurie, a student at the Homoeopathic Medical College of Pennsylvania, wrote in his 1851 MD thesis. 'They consider him as the man who first placed the study of medicine on its correct basis.' He continued:

> A learned medical authority has observed that he [Hippocrates] had the sagacity to discover the great and fundamental truth, that in medicine probably more than in any other science, the basis of all our knowledge is the accurate observation of actual phenomena.[96]

Indeed, while homoeopathic accounts of history ordinarily presented the law of similars as the new discovery by Hahnemann of a fundamental truth, they often depicted Hahnemann's allegiance to direct empirical observation of nature as a return to an older Hippocratic ideal. As Laurie, quoting from his own thesis, wrote in praising Hahnemann some years later:

> No practitioner better understood or more perseveringly acted upon the fundamental truth of Hippocrates, 'that the only sound basis of medical science is the accurate observation of actual phenomena.'[97]

Hahnemann had recovered what was to be valued and salvaged from the past, bypassing two millennia of allopathic corruptions to reinstate a commitment to empirical observation as the cardinal source of medical knowledge. In this scheme of things, Hippocrates was invoked not only as an ancestral figure worthy of veneration but as sanction for the primacy of homoeopathic *provings* — that is, tests of the actions of drugs on the human body – the empiricist method at the very heart of homoeopathic epistemology.

Hippocrates, Greek revival medicine, and the crusade for southern nationalism

The broad narrative of medical history was not told with a single voice even by those who shared a common discipleship to French medicine. While their historical account uniformly urged the animus against the spirit of system, it could simultaneously be adapted to the circumstances and needs of various groups within the orthodox medical profession, who placed history-telling in the service of their own particular ends. Nor did the theme of return to certain Hippocratic ideals that was a common corollary to their story of the French empiricist revolt necessarily promote a uniform plan for medical reform.

One powerful variation on the historical story that proclaimed medicine's liberation by the empiricist spirit of the Paris School is clearly displayed in the antebellum drive by southern physicians for regional medical separatism. Leading southern physicians, many of whom had studied in Paris, found in the account of the revolt against system and return to Hippocrates both support for their intellectual and political aspirations and a framework for defining their medical programme. In this case, an historical narrative shared by physicians in all parts of the United States was partly rescripted in ways that made Hippocrates a sanction of southern cultural separatism, the figurative cornerstone of a Greek revival medicine that could be used to support the larger crusade for southern nationalism.

Especially from the 1830s, and intensifying in the 1840s and 1850s, the Parisian call for empirical observation of disease that was a hallmark of the French impulse throughout the United States was echoed in the American South by a mounting call for the empirical observation of *southern* diseases. The starting premise, fundamental to the programme of the Paris School, was that only direct observation of concrete individual patients, at the bedside and at the autopsy table, could generate valid knowledge about morbid natural history. Therefore, southern physicians reasoned, with a logic entirely in keeping with French precepts, any authentic knowledge of the diseases of the South could be derived only from close study of the peoples of that region pursued within the context of its peculiar environments. A South Carolina physician who, in 1848, enthusiastically reviewed Elisha Bartlett's *History, Diagnosis and Treatment of the Fevers of the United States* (1847), went on to note that the natural history of 'our remittent and congestive fevers of the South' had yet to appear. 'Much original work remains to be done by those residing in malarious regions before a complete history of their fevers can be written. Their Louis has not yet appeared.'[98]

More than just a call for the study of southern diseases, however, this logic equally demanded the rejection of all rules for their diagnosis and treatment that had not stemmed from direct observation; it demanded, in other words, the overthrow of northern American and northern European authority over southern medicine. Overturning rationalistic systems and overturning northern authority, both equally misleading in the practice of medicine in the South, were projects that, in the eyes of many southern physicians, went hand-in-hand. Rejecting 'fashionable dogmas' and 'hypotheses' would be the first step toward preparing a treatise on fevers, one physician in Memphis considering such an undertaking told a Philadelphia editor in 1857, and in the process such a work 'would open the eyes of southern practitioners, and confirm them in the disposition now manifested by many, to cut loose from and declare their independence of, all northern and European authors on this subject'.[99] Expressing a similar animus against established authority, a New Orleans physician urged in 1856:

The day is coming when the folly of treating the diseases of negroes by books written by authors who have never seen a negro, and know nothing of his anatomical and physiological peculiarities, and who have never been in a cane or cotton field, or in a negro quarter, will be apparent.

That, he continued:

... will prepare the way for seeing the folly of treating white people, in a Southern climate, by the remedies found most appropriate for the same people in a Northern climate.[100]

Signalled by a revolt against authority in favour of empirical observation, an Atlanta physician asserted in 1855, that 'a new era has dawned upon the profession of Medicine in the South'.[101]

Like the broader narrative about the overthrow of systems, this southern story of revolt also invoked a theme of return. And as in the broader narrative, the return was to be to Hippocrates, depicted, however, to highlight not just his allegiance to observation but also his standing as a model southern physician. During the 1850s the most strident leaders of the movement for southern medical separatism, such as Samuel Cartwright, Erasmus Darwin Fenner, Josiah Nott and Alexander Means, used the theme of return in an account of history that was yet another way of calling for the overthrow of northern authority.

The 'true regular science of medicine', this history held, originated in a southern climate, the Greece of Hippocrates, and in this southern cradle it approached perfection. Constructed from observations of southern climates, constitutions and diseases, the principles of this medicine were matched to southern needs and remained suited to many of the medical needs of the American South. But southern medicine, boasting an unrivalled intellectual vitality at a time when, according to the New Orleans medical professor and editor Erasmus Darwin Fenner, 'London and Paris, Edinburgh, Dublin and Vienna, were in a state of barbarism', did not retain its dominance.[102] Medicine flourished in the southern latitude of Rome 'until', as one Atlanta professor told an entering class of medical students, 'the floods of vandal barbarism poured down upon the doomed city, from the plains of the North, and bore off upon their dark and turbid bosom, almost every trace of learning and refinement'.[103] The looted remains of an authentic southern medicine were taken to cold latitudes and, there, were distorted to meet northern needs.

Just as Hippocratic observation of nature had been subverted by centuries of speculative system-making, according to this historical account, so Hippocratic knowledge of southern diseases and their treatment had been corrupted when medical authority shifted to northern centres. Moreover, the medicine which some regular southern physicians practised in mid-nineteenth-century America, and learned though northern institutions such as textbooks, journals and schools, was not true regular medicine but rather a 'reformed' system better suited to the climate of the northern parts of America and Europe. According to this narrative, which was cast in a loose temporal framework typical of myth, medical sovereignty passed almost directly from Rome to Edinburgh, a city characterised as a cold, desolate outpost on the northernmost boundary of civilisation. There, medicine was transformed to suit the peculiar requirements of the Edinburgh environment; according to the physician and ardent southern nationalist Samuel Cartwright, 'a new nomenclature was there made to embrace the new order of diseases observed, new theories invented, and a new practice adopted to suit the diseases in that little hyperborean corner of the globe'. This reformed system of medicine was transplanted to America when pupils of the Edinburgh School established what Cartwright called a 'branch school' in Philadelphia and taught Edinburgh medicine until it attained national dominance.[104]

This reformed system, however, was a delusory guide for southern medical practice. Treatment, transformed as it was to suit a northern climate 'under the auspices of Cullen and his followers', one Alabama physician asserted, 'became quite too frigid for the ardent temperament and more relaxed system of our "Sunny south"'.[105] Therefore, adherence to Cullen's system, or to the system of any northern teacher, led southern physicians to practise in ways fundamentally unsuited to the realities of their region. Many of the therapeutic and social failings of the southern medical profession were due to their misplaced faith in an improper northern authority, a continual source of corruption, rather than on the observation and experience of physicians practising in the South. The lesson of this version of medical history was that physicians of the South could elevate their collective professional standing and regain for their region its position of leadership by throwing off the hegemony of a system of medicine never designed for use in the South, by studying southern diseases and treatments for themselves, and by restoring true regular medicine through an active allegiance to direct, empirical observation at the southern bedside.

As a stylised narrative recounted as a preface to calls for professional vigour and improvement in a region increasingly self-conscious and defensive about its perceived dependency, isolation and inferiority, this historical story served functions conventionally attributed to myth. It explained why medicine in the antebellum South occupied a degraded status and how this had come to be. Further, it encouraged efforts to develop or redevelop a distinctive, authentic southern medicine by demonstrating its ancient roots and modern corruptions. Like other master narratives prominent in antebellum American medicine, it fostered a campaign to seek truth and expose falsehood that had both social and moral meaning for reformers. Finally, it exemplified proper values for the professional culture, clarifying what was important, and set role models.

The message conveyed by this story about 'the father of medicine', moreover, was clear. Hippocrates was the archetype of the true southern physician, for rather than relying on established wisdom he observed for himself southern diseases, peoples and environments, developing morbid natural histories and therapeutic strategies appropriate to southern patients. As one physician told delegates gathered for the annual meeting of the Medical Association of the State of Alabama in 1855, 'Hippocrates lived in a southern climate, presenting diseases similar to our own, and his practice points out the true treatment of southern diseases'.[106] Southern physicians, in turn, needed to follow the Hippocratic example, recognise the distinctive character of southern medicine, and liberate themselves from the domination of northern and European systems. What those who advocated this revolt from false authority and return to Hippocrates envisaged was nothing less than a Greek revival medicine, confluent with other streams in antebellum southern culture, ranging from architecture to politics, yet informed by the epistemological lessons of the Paris School.

Conclusion

The variety of depictions of Hippocrates that were put on the market in antebellum America and the meanings attached to them deserve much more attention than they have received from historians or can receive in this essay. We need a much fuller mapping of the representations of Hippocrates Americans produced and of what, collectively, characterised those medical practitioners who promoted or contested one or another of these images. Equally, we need to trace how American depictions of Hippocrates changed over time (including periods that preceded and followed the antebellum decades), correlating permutations with broader transformations in the culture of American medicine and American culture in general. We also need to explore how other medical figures – Galen, for example – were represented, paying attention to shifting American sensibilities to Greek and Roman antiquity, as well as to the changing place of classical studies in revolutionary, early republican and antebellum American intellectual life. Precisely how much American physicians seriously engaged with the Hippocratic writings, and to what extent they merely appropriated a convenient image of Hippocrates for their own programme, merits close exploration. In addition, we need to compare American attitudes towards Hippocrates with those of other societies, a task this volume will inform. Finally, not least of all, we need to learn a great deal more about the telling of historical stories as a medical practice.

Writing about his fellow classicists rather than about medical historians, Meyer Reinhold proposed in 1984 that:

> ... it is now acknowledged that the *function* that knowledge of classical antiquity served should be our prime concern: how the classics functioned in early America, how Americans used, even misused and abused antiquity.[107]

In antebellum American medicine, the predominant image of an empiricist Hippocrates was actively used as a tool in promoting a wide range of reforms. The account of history deployed by the American disciples of the Paris School that has been my main focus here, but also historical stories told by homoeopaths and by orthodox southern physicians that I have sketched briefly, were designed both to persuade and reassure and to promote action. A recent empiricist revolt had broken medicine free from traditional authority, they all argued, and had initiated an ongoing battle against system (in its many guises) that would inaugurate a new era. Conjuring up the image of Hippocrates as archetypal empiricist could either soften the unsettling radicalness of the new departure, as was the case for Americans who celebrated the newness of the French empiricist revolution or, conversely, could radicalise calls for change, as in the example of southern separatist physicians who found in Hippocrates a sanction for throwing off the domination of northern and European authority. In all these instances, Hippocrates was brought forward to second calls for reform, sanctifying programmes for radical change by invoking authority that bore compelling hallmarks of authenticity.

In investigating the uses of Hippocrates, however, it is important to keep in mind that function is not meaning, or at least does not exhaust it. Hippocrates – who by the nineteenth century, was Western medicine's most renowned mythical figure – was an obvious candidate for veneration, and it is hardly surprising that physicians laid claim to him not merely by drawing attention to how they resembled Hippocrates but also by representing him in ways that made 'the father of medicine' resemble themselves as much as possible. Stories about Hippocrates were largely stories about identity – vehicles for displaying conceptions of self and for clarifying the social, moral and epistemological boundaries that distinguished self from the other. Furthermore, the peculiar preoccupations and apprehensions of antebellum American life – for example, concerns about authenticity and counterfeit, as well as about simple truth and deluding mystification – gave the divergent uses of an empiricist Hippocrates a set of cultural meanings that were shared by a diverse array of medical Americans. It was, in turn, the particular ways in which an ideal of empirical truth was valorised in American society that both empowered narratives scripted around the dual theme of revolt and return and gave such force to the representation of Hippocrates as an empiricist hero in antebellum medical culture.

Acknowledgements

Research for this essay was supported in part by National Institutes of Health Publication Grant LM 05013 from the National Library of Medicine. In some sections I draw heavily from John Harley Warner, *Against the Spirit of System:*

The French Impulse in Nineteenth-Century American Medicine (Princeton, NJ: Princeton University Press, 1998).

Notes

1. Gerald L. Geison, 'The myth of Pasteur', in Gerald L. Geison, *The Private Science of Louis Pasteur*, Princeton, NJ: Princeton University Press, 1995, pp. 259–78; L.S. Jacyna, 'Images of John Hunter in the nineteenth century', *History of Science*, 21, 1983, pp. 85–108; Susan E. Lederer and John Harley Warner, 'The memorialization of Walter Reed: constructing and reconstructing an American medical imperialist hero', paper for 'Medicine and the Colonies', annual conference of the Society for the Social History of Medicine, University of Oxford, 19–21 July 1996; J.P. Vandenbroucke, H.M. Eelkman Rooda and H. Beukers, 'Who made John Snow a hero?' *American Journal of Epidemiology*, 133, 1991, pp. 967–73; Loraine Ward, 'The cult of relics: Pasteur material at the science museum," *Medical History*, 38, 1994, pp. 52–72; and George Weisz, 'The posthumous Laënnec: creating a modern medical hero', in George Weisz, *The Medical Mandarins: The French Academy of Medicine in the Nineteenth and Early Twentieth Centuries*, New York and Oxford: Oxford University Press, 1995, pp. 189–211. Remembrances and commemorations of a scientific or medical centre can be analysed taking a similar historiographical line; see, for example, John Harley Warner, 'Remembering Paris: memory and the American disciples of French medicine in the nineteenth century', *Bulletin of the History of Medicine*, 65, 1991, pp. 301–25. Recent explorations of commemoration in science, which appeared after this essay was in the press, include William Ashworth, Jon Agar and Jeff Hughes (eds), *On Time: History, Science, and Commemoration*, special issue of the *British Journal for the History of Science*, 33, 2000; and Pnina G. Abir-Am and Clark A. Elliot (eds), *Commemorative Practices in Science:Historical Perspectives on the Politics of Collective Memory*, *Osiris*, n.s., 14, 1999. Quotation from Jacyna, 'Images of John Hunter', p. 86.
2. B. Bham, 'Notes taken on lectures delivered by Theodore Woodward', Lecture 1st, 1820, Vermont Academy of Medicine, Castleton, Vermont Historical Society, Montpelier, Vermont.
3. A.M. Cushing, 'Progress of Medicine', MD thesis, Homoeopathic Medical College of Pennsylvania, 1856, Hahnemann University Archives and Special Collections at the Allegheny University of the Health Sciences, Philadelphia, Pennsylvania. And see, for example, the assertion that 'the great Hippocrates has the honor of being called the Father of Medicine' in N. Bedortha, 'Medical Reform,' *The Water-Cure Journal, and Herald of Reforms*, 16, 1853, pp. 28–32 at p. 28.
4. John Redman Coxe, *The Writings of Hippocrates and Galen. Epitomised from the Original Latin Translations*, Philadelphia: Lindsay and Blakiston, 1846, pp. iii–iv. Coxe recognised the problem of authorship in the Hippocratic writings, noting, 'What actual portion of those writings that have reached us under his name, belonged exclusively to him, it is impossible to say. I should myself judge but few, and that one of his chief merits consists in having afforded them, through his writings, a "local habitation and a name"' (p. 19).
5. John Redman Coxe, 'An Introductory Lecture, in Vindication of Hippocrates, Delivered in the University of Pennsylvania, 3 November 1829', in John Redman

Coxe, *An Inquiry into the Claims of Doctor William Harvey to the Discovery of the Circulation of the Blood; with a More Equitable Retrospect of that Event. To Which is Added, an Introductory Lecture, Delivered on the Third of November, 1829, in Vindication of Hippocrates from Sundry Charges of Ignorance Preferred against Him by the Late Professor Rush*, Philadelphia: C. Sherman & Co., 1834, pp. 219–45 at p. 220.

6. See 'Attitudes toward Change', in John Harley Warner, *The Therapeutic Perspective: Medical Practice, Knowledge, and Identity in America, 1820–1885*, Cambridge, Mass. and London: Harvard University Press, 1986, pp. 162–84.
7. B.B. Smith, 'What of theory?', MD thesis, University of Nashville, 1857, Historical Collection, Eskind Biomedical Library, Vanderbilt University, Nashville, Tennessee.
8. Victor J. Fourgeaud, 'An Introductory Lecture on the History of Medicine, Delivered on the 23d December, 1845, before the Medico-Chirugical [sic] Society of St. Louis, Mo.', *Saint Louis Medical and Surgical Journal*, 4, 1847, pp. 481–96 at p. 482.
9. 'Review of *The Writings of Hippocrates and Galen*. Epitomised from the Original Latin Translations. By John Redman Coxe', *Western Journal of Medicine and Surgery*, s. 2, 5, 1846, pp. 485–515 at pp. 485, 497.
10. Quoted in Coxe, 'Introductory Lecture', (n. 5), p. 221.
11. Coxe, 'Introductory Lecture', (n. 5), p. 237.
12. Ibid., p. 245.
13. Elisha Bartlett, *An Essay on the Philosophy of Medical Science*, Philadelphia: Lea and Blanchard, 1844, p. 296; in the second quotation (italics removed), Bartlett is citing the words a British medical practitioner.
14. R. La Roche, 'Remarks on French practice. Communicated in a letter to Charles D. Meigs' (Paris, 28 February 1829), *North American Medical and Surgical Journal*, 8, 1829, pp. 293–318 at p. 298. On the context for this therapeutic reasoning, see Charles E. Rosenberg, 'The therapeutic revolution: medicine, meaning, and social change in nineteenth century America', in Morris J. Vogel and Charles E. Rosenberg (eds), *The Therapeutic Revolution: Essays in the Social History of American Medicine*, Philadelphia: University of Pennsylvania Press, 1979, pp. 3–25; and Warner, *The Therapeutic Perspective* (n. 6), esp. pp. 58–80.
15. 'Notes taken on John Eberle, lectures on the theory and practice of medicine', 3 vols, 1827–1828, Vol. 1, History of Medicine Division, National Library of Medicine, Bethesda, Maryland. Likewise, Nathaniel Chapman told his students, 'In the days of Hippocrates, the habits of the people were distinguished by their great simplicity; the climate of Greece was mild; & the remedies then used were a simple & more lenient kind' (Samuel Barrington, 'Notes taken on lectures given by Nathaniel Chapman on the practice of medicine, University of Pennsylvania, 1818–1819, 1820–1821, 1821–1822', notes for 1818–1819, History of Medicine Division, National Library of Medicine.
16. Fourgeaud, 'Introductory Lecture', (n. 8), p. 482.
17. Henry Gilson, 'Medical Science', MD thesis, Albany Medical College, 1840, Archives, Albany Medical Center, Schaeffer Library of Health Sciences, Albany, New York.
18. The larger context for the representations of Hippocrates that I explore here is drawn heavily from my book *Against the Spirit of System: The French Impulse in Nineteenth-Century American Medicine*, Princeton, NJ: Princeton University Press, 1998.
19. George H. Daniels, *American Science in the Age of Jackson*, London and New

York: Columbia University Press, 1968, esp. pp. 63–85; Theodore Dwight Bozeman, *Protestants in an Age of Science: The Baconian Ideal and Antebellum American Religious Thought*, Chapel Hill: University of North Carolina Press, 1977.
20. John P. Barratt, 'An Address delivered before the Medical Society, of Abbeville District, S.C. at their second anniversary, in May, 1837', *Southern Medical and Surgical Journal*, **2**, 1838, pp. 585–94 at p. 588.
21. L.M. Whiting, 'Investigation of disease', *Boston Medical and Surgical Journal*, **14**, 1836, pp. 181–90 at p. 181 (emphasis removed). See also C.D., 'Review of *A Treatise on Pathological Anatomy*. By G. Andral', *American Journal of the Medical Sciences*, **9**, 1831, pp. 389–419 at p. 389.
22. Alfred Stillé, *Elements of General Pathology: A Practical Treatise*, Philadelphia: Lindsay and Blackiston, 1848, p. 27.
23. Ibid., p. 34.
24. Ibid., p. 35.
25. Ibid., pp. 31, 163.
26. Lundsford P. Yandell, 'Notes taken on lectures given at Transylvania University, introductory lecture of Caldwell, 7 Nov. 1825', *Daniel Drake Papers*, Emmet Field Horine Collection, Division of Special Collections and Archives, Margaret I. King Library, University of Kentucky Library, Lexington, Kentucky.
27. John A. Lyle, 'Exclusive systems of medicine', MD thesis, Transylvania University, 1841, Special Collections, Library, Transylvania University, Lexington, Kentucky.
28. John Williams, 'Systems of Medicine', MD thesis, Transylvania University, 1842, Special Collections, Transylvania University.
29. Brett Randolph, 'Violation of the Natural Laws', MD thesis, Transylvania University, 1848, Special Collections, Transylvania University. A medical student in South Carolina urged in his thesis that ' "the spirit of system" ... has greatly retarded the progress of medicine'; but while he held that 'the spirit of system is a propensity belonging to the human mind', the modern recognition that the medical profession faced 'no greater enemy' offered hope in the struggle to overcome it: S.C. Furman, 'The impediments to the progress of medical science', MD thesis, Medical College of the State of South Carolina, 1852, Waring Historical Library, Medical University of South Carolina, Charleston, South Carolina. And see D. Bryan Baker, 'Medical reform', MD thesis, Albany Medical College, 1843, Archives, Albany Medical Center; and George K.G. Todd, 'Young physic', MD thesis, Transylvania University, 1848, Special Collections, Transylvania University.
30. Letter from Robert Peter to Frances Peter, London, 11 August 1839, *Evans Papers*, Special Collections, University of Kentucky Library.
31. Smith, 'What of theory?' (n. 7).
32. Austin Flint, 'Foreign correspondence' (Paris, 18 June 1854), *Western Journal of Medicine and Surgery*, **2**, 1854, pp. 89–99 at p. 98.
33. Gilson, 'Medical science' (n. 17).
34. Fourgeaud, 'Introductory Lecture' (n. 8), p. 482.
35. 'Review of *The Writings of Hippocrates*' (n. 9) p. 507; and see p. 497.
36. Eugene Henderson, 'Honorable medicine', MD thesis, University of Nashville, 1858, Historical Collection, Eskind Biomedical Library, Vanderbilt University.
37. Letter from [P.C.A.] Louis to [H.I.] Bowditch, Paris, 5 February 1840, Oliver Wendell Holmes Hall, Francis A. Countway Library of Medicine, Harvard Medical School, Boston, Massachusetts.

38. Marvin Meyes long ago made this suggestion in *The Jacksonian Persuasion: Politics and Belief*, Stanford, Conn.: Stanford University Press, 1951.
39. Erwin H. Ackerknecht, 'Elisha Bartlett and the philosophy of the Paris clinical school', *Bulletin of the History of Medicine*, **24**, 1950, pp. 43–60 at pp. 43, 60. See also William Osler, 'Elisha Bartlett, a Rhode Island philosopher', in *An Alabama Student and Other Biographical Essays*, London: Oxford University Press, 1908, pp. 108–58.
40. Elisha Bartlett, address that begins 'Gentlemen of the Class', nd, *Bartlett (Elisha) Family Papers*, Department of Rare Books and Special Collections, Rush Rees Library, University of Rochester, Rochester, New York.
41. Bartlett, *Philosophy of Medical Science* (n. 13), p. 182. On the distribution of the text, including three copies sent to Louis, see Elisha Bartlett to Gentlemen [his publishers], Lowell, 3 September 1844, *Gratz Collection*, Manuscripts Department, The Historical Society of Pennsylvania, Philadelphia, Pennsylvania.
42. Bartlett, *Philosophy of Medical Science*, (n. 13), p. 218.
43. Ibid., pp. 201, 290.
44. Ibid., p. 205.
45. Ibid., p. 224 (upper case lettering removed).
46. E. Leigh, 'The Philosophy of Medical Science, Considered with Special Reference to Dr. Elisha Bartlett's "Essay on the Philosophy of Medical Science"', *Boston Medical and Surgical Journal*, **48**, 1853, pp. 69–74, 89–95, 115–121 at p. 71; 'Review of Elisha Bartlett, *An Essay on the Philosophy of Medical Science* (1844)', *Western Lancet*, **3**, 1844–45, pp. 386–88 at p. 387.
47. J[osiah] C[lark] N[ott], 'Review of "An Essay on the Philosophy of Medical Science", by Elisha Bartlett', *New Orleans Medical Journal*, **1**, 1844, pp. 490–94 at pp. 491, 492.
48. Letter from A. Stillé to G.C. Shattuck, Philadelphia, 24 October 1844, *Shattuck Papers*, Vol. 18, Massachusetts Historical Society, Boston, Massachusetts.
49. Bartlett, *Philosophy of Medical Science* (n.13), p. 179.
50. Ibid., p. 178.
51. Elisha Bartlett, *A Discourse on the Times, Character and Writings of Hippocrates. Read before the Trustees, Faculty and Medical Class of the College of Physicians and Surgeons, at the Opening of the Term of 1852–3*, New York: H. Bailliere, 1852, pp. 23, 23, 24, 25, 25, 25–26.
52. Ibid., pp. 47, 35, 47.
53. John Harley Warner, 'The fall and rise of professional mystery: epistemology, authority, and the emergence of laboratory medicine in nineteenth-century America', in Andrew Cunningham and Perry Williams (eds), *The Laboratory Revolution in Medicine*, Cambridge: Cambridge University Press, 1992, pp. 310–41.
54. Karen Halttunen, *Confidence Men and Painted Women: A Study of Middle-Class Culture in America, 1830–1870*, New Haven and London: Yale University Press, 1982; Neil Harris, *Humbug: The Art of P.T. Barnum*, Boston: Little, Brown and Co, 1973; Lawrence Frederick Kohl, *The Politics of Individualism: Parties and the American Character in the Jacksonian Era*, New York and Oxford: Oxford University Press, 1989; Lewis Perry, *Boats against the Current: American Culture between Revolution and Modernity, 1820–1860*, New York: Oxford University Press, 1993.
55. Benjamin G. Bruce, 'Medical science, its improvements: and the spirit of progress', MD thesis, Transylvania University, 1850, Special Collections, Transylvania University.

56. Letter from Alfred Stillé to George C. Shattuck, Philadelphia, 8 July 1848, *Shattuck Papers*, Vol. 21, Massachusetts Historical Society, Boston, Massachusetts.
57. Letter from Alfred Stillé to [George Cheyne] Shattuck, Philadelphia, 5 October 1857, Holmes Hall, Countway Library.
58. Letter from A. Stillé to Geo. C. Shattuck, Philadelphia, 3 June 1840, *Shattuck Papers*, Vol. 16, Massachusetts Historical Society, Boston, Massachusetts.
59. Alfred Stillé, *An Introductory Lecture Delivered at the Pennsylvania College, – Medical Department, Philadelphia, October 13th, 1854*, Philadelphia: C.K. Kind & Baird, 1854, p. 13.
60. James R.R. Horne, 'Specifics in medicine', MD thesis, University of Nashville, 1857, Historical Collection, Eskind Biomedical Library, Vanderbilt University.
61. Stillé, *Elements of General Pathology* (n. 22), pp. 165, 166.
62. Ibid., p. viii.
63. M.C.R. to [Elisha Bartlett], Hanover, 6 September 1847, *Bartlett Family Papers*.
64. Orthodox physicians sometimes explicitly urged their colleagues to call unqualified healers and mountebanks something else. Thus, a medical student at the University of Pennsylvania wrote his MD thesis to assert 'the importance of Empiricism to the Scientific Physician' and 'to protest against the use of a word whose definition comprehends so much that is useful, and which defines the very foundation of true Medical Knowledge' – 'that word is Empiric, and is used in this sense as synonymous with Quack, Charlatan, Imposter &c.'. He urged that empiricism be reserved for regular medicine and, as for the irregular physician, 'call him ignoramus, but not an Empiric': Jamie V. Ingham, 'An essay on empiricism', MD thesis, University of Pennsylvania, 1866, Special Collections, Van Pelt Library, University of Pennsylvania, Philadelphia, Pennsylvania. For a fuller discussion of the use of the terms 'rational', 'empirical', and 'rational empiricism' in antebellum American medical rhetoric, see Warner, *The Therapeutic Perspective* (n. 6), pp. 41–46.
65. Sam[ue]l Clark, 'Medical science in the United States', MD thesis, University of Pennsylvania, 1820, Special Collections, Van Pelt Library, University of Pennsylvania.
66. Letter from Stillé to Shattuck (n. 48).
67. W.C. Smith, 'Remarks on empiricism', MD thesis, Medical College of the State of South Carolina, 1850, Waring Historical Library.
68. Augustus Kinsley Gardner, *Old Wine in New Bottles; or, Spare Hours of a Student in Paris*, New York: C.S. Francis and Co., 1848, p. 160.
69. R.F. McGuire, Diary, 1818–1852, Ouachita Parish, Monroe, Louisiana, entry for July 1837, Louisiana and Lower Mississippi Valley Collections, Louisiana State University Libraries, Louisiana State University, Baton Rouge, Louisiana.
70. Letter from J.D.B. Stillman to Dear Brother, San Antonio, [Texas], 1 June 1855, *Jacob Davis Babcock Stillman Correspondence*, California Historical Society, Manuscript Collection (MS 3126), San Francisco, California. The best known articulation of this theme is Oliver Wendell Holmes, *Homeopathy and its Kindred Delusions: Two Lectures Delivered before the Boston Society for the Diffusion of Useful Knowledge*, Boston: William D. Ticknor, 1842.
71. Charles A. Lee, *Homeopathy. An Introductory Address to the Students of Starling Medical College, November 2, 1853*, Columbus: Osgood, Blake and Knapp, 1853, pp. 30, 31.
72. *The Anatomy of a Humbug, of the Genus Germanicus, Species Homeopathia*, New York: printed for the author, 1837, pp. 8, 7, 15, 16.

73. Stillé, *Introductory Lecture* (n. 59), p. 13.
74. Letter from James Jackson jr, to James Jackson sr, Paris, 18 March 1832, and ibid., 21 October 1832, *James Jackson Papers*, Holmes Hall, Countway Library; and see ibid., Paris, 24 November 1832; ibid., Paris, 22 February 1833. 'In the notes of the introductory part of my course of Lectures', Stillé told Shattuck, 'I had developed the idea of Rousseau used by Louis as an epigraph, to this effect, that "truth resides in the subject not in us," consult Nature honestly & she will reply truly: – an idea which is the *Resumé* of Bartlett's treatise': letter from Stillé to Shattuck (n. 48).
75. Elisha Bartlett, 'Letter from Paris' (Paris, 4 May 1846), *Western Lancet*, 5, 1846–47, pp. 172–76 at p. 174.
76. A helpful study of the *Oath* is Dale C. Smith, 'The Hippocratic oath in modern medicine', *Journal of the History of Medicine and Allied Sciences*, 51, 1996, pp. 484–500.
77. Letter from Samuel Brown to Orlando Brown, Lexington, 20 January 1821, *Orlando Brown Papers*, Manuscript Department, Filson Club, Louisville, Kentucky.
78. Stillé, *Elements of General Pathology* (n. 22), p. 46.
79. Samantha S. Nivision, 'Priest of nature and her interpreter', MD thesis, Female Medical College of Pennsylvania, 1855, Archives and Special Collections on Women in Medicine of Allegheny University of the Health Sciences, Philadelphia, Pennsylvania.
80. Joseph P. Logan, 'Medicine as it is', *Atlanta Medical and Surgical Journal*, 1, 1855, pp. 1–11 at pp. 1–2, 3, 6, 10.
81. Richard M. Jones, 'The moral responsibilities and the proper qualifications of the physician', MD thesis, Transylvania University, 1844, Special Collections, Transylvania University.
82. As Josiah Clark Nott wrote in reviewing Bartlett's treatise, praising it for exposing evil and for showing the profession the right path, 'It tears off the veil which has been thrown over false science, and exposes it in all its deformity': J.C. N[ott], '[Review of] An Essay on the Philosophy of Medical Science, by Elisha Bartlett ...' *New Orleans Medical Journal*, 1, 1844–45, pp. 490–94 at p. 491.
83. Joshua B. Flint, *Address Delivered to the Students of the Louisville Medical Institute, in Presence of the Citizens of the Place, at the Commencement of the Second Session of the Institute, November 13th, 1838*, Louisville: Prentice and Weissenger, 1838, p. 20.
84. Ibid., p. 20.
85. Ibid., p. 21.
86. Ibid.
87. Ibid., pp. 21, 23, 22.
88. Ibid., pp. 26, 27.
89. Ibid., pp. 28, 21.
90. H[enry] I[ngersoll] B[owditch], 'Medical and physiological commentaries', *Boston Medical and Surgical Journal*, 23, 1840–41, pp. 73–84, 89–98, 106–10 at p. 73.
91. 'Dr. Paine's reply to H.I.B.', *Boston Medical and Surgical Journal*, 23, 1840–41, pp. 185–93, 201–10, 217–21, 233–39, 269–78, 329–31 at p. 235. See also Martyn Paine, *Medical and Physiological Commentaries*, 2 Vols, New York: Collins, Keese and Co.; London: John Churchill, 1840, and a third volume bearing the same title, New York: printed for the author, 1841–44.
92. 'Preface', *North American Homoeopathic Journal*, 1, 1851, pp. v–vi at p. vi.

93. J.H.P. Frost, 'Introductory address delivered at the opening of the Eighteenth Annual Session of the Homoeopathic Medical College of Pennsylvania', *Hahnemannian Monthly*, **1**, 1865, pp. 147–70 at p. 166.
94. William H. Holcombe, *How I Became a Homoeopath*, New York and Philadelphia: Boericke and Tafel, 1877, pp. 12, 4. For a more contemporary account of his perceptions and struggles, see William Henry Holcombe, Diary and Notes, 1855–1857, Manuscripts Department, Southern Historical Collection, Library of the University of North Carolina at Chapel Hill, Chapel Hill, North Carolina.
95. J.H. Pulte, 'Progress of homoeopathy', *American Magazine of Homoeopathy*, **2**, 1853, pp. 141–47 at p. 144.
96. Joseph Laurie, 'A thesis on the antagonism to new medical theories and to the doctrines of Hahnemann in particular. Presented to the Faculty of the Homoeopathic Medical College of Pennsylvania, March, 1851', *Hahnemannian Monthly*, **1**, 1866, pp. 227–40 at p. 230.
97. Joseph Laurie, 'Antagonism to new medical theories', *Hahnemannian Monthly*, **1**, 1866, pp. 280–84 at p. 283. See also Henry C. Knight, 'Bartlett's philosophy of medical science', *American Journal of Homoeopathy*, **2**, 1847, pp. 162–66, and J. Rutherfurd Russell, 'Homoeopathy *via* young physic', *American Journal of Homoeopathy*, **7**, 1853, pp. 134–36.
98. 'Review of *The History, Diagnosis and Treatment of the Fevers of the United States*. By Elisha Bartlett', *Charleston Medical Journal and Review*, **3**, 1848, pp. 171–85 at p. 171.
99. Letter from A[yres] P[hillips] Merrill to R. La Roche, Memphis, 15 January 1857, and Memphis, 15 May 1857, *La Roche Correspondence*, Historical Collections, Library, College of Physicians of Philadelphia, Philadelphia, Pennsylvania.
100. 'Letter from Dr. Cartwright' (Samuel A. Cartwright to Rezin Thompson, New Orleans, 15 June 1856), *Nashville Journal of Medicine and Surgery*, **1**, 1851, pp. 212–16 at p. 213. See also S.P. Crawford, 'Southern medical literature', *Nashville Medical and Surgical Journal*, **18**, 1860, pp. 195–98.
101. Alexander Means, 'An address, introductory to the second course of lectures in the Atlanta Medical College', *Atlanta Medical and Surgical Journal*, **1**, 1855–56, pp. 707–23 at p. 707. This section draws heavily from John Harley Warner, 'The idea of southern medical distinctiveness: medical knowledge and practice in the old South', in Ronald L. Numbers and Todd L. Savitt (eds), *Science and Medicine in the Old South*, Baton Rouge and London: Louisiana State University Press, 1989, pp. 179–205, esp. pp. 199–203; and from idem, 'A southern medical reform: the meaning of the antebellum argument for southern medical education', *Bulletin of the History of Medicine*, **57**, 1983, pp. 364–81, both of which explore the larger animus and expressions of the movement for southern medical separatism.
102. E.D. Fenner, 'Introductory lecture delivered at the opening of the New Orleans School of Medicine, on the 17th Nov., '56', *New Orleans Medical News and Hospital Gazette*, **3**, 1856–57, pp. 577–600 at p. 597.
103. Means, 'Address', (n. 101), p. 708.
104. Samuel A. Cartwright, 'Malum Egyptiäcum, cold plague, diphtheria, or black tongue', *New Orleans Medical and Surgical Journal*, **16**, 1859, pp. 378–88, 797–821 at pp. 380, 815.
105. W. Taylor, 'Annual oration', *Transactions of the Medical Association of the State of Alabama at Its Eighth Annual Session, Begun and Held in the City of Mobile, February 5,–6,–7, 1855*, Mobile: Middleton, Harris and Company, 1855, p. 120.
106. Ibid.

107. Meyer Reinhold, *Classica Americana: The Greek and Roman Heritage in the United States*, Detroit, Michigan: Wayne State University Press, 1984, p. 19.

Part IV

Twentieth-century Hippocratic Revivals

CHAPTER ELEVEN

Hippocrates American Style: Representing Professional Morality in Early Twentieth-century America

Susan E. Lederer

In the twentieth-century edition of his enormously popular guide to success in medical practice, D.W. Cathell and his son William offered practical advice to physicians setting up their professional offices. They stressed the importance of a comfortable waiting area, an airy consulting room, and at least two doors, enabling patients to escape the gaze of waiting patients. In addition to producing a 'snug, bright, and cosy medical tone inside', the Cathells urged physicians to ensure that the arrangement of the offices established the physician as 'possessed of good breeding and cultivated taste, as well as learning and skill'. The doctor's offices, the Cathells characteristically observed:

> ... are not a lawyer's consulting-rooms, nor a clergyman's sanctum, nor an instrument-maker's shop, nor a smoking-club's headquarters, – with a vile smell of stale cigars or pipes, – nor a sportsman's rest nor a loafing room for the idle, the dissipated, and the unemployed; nor a family parlor, nor a social meeting-place of any kind; but the office of an earnest, working, scientific physician, who has a library, takes the journals, and makes full use of the instruments of precision, and the various methods that science has devised for doing different kinds of medical and surgical work, and regards his office as the twin sister to the sick-room.[1]

Unlike 'quackish' practitioners who adopted such tasteless features of office decoration as 'grinning skulls, jars of amputated extremities, tumors, manikins, the unripe fruit of the uterus', the Cathells argued that a respectable physician could display the technologies – the microscope, stethoscope and ophthalmoscope – that distinguished modern, scientific medical practice. The exhibition of diplomas and certificates of society membership further confirmed the physician's credentials, but medicine's history could also be appropriated in establishing the modern practitioner. Portraits or busts and statues situated the doctor within a tradition of distinguished doctors.[2]

This essay examines how one of Cathell's medical celebrities, Hippocrates, and his multiple representations in the first half of the twentieth century served to define the public image of the ideal physician in American society. The Hippocratic heritage had long provided a source of both learning and solace for American physicians. In the early nineteenth century, even such indigenous American healing systems as Thomsonianism relied extensively on concepts that had been associated with the Hippocratic tradition since the fifth century BC. In his *New Guide to Health, Or Botanic Family Physician* (1822), Samuel Thomson often made reference to Hippocrates, the 'acknowledged father of physicians', in challenging the therapeutic practices of regular or orthodox physicians.[3] By the mid-nineteenth century, as historian John Harley Warner makes clear, regular physicians invoked Hippocratic medicine as a means of diffusing the disturbing claim that the science of medicine was only in its infancy. Through their appeals to the Hippocratic tradition, physicians sought to preserve what was best in medicine's distinguished lineage, while simultaneously advancing a new, scientific medicine.[4]

In 1882, when physician D.W. Cathell first compiled his professional manual on 'the personal questions in medical practice', he advised physicians to 'show aesthetic cultivation' in the arrangement of their offices, encouraging young doctors to make their offices 'fresh, neat, clean and scientific'. Flower arrangements, Cathell suggested, were 'pleasing to the eye', and also served to manifest the 'culture and refined taste on the part of the physician and those about him'.[5] In this first edition and in several subsequent editions, Cathell did not elaborate on the medical celebrities whose pictures or busts would further serve to mark the physician as a man of culture and learning. By 1890, the revised and enlarged ninth edition of Cathell's advice manual offered physicians a listing of the medical celebrities whose faces would enhance their professional standing.[6] Deleting his earlier advice about using flowers to decorate the office and reiterating the recommendation that doctors avoid displaying on their desks jars of amputated body parts and using human bones as paperweights, Cathell described how portraits and busts of Hippocrates, Galen, Harvey and Gross could be used to establish the doctor as one of a distinguished line of physicians. In twentieth-century editions of the book, Cathell, now aided by his son, continued to offer the same counsel about displaying medical celebrities and, in acknowledgement of the increasing importance of bacteriology, the two Cathells added French chemist Louis Pasteur to their shortlist.

In the early twentieth century Hippocratic medicine and the oath associated with the healer gained a new resonance in American society. For American physicians the revival of Hippocratism afforded both intellectual and material comforts in light of the rapid and drastic changes confronting the profession and the nation at large. Within American popular culture the renewed interest in the Hippocratic oath contributed to a greater public discussion of certain elements of the cultural crisis of the 1920s and 1930s, especially as they related to the professional character and integrity of the medical profession.

Material Hippocratism

The medical world of the nineteenth and twentieth centuries was made up 'not only of ideas but things'.[7] Such material objects as stethoscopes and microscopes functioned as both instruments of medical diagnosis and emblems of modern medical science. As the Cathells suggested, other things could be self-consciously deployed to establish the physician as a member of a learned profession. Through the acquisition and display of such material objects as flower arrangements, potted plants and busts of medical luminaries, physicians sought to create a particular environment for themselves as professionals and for the public, especially patients and their families who experienced medical care in this intentionally constructed space.

Statuary, especially busts of the Greek physician, made the Hippocratic countenance a feature of physicians' schools, libraries, homes and offices. In the early nineteenth century, Nathaniel Hawthorne summoned the 'brazen head of Hippocrates' in his short stories. In 'Dr. Heidegger's Experiment' (1837), for example, Hawthorne described the curious study of the singular old physician, which included not only an oaken closet containing a skeleton but a bookcase displaying 'a bronze bust of Hippocrates, with which, according to some authorities, Dr. Heidegger was accustomed to hold consultations in all difficult cases of his practice'.[8] In an earlier short story, 'The Haunted Quack' (1831), Hawthorne's character, a young man bearing the name Hippocrates Jenkins, becomes apprenticed to a quack physician, whose office, perhaps befitting his questionable professional qualifications to medicine, includes a few bottles of pickled morbid anatomy and a 'mouldy plaster bust of some unknown worthy'. In 1854 Hawthorne once again invoked Hippocrates in a story about a young wood carver whose skill in rendering the human image was such that no apothecary would set up his trade without purchasing a head of Hippocrates or Galen from him.[9]

In the late nineteenth and early twentieth centuries, as part of a neo-classical revival, middle- and upper-class Americans decorated their homes with busts of eminent politicians, artists, musicians, writers and other distinguished individuals. For the decor of their homes, hospitals, and schools, physicians and hospital administrators could purchase busts of Hippocrates of varying sizes and quality from several sources. The 1915–1916 catalogue of the Florentine Art Plaster Company of Philadelphia, for example, advertised plaster casts of reproductions from antique, Renaissance and modern sculpture for the interior decoration of schools, homes, and offices. Available for $2, a 12-inch cast of Hippocrates appeared sandwiched between novelist Walter Scott and author Mark Twain. Hippocrates was not the only physician available as a bust. The company offered two other 'fathers of medicine' for purchase – German physician Samuel Hahnemann, the founder of homoeopathy, and American Andrew Taylor Still, the founder of osteopathy.

In addition to busts, physicians had access to Hippocrates in printed form. Although such prominent physicians as William Osler and Baltimore gynaecologist Howard A. Kelly amassed collections of rare medical books and manuscripts including Hippocratic texts, a new two-volume English edition of Hippocrates from the Loeb Classical Library, published in 1923, made the Hippocratic texts both inexpensive and accessible to many physicians. The small size of this edition – the book could fit easily into a pocket – may have encouraged its use. In 1925 physician John Rathbone Oliver, describing an eminent Baltimore physician 'who never goes to a football match or a baseball game, without putting [the edition] into his pocket', speculated that there would 'doubtless be more like him, if the Loeb volumes were better known'.[10]

More costly than the purchase of books and busts of Hippocrates was the excursion undertaken by some physicians to the font of Hippocratism, the Aegean island of Cos where the Greek physician lived in the fifth century BC. Philadelphia surgeon William Williams Keen was among those who travelled to Greece where he photographed the plane tree planted on the site where Hippocrates taught his students. Keen returned to Philadelphia with tangible reminders of his odyssey abroad; he brought planks taken from the temple of Asclepius on the island of Cos, as well as wood removed from the floor of the upper step of the famous Anatomical Theatre in Bologna. In his autobiography, surgeon Hugh Young recalled his cruise in the Aegean in 1929, during which he visited Cos: 'Here were written those immortal works which for centuries were the foundation stones of medicine and still contain many golden truths by which we moderns may well profit'.[11] Like other medical tourists, Young described the great tree reputedly dating from the time of Hippocrates and under whose branches the great physician instructed his pupils. Physician Ralph Major made the journey to the island in 1934. As a medical student at Johns Hopkins University, Major had heard William Osler express the wish that he had lived during the fifth century BC so that he might have sat at the feet of Hippocrates under the old plane tree on the island of Cos. Thus, more than two decades later, Major made Cos his destination, where his 'first pilgrimage' was to the Tree of Hippocrates. 'The tree itself', Major informed his guide, 'could not possibly have been there at the time of Hippocrates, since these trees do no live as long as 2000 years'.[12] The guide explained that it was not the original tree, but a descendant of the tree under which Hippocrates sat. Such pilgrimages and mementoes of the journeys – photographs, leaves, or branches taken from the Tree of Hippocrates – provided palpable links to medicine's illustrious past and to the physician who had come to symbolise the ideal healer.

How did Hippocrates come to embody the ideal in American medicine? The heyday of material Hippocratism in the 1920s and 1930s coincided with a revival of interest in Hippocratic medicine in general and the Hippocratic oath in particular. In the United States, as well as in the United Kingdom, France and Germany, Hippocratic holism offered an attractive antidote to the cultural crisis of the interwar period – a crisis fostered by recurrent economic and social instability in Europe and America, including the Bolshevik Revolution, the rise of fascism and the worldwide depression.[13] Amid the bewildering social dislocations of the 1920s and 1930s, such leading American medical scientists as Walter Bradford Cannon and Lawrence J. Henderson identified the Hippocratic principle of the 'vis medicatrix naturae', the healing power of nature, as central to understanding both the human body and the body politic. The emphasis on organic stability in the influential works of both physiologists, as historians Stephen Cross and Randall Albury have noted, 'was in part the product of a peculiarly Hippocratic interpretation of the significance of physiological constancy, which in turn was nurtured by anxieties about social instability'.[14]

Within the medical community, structural changes in the profession, especially the growth of specialisation and group practice, encouraged the renewed embrace of Hippocratic principles – what physicians identified as the classical values of the profession. As urologist J. Bentley Squier explained in 1934, in a time of 'rapid and disconcerting' changes, the enduring values identified by Hippocrates, enabled the medical profession to stand apart:

> ... in the effort to revive our failing economic system, codifying every branch of human endeavor has become a national pursuit, but the medical code need not be altered for it was not reared on competitive gain. The moral debacles which have occurred in industry, public utilities, banking and so on, have not taken place in medical practice, and will never take place as long as physicians follow the precepts of the Hippocratic code.[15]

For Squier, the Hippocratic heritage provided a classical argument against collectivism in medical practice and for the integrity of the individual physician. These Hippocratic principles were malleable enough, however, to support very different positions. Writing on the economic organisation of medical care in the 1930s, economist L.W. Jones identified the resistance to group practice as contrary to Hippocratic ideals:

> The opposition of certain organized sections of the medical profession to all forms of medical service, however desirable from the point of view of the public, which threaten in any way the business of the private practitioner often emphasizes the un-hippocratic, craft aspects of medical ethics.[16]

Physicians appropriated incidents from the life of Hippocrates to instruct the public and practitioners about professional commitments. The dearth of historical information about the Greek physician's life did not deter such uses; even apocryphal stories could be pressed into service to make the point about professional ethics. American physicians – as did British physicians in the nineteenth century – highlighted the healer's detachment from material reward and his commitment to higher morality by retelling Hippocrates's refusal to serve the King of the Persians despite the offer of great wealth.[17] As one American physician explained:

> Hippocrates's disdain for pecuniary rewards was well shown in his refusal of a royal fee, tendered him by Perdiccas, King of Macedonia, and by his declination to go into Persia at Artaxerxes' bidding, even though he accompanied his invitation by 100 talents of silver and the promise of the gift of certain cities.[18]

Amid charges in the 1920s and 1930s that many Americans could not afford health care, the Hippocratic example illustrated the professional's duty to act in the best interests of their patients, without regard to their ability to pay for medical services.

The Hippocratic oath itself continued to be a particularly public and powerful embodiment of classical values. As physicians Samuel Lambert and George Goodwin explained in their popular book *Minute Men of Life* (1929), 'the medical student to-day, upon graduation, subscribes to a modification of the Hippocratic Oath, which, if not original with Hippocrates, embodies the ideals for which he stood'.[19] In 1935, also writing for a popular audience, physician James Warbasse noted how American universities administered the Hippocratic oath to all graduates in medicine. The oath, he explained:

> has been pledged by doctors in all lands through the ages. And now, after twenty five hundred years, it is still used in the medical schools throughout the world. I took it. My sons will take it. Medical practice has changed, the technique of medicine is transformed, science has grown into new avenues, but the fundamentals of ethical conduct are the same as of old.[20]

In fact, Warbasse overstated the extent of the Hippocratic presence in American medicine. Eben Carey's 1928 survey of medical schools in the United States provided little support for the popular view that all medical students routinely swore the Hippocratic oath at graduation, he reported that only 14 of the 79 schools he surveyed administered the oath at this occasion.[21]

If most schools did not formally administer the oath to graduates, the oath nonetheless appeared in various aspects of the medical curriculum. Carey noted that some deans mentioned the incorporation of the oath into medical history and medical ethics courses, or displayed it prominently and conspicuously in the medical school. Some medical schools, such as the University of Michigan, reserved the oath for members of the honorary medical fraternity, Alpha Omega Alpha, whose initiates were required to take it. Students heard references to the Hippocratic oath in lectures at schools where the oath was not part of the formal curriculum. At Harvard Medical School, physician Stephen Rushmore, addressing Harvard medical students on 'the Care of the Patient' in 1934, quoted precepts from the oath explaining:

> Though we no longer subscribe formally to the Hippocratic Oath we are nevertheless bound together by a common devotion, expressed so well in

those words which have come down to us through the ages, – according to our ability and judgment ... for the benefit of our patients ... passing our lives and practicing our art with purity and holiness ... with the seal of silence set upon our lips, so that whatever we see or hear in the life of man, which ought not to be spoken of abroad, we will not divulge.[22]

In 1935, Harvard students heard physicians James B. Herrick, the George W. Gay Lecturer on 'Medical Ethics', and Lincoln Davis, who delivered the lecture the following year, similarly invoke the Hippocratic oath as 'an inspiring document which can hardly be improved upon today'.[23]

The medical schools that administered the oath to their graduates preferred to use a version appropriately modified to American circumstances. In Carey's survey, he discovered only one school, the Women's Medical College of Pennsylvania, which administered a classical version. This reformulated oath did not invoke the gods and goddesses of the Greek pantheon; medical graduates instead swore by whatever they held most sacred. Statements in the classical oath against cutting for the stone were deleted. In light of the statutes criminalising abortion which had been enacted by most American states by the 1920s, oath-takers promised 'to give no drug, perform no operation for a criminal purpose, even if solicited'. These changes, as historian Dale Smith noted, enabled physicians 'to swear a meaningful oath and avoid a difficult and potentially divisive social issue'.[24]

Such difficult and potentially divisive social issues not surprisingly attracted the most attention from novelists, playwrights and film-makers who used doctors as characters in their work. In popular books and films of the 1930s, certain features of the Hippocratic oath received greater attention than others. Two precepts in particular had great appeal: the imperative against abortion and the injunction to keep secret things that the physician might learn in connection with his or her professional practice. The representations of the oath in popular culture suggests that issues of trust and character interested artists and audiences. At a time when the medical profession was rising in American popular esteem, concerns about the trustworthiness of individual physicians may have also been increasing.

The oath in 1930s popular culture

In 1933, playwright Sidney Kingsley invoked the Hippocratic oath in his dramatic play *Men in White*.[25] One of the few plays at the time to focus on hospital life and the professional activities of physicians, this Broadway production, which ran for 367 performances, earned Kingsley the Pulitzer Prize for drama.[26] Set in the fictional St George's Hospital, *Men In White* highlighted the conflict between a young surgical intern's desire to devote himself selflessly to surgical research and his love for a young woman. From the start, Kingsley called on Hippocratic images to set the requisite tone. For the opening scene of the play, the playwright's description of the hospital library called for ceiling-high bookcases, bulletin boards, plump leather chairs and tables strewn with professional journals. The playwright further specified that:

> Niched high in the wall is a marble bust of Hippocrates, the father of medicine, his kindly, brooding spirit looking down upon the scene. At the base of the bust is engraved a quotation from his Precepts: 'Where there is love of man there also is the love of the art of healing.'[27]

Photographs from the original Broadway production reveal that set designers used the bust of Hippocrates on stage. When Kingsley published his play in 1933, he prefaced the book with the Hippocratic Oath.[28]

In addition to the material invocation of Hippocratic idealism, the play explicitly addressed one of the ethical precepts of the oath – namely, the proscription on abortion. In a moment of weakness, George Ferguson, the surgical intern at the centre of the play, has a sexual encounter with Barbara Dennin, a student nurse, who becomes pregnant as a result. After a criminal abortion, the nurse develops sepsis and is taken into the operating room for an emergency hysterectomy. Ferguson's mentor, the kindly, if demanding, Dr Hochberg, asks aloud why young women go to butchers to solve their problems. One of his young interns solemnly reminds him that physicians and surgeons are precluded from helping these unfortunate young women. Although the abortion occurs off-stage, the nurse's emergency surgery is portrayed on-stage in what medical journalist Morris Fishbein described as the 'most authentic and dramatic operating scene ever put into a play'.[29] Despite the efforts of the surgeons to save her, the nurse dies. Her death leads Ferguson to renounce his marriage plans and to pursue without distractions the harsh discipline of a surgical career. His mentor offers him gentle comfort: 'It is not easy for any of us. But in the end our reward is something richer than simply living. Maybe it's a kind of success that world out there can't measure ... maybe it's a kind of glory, George.'[30] The playwright's reference to glory suggests not only fame but a higher calling. 'It is Kingsley's thesis', explained *New York Times* critic Brooks Atkinson, 'that medicine is a ruthless master. Those who take the Hippocratic Oath are embracing a religion.'[31]

Kingsley's explicit discussion of abortion linked the Hippocratic oath to a pressing contemporary issue confronting doctors and women – the increased demand and availability of abortion services. Historian Leslie Reagan has documented the pattern of expanded medical involvement in illegal abortion in the 1930s, when American women had abortions on a massive scale.[32] As the Depression adversely affected physicians' earnings, more became interested in providing abortion services, although the procedure remained risky for both physicians and patients. As part of his research, Kingsley accompanied a physician friend to the Bellevue Hospital morgue where he witnessed an autopsy on a young woman dead as a result of a septic abortion. Later, in 1995, Kingsley recalled how he had been 'horrified to learn there were more than a million abortions being performed every year in this country – all illegal and mostly done by incompetents in septic, crude circumstances'.[33] Despite Kingsley's horror at the personal and social costs of criminal abortion, the fact that the young nurse dies from complications of her illegal operation reminded audiences and theatre critics that sins of the body are likely to be punished, even by death.

Despite Kingsley's explicit discussion of abortion in the play, most theatre critics ignored the issue of the nurse's illegal operation. However, when the Metro-Goldwyn-Mayer studios acquired the film rights to the play, censors at the Production Code Administration in Hollywood insisted that all references to the abortion be removed from the screenplay, including such details as the use of the word 'peritonitis' which they deemed too suggestive of the failed, illegal operation. In spite of the censors' efforts to rid the film of its objectionable content, the Legion of Decency labelled *Men In White* 'unfit for public exhibition', and encouraged American Catholics to boycott the movie.[34]

Despite the difficulties with censors over the issue of abortion in the film, the studio publicity department specifically invoked the Hippocratic oath in its efforts to market the film. In addition to suggestive catchphrases ('Medicine versus Morals', 'Miracle Men! Ministers of Mankind!') and such novelty items as prescription pads advertising 'Men in White', the publicity department furnished a partial text of the Hippocratic oath for use by reporters. Identified as the 'keynote' of the film, the studio used the same version of the oath as Kingsley had in the play – one that did not include the explicit stipulation against giving a woman a pessary to produce abortion. Instead, the studio version offered the following: 'To none will I give a deadly drug even if solicited, nor offer counsel to such an end; but guiltless and hallowed will I keep my life and mine art.' In a more humorous vein, the publicity department made light of the fact that the set designers had encountered difficulties in securing busts of Hippocrates and such medical luminaries as Jenner, Metchnikoff and Pasteur in Hollywood. Publicity for the film included an article which explained how, at the director's suggestion, studio sculptors applied plastic clay to six busts of Voltaire to create the 'famous figures in medicine for the hospital library scene' in the film.[35]

In 1938 Edgar Dittler followed Kingsley's lead in using the Hippocratic oath to explore the medical profession's stance on abortion and other ethical issues. In a novel entitled *The Hippocratic Oath*, Dittler, a physician at the New York Medical College, focused on the experiences of a young intern and his encounters with the medical system at a large urban hospital.[36] The oath of Hippocrates, the book jacket informs readers, was formulated more than 2000 years ago and remains the code of ethics followed by physicians. 'Is it possible', the author asks, 'for a young man to remain true to this Oath when faced with the law of self-preservation, the lust for flesh, and the desire for success and prestige?' The author was not hopeful. 'The need for money and the urge of unfilled desires bring about debauchery and evil practices that inevitably leave tell-tale scars on character and destroy honor.'[37]

Dittler's book, unlike *Men in White*, begins with the full text of the oath of Hippocrates, which the author uses to examine a number of medical ethical issues that arise at the fictional Hippocrates General Hospital. In the novel, the tension between the proscription against abortion in the Hippocratic oath and the financial needs of young doctors receives special attention. As two interns discuss the framed copy of the Hippocratic oath on the wall of the doctor's lounge, one recalls that 'The dean of our medical school read it to us. Just in case we remembered to forget'. After Frank Durbin, the lowly junior intern and the novel's main protagonist, reads the oath's proscription on abortion ('in like manner I will not give to a woman a pessary to produce abortion'), his fellow intern advises him that 'Hippocrates was very old-fashioned. Either that, or perhaps in those days with the little they knew about sterilization, the interference with pregnancy carried with it a death sentence for the expectant mother'.[38] The same intern, newly married and barely able to support his family, goes on to explain that he has taken money for referring 'fair ladies of considerable means' to practitioners willing to perform abortions.

Durbin takes a strong stand against such referrals because of the illegal nature of the procedure. However, he has no such scruples about receiving financial compensation for referring parents desiring circumcisions for their newborn sons to a mohel (a person trained to perform Jewish ritual circumcision) at the hospital or about receiving similar kickbacks for prescribing surgical belts.[39] Although professional societies like the American Medical Association and the American College of Surgeons condemned such fee-splitting – 'the sharing by two or more men in a fee which has been given by the patient supposedly as the reimbursement for the services of one man alone' – the practice remained pervasive in the 1920s and 1930s.[40] The discrepancy between professed standards of the medical profession which strenuously condemned fee-splitting or rake-offs and the actual practices of physicians created significant tension in the medical and surgical communities. Although the Hippocratic oath says nothing about fee-splitting, Dittler explored these tensions over financial reimbursement against the backdrop of Hippocratic idealism, especially the commitment to place the patient's needs first.

In light of this professed allegiance to patient welfare, Dittler reserved harsh criticism for the medical profession's 'ethical or gentlemanly way' of one doctor not intruding in a case under the direction of a fellow physician. This practice, Dittler suggested, did not conform to the pledge in the Hippocratic oath to practise the art for the benefit of the sick; rather, such behaviour directly endangered patients' lives. In the novel, medical incompetence leads to the death of a beautiful young female patient. The young intern, compelled by medical ethics to remain silent about the blunders of his superiors, is required to obtain consent from the dead girl's mother for an autopsy in which the young woman is 'stretched out nude on a marble table surrounded by men and women dressed in white'.[41]

The book reviewer for the *New Yorker*, who described the book as 'frank and lively', was proven right in his prediction that 'the doctors probably won't like it much'.[42] Physicians did not enjoy the graphic depictions of issues of medical competency, abortion and questionable financial arrangements, nor did they welcome the portrayal of the hospital staff's sexual antics. Whereas *Men in White* had addressed the troubling issue of abortion in an environment blessed by Hippocratic wisdom and idealism, Dittler's novel portrayed medical ethics corrupted by greed and arrogance. The Book Notices column of the *Journal of the American Medical Association*, rejecting the novel's focus on the 'old question' whether a physician or intern could resist the temptations of money while remaining true to the profession's ideals, dismissed the book: 'Obviously there are a few that cannot, but the vast majority can. All the old situations of life and love in the hospital are here reflected without much literary quality.'[43]

Such old situations of life and love in the hospital remained intensely interesting to writers and readers in the 1930s. Three years before Dittler's novel, American author Sinclair Lewis had used the Hippocratic oath as both a title and a framework for juxtaposing the tensions between the personal desires and professional responsibilities of physicians. In 1935 Lewis authored a short story entitled 'The Hippocratic Oath' for *Hearst's International-Cosmopolitan*, a popular literary magazine with a circulation, in 1931, of more than 1.7 million readers. In addition to serialising Lewis's novels, the journal published fiction by such popular writers as S.S. Van Dine, Agatha Christie, Lloyd C. Douglas (including a serialisation of the novel *Green Light* discussed later in this essay), and British physician-author A.J. Cronin.[44] Much of the short fiction that appeared in the magazine explored sexual themes and, despite its title, so did Lewis' short story.

Lewis had already extensively dealt with medical experience in his Pulitzer-Prize winning novel, *Arrowsmith* (1925), which featured a young physician's eventual triumph in his struggles to pursue research amid a series of material temptations.[45] In his short story, Lewis adopted a sardonic tone as he explored the dilemma of a middle-aged clinician who wonders whether the Hippocratic oath would prevent him from going to the police if he ever caught a patient in a murder. For readers perhaps unfamiliar with this aspect of the oath, the magazine's illustrator used large letters to identify the specific precept: 'Whatsoever in my practice I shall see or hear amid the lives of men, which ought not to be noised abroad... as to this I will keep silence' (see Figure 11.1).

Given Lewis' description of the saliency of the oath for modern physicians, the reader may have wondered just how pressing the physician's concern was. The oath of Hippocrates, the author irreverently observed:

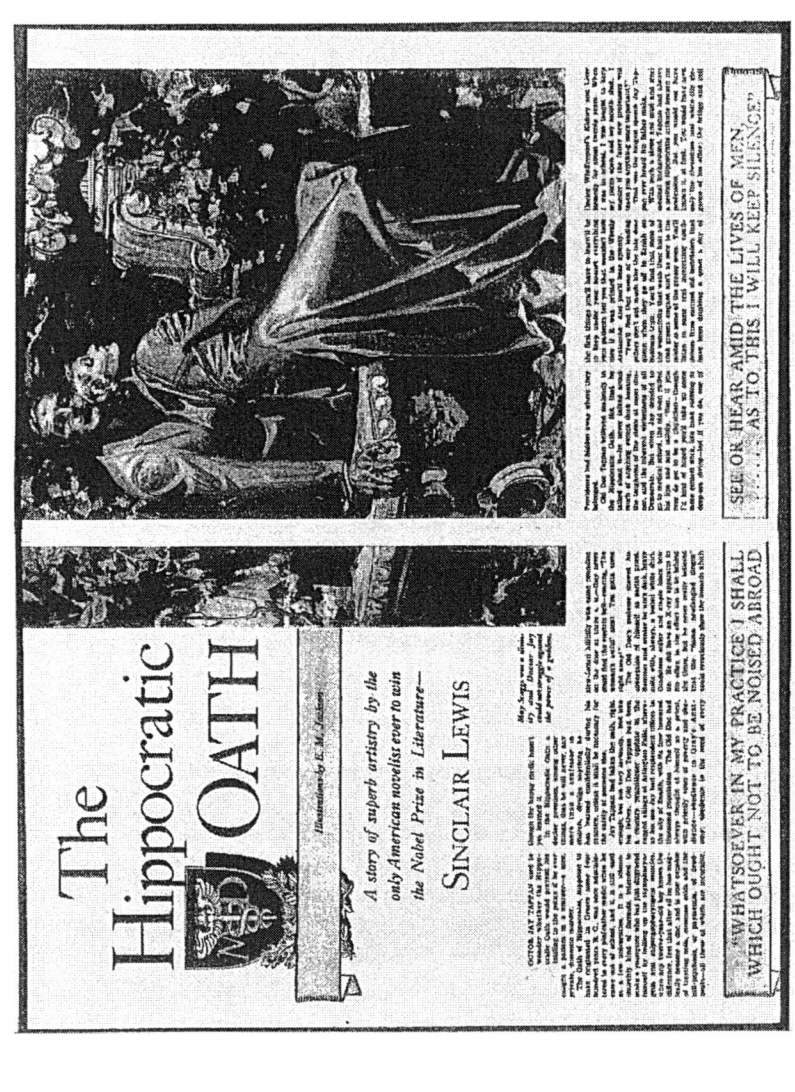

Figure 11.1 The front page of Sinclair Lewis's 'The Hippocratic Oath'

... supposed to have originated in Greece some four hundred years B.C., was once administered to every pinfeather medic when he came out of school, and it is still used at a few universities. It is a solemn, churchly kind of formula, intended to make a youngster who has just disgraced himself by balling up the stylopharyngeus and salpingopharyngeus muscles, when any twelve-year-old boy knows the difference, feel that after all he has magically become a doc, and is now capable of treating boils, common colds and the bill-psychosis, or paymentia, of dead-beats – all three of which are incurable, though the happy medic hasn't yet learned it.[46]

Albeit with considerable flippancy, the solemn and churchly formula gives the physician in the story the opportunity to evaluate both his professional conduct and his personal commitments. In the story, Tappan, who, the readers learn, had taken the oath at graduation but not very seriously, recalls that his father, also a doctor, had warned him that as a physician, he would hear much about his patients that wouldn't look very good if publicly repeated – for example, information about teetotallers addicted to patent medicines containing alcohol, about rich women mistreating their husbands, and about the conduct of leading pillars of society when away from home on business trips.

Tappan's dilemma about disclosing a patient's confidence initially arises in the care of 'the highest ranking pest' at the country club, a speculator in real estate and constructor of jerry-built houses. In the course of caring for the vulgar and unpleasant Scaggs, Tappan learns that this 'human sarcoma' is cheating on his wife – a woman for whom Tappan experiences a growing sexual attraction. Amid increasingly frequent visits ostensibly to check on his patient, Tappan fights the impulse to tell May the truth about her husband:

> Oh, it wasn't the Hippocratic Oath in itself that kept Tappan from telling May the sickbed confidences that would have encouraged her to seek divorce and a cleansed existence. In itself an Oath is nothing, as in itself a Cross is only a trick of ebony and silver, and a Flag a streaky swatch of cotton or wool. It was the feeling behind the Oath: that a doctor must never betray anyone who depends upon him, no matter how vile.[47]

In his musings, other features of the Oath receive consideration, including the clauses about a doctor's obligation not to bring harm to any house in which he enters and to avoid the seduction of women in the household. Tappan eventually confronts the injunction about killing, when he begins to fantasise about murdering Scaggs. Realising that his profession is more sacred to him than he had previously thought, Tappan resolves to kill Scaggs not in his capacity as a physician (which for a doctor would be so easy, in the slip of the knife on the operating table, for example) but as a private citizen. To his horror, however, Tappan discovers that his patient's severe gastritis results from the arsenic that his wife has been feeding him. After an ugly confrontation between the doctor and May, the husband informs Tappan that he knows his wife is trying to poison him. The physician, consistent with the oath, angrily refuses to allow his patient to die – at least until he pays his bill.

This story offered readers a somewhat different view of physicians and medical ethics than might otherwise have been expected from the title. Although he dismissed the oath on one level as a mere ritual, Lewis nonetheless employed it to symbolise the ethical standards of the medical profession and to explore the tension between these professed standards and the temptations experienced by fallible human beings in their daily lives.

In contrast to Lewis' use of the oath to examine sexual temptations in medical practice, novelist Lloyd Douglas emphasised the tensions physicians experienced in reconciling professional ethics with personal beliefs. Published in the same year as Lewis' short story, Douglas's novel, *Green Light*, first appeared as a serial in *Hearst's International* before it became the best-selling novel in America in 1935.[48] The book was not Douglas' first foray into medical fiction. Six years earlier the university pastor enjoyed tremendous success with his first novel, the story of a brain surgeon who makes 'personality investments' as a form of private philanthropy. *Magnificent Obsession* eventually went through more than 50 editions and three film versions, enabling Douglas to retire from active religious duty to become a full-time writer.[49]

In *Green Light*, Newell Paige, a rising young surgeon, takes the blame for a patient's death when his surgical mentor, Dr Endicott, frantic after learning about the collapse of his fortune in the stock market, mistakenly cuts an artery too short during surgery. Endicott allows the hospital to dismiss Paige, who rages about the gap between the doctor's invocation of Hippocratic standards and his own self-serving behaviour:

> All that noble talk in his sumptuous library of an evening about professional ethics, good sportsmanship, the inviolability of the Hippocratic (or was it hypocritic?) oath, the devotion to duty that demanded precedence over any and all ambition – bah! – and to hell with it.[50]

Nonetheless, bound by the injunction not to divulge the shortcomings of a fellow physician, Paige abandons his career as a surgeon, and eventually ends up in western Montana, where he joins a bacteriologist seeking a cure for Rocky Mountain spotted fever and falls in love with the daughter of his dead patient. The novel ends on a happy note. Paige's mentor recognises his moral cowardice and reluctantly confesses to the hospital board that he, not the young surgeon, was responsible for the death of the patient.[51]

The American reading public avidly embraced Douglas' presentation of medical ethics and the details of the oath that bound physicians. Although, to some readers, the idea that Paige and the other physicians and nurses in the operating room would not speak out against Endicott may have seemed strange and even disturbing, Douglas offered a reassuring view of the higher calling of medicine. Endicott's failure to rise to the idealism embodied in the Hippocratic oath enables Paige to endure his own form of Christ's passion (Paige uses his own body in experiments with infected ticks, becomes sick, but does not die).

Like many of Douglas' novels, *Green Light* became a major studio film. Released in 1937, the screen adaptation, which starred popular actor Errol Flynn as the young surgeon, gave even greater prominence to the Hippocratic oath. In the dramatic scene in which the senior surgeon allows his young colleague to take the blame for the patient's death, the film-makers filled the entire screen with the Hippocratic oath chiselled into stone, gradually focusing on the specific precept enjoining physicians to keep silent about things they learn in the course of their professional duties. Given the prominence of the Hippocratic oath in popular fiction, film and in physicians' writings, it was hardly surprising, as physician J.G. Avery observed in 1936, that it was 'common knowledge that the public believes that doctors are bound by some such oath [the Hippocratic Oath] to keep their patients' secrets inviolate, even in a court of law'.[52]

In the early twentieth century, the Hippocratic oath and the Hippocratic heritage resonated within American popular culture, offering a standard by which to judge physicians' beliefs and behaviour. These popular stories, novels, plays and films did not expand the knowledge or understanding about the Greek physician as a historical figure, but instead served a symbolic function, linking contemporary medical practice and concerns to an illustrious past and a high moral calling. At the same time, the oath enabled authors and film-makers to explore the tensions between professional idealism and the actual practice of medicine. In so doing, such representations about professional morality in film and fiction influenced not only popular notions about medicine and medical ethics, but those of doctors as well. Despite its 'unsparing onslaught on the healing art as practiced in America', for example, American physicians identified Sinclair Lewis's novel *Arrowsmith* as 'their chief literary inspiration' for the decision to enter the medical profession.[53] Thus, popular culture and professional aspirations participated in a complex and dynamic fashion to create the public face of American medicine and medical ethics in the early twentieth century.

Notes

1. Daniel Webster Cathell and William T. Cathell, *Book on the Physician Himself and Things that Concern his Reputation and Success*, Philadelphia: F.A. Davis Co., 1906, pp. 9–10. For more on the popularity of these manuals, see Joel D. Howell, 'Making a medical practice in an uneasy world: some thoughts from a century ago', *Academic Medicine*, 72, 1997, pp. 977–81.
2. By the 1930s the Walters Surgical Company offered physicians a complete consultation service with an interior decorator to help physicians achieve 'a beautiful artistic office at a minimum of expense'. See Neil L. Shumsky, James Bohland and Paul Knox, 'Separating doctors' homes and doctors' offices: San Francisco, 1881–1941', *Social Science and Medicine*, 23, 1986, pp. 1051–57.

3. J. Worth Estes, 'Samuel Thomson Rewrites Hippocrates', in Peter Benes (ed.), *Medicine and Healing*, Boston: Boston University Press, 1992, pp. 113–32.
4. John Harley Warner, Chapter Ten in this volume; see also Warner, *Against the Spirit of System: The French Impulse in Nineteenth-Century American Medicine*, Princeton, NJ: Princeton University Press, 1998, pp. 174–75.
5. D.W. Cathell, *The Physician Himself And What He Should Add to the Strictly Scientific*, Baltimore: Cushings and Bailey, 1882, pp. 10–11.
6. D.W. Cathell, *Book on the Physician Himself and Things that Concern His Reputation and Success*, Philadelphia: F.A. Davis, 1890.
7. Colleen McDannell, *Material Christianity: Religion and Popular Culture in America*, New Haven, CT: Yale University Press, 1995, p. 2.
8. Nathaniel Hawthorne, 'Dr. Heidegger's Experiment', in *Hawthorne's Short Stories*, ed. Louis B. Salomon, New York: Dodd, Mead & Co., 1962, pp. 99–107 at p. 100.
9. Nathaniel Hawthorne, 'The Haunted Quack' (1831), *Tales of Honor*, Boston: E. Littlefield, 1840 and 'Drowne's Wooden Image', from *Mosses from an Old Manse* (1854), ed. George Parsons Lathrop, Boston: Houghton Mifflin, 1883.
10. John Rathbone Oliver, ' "Hippocrates": a medico-historical note on the Howard A. Kelly collection', *Bulletin of the Johns Hopkins Hospital*, **37**, 1925, pp. 189–202 at p. 201.
11. Hugh Young, *A Surgeon's Autobiography*, New York: Harcourt Brace, 1940, p. 406.
12. Ralph H. Majors, 'Hippocrates and the island of Cos', *Yale Journal of Biology and Medicine*, **14**, 1941–42, pp. 1–11 at p. 7.
13. See the essays by George Weisz, David Cantor and Carsten Timmerman, Chapters 12, 13 and 14, in this volume.
14. Stephen J. Cross and William R. Albury, 'Walter B. Cannon, L.J. Henderson, and the organic analogy', *Osiris*, **3**, 1987, pp. 165–92 at pp. 187–88. For a recent challenge to their interpretation, see Allan Young, 'Walter Cannon and the psychophysiology of fear', in Christopher Lawrence and George Weisz (eds), *Greater than the Parts: Holism in Biomedicine, 1920–1950*, Oxford: Oxford University Press, 1998, pp. 234–56.
15. J. Bentley Squier, 'The Hippocratic code and the new deal', *Surgery, Gynecology, and Obstetrics*, **58**, 1934, pp. 407–9 at p. 407.
16. Quoted in 'Study Guide to Men in White', Human Relations Series of Films, Commission on Human Relations, Progressive Education Association, New York City, 1939.
17. See Jody Rubin Pinault, *Hippocratic Lives and Legends*, Leiden: E.J. Brill, 1992 for details about the legends surrounding the life of Hippocrates.
18. 'The Boston medical library: Hippocrates', *New England Journal of Medicine*, **204**, 1931, pp. 569–71 at p. 570.
19. Samuel W. Lambert and George M. Goodwin, *Minute Men of Life*, New York: Grosset and Dunlap,1929, p. 24.
20. James P. Warbasse, *The Doctor and the Public*, New York: Paul B. Hoeber, 1935, p. 70. The frontispiece of the book features a photograph of a bust of Hippocrates.
21. Eben Carey, 'The formal use of the Hippocratic Oath for medical students at commencement exercises', *Bulletin of the Association of American Medical Colleges*, **3**, 1928, pp. 159–66.
22. Stephen Rushmore, 'The care of the patient as the religion of the physician', *New England Journal of Medicine*, **211**, 1934, pp. 1081–87 at p. 1187.
23. James B. Herrick, 'The George W. Gay lecture on "medical ethics"', *New*

England Journal of Medicine, **214**, 1936, pp. 9–15; and Lincoln Davis, 'George Washington Gay Lecture: medical ethics and the art and practice of medicine', New England Journal of Medicine, **217**, 1936, pp. 206–12 at p. 206.
24. Dale C. Smith, 'The Hippocratic oath and modern medicine', Journal of the History of Medicine, **51**, 1996, pp. 484–500 at p. 494.
25. Estelle Manette Raben, '*Men in White* and *Yellow Jack* as Mirrors of the Medical Profession', Literature and Medicine, **12**, 1993, pp. 19–41.
26. Nena Couch (ed.), Sidney Kingsley: Five Prizewinning Plays, Columbus: Ohio State University Press, 1995, pp. xvii.
27. Sidney Kingsley, Men in White, in Three Plays about Doctors, ed. Joseph Mersand, New York: Washington Square Press, 1961, p. 101.
28. Raben, '*Men In White*' (n. 25), p. 30.
29. Morris Fishbein, 'New books on health: *Men in White*', Hygeia, **12**, 1934, pp. 358–60. Physician George W. Corner praised *Men in White* as 'the best play about doctors'; see 'Medicine in the modern drama', Annals of Medical History, **10**, 1938, pp. 309–17.
30. *Men in White* is briefly discussed in Edward Shorter, Bedside Manners: The Troubled History of Doctors and Patients, New York: Simon and Schuster, 1985, pp. 135–36.
31. Brooks Atkinson, 'Men of medicine', New York Times 27 September 1933; and 'Medicine men', ibid., 1 October 1933.
32. Leslie J. Reagan, When Abortion was a Crime: Women, Medicine, and Law in the United States, 1867–1973, Berkeley: University of California Press, 1997, p. 133.
33. Couch, Sidney Kingsley (n. 26), p. 6.
34. Susan E. Lederer, 'Repellent subjects: Hollywood censorship and surgical images in the 1930s', Literature and Medicine, **17**, 1998, pp. 91–113. Both the play and the film were banned in Nazi Germany as 'not consistent with Nazi philosophy'.
35. Studio Publicity, Men in White file, Margaret Herrick Library, Academy of Motion Pictures Arts and Sciences, Beverly Hills, California.
36. Dittler is identified in an article published with Thomas H. McGavack, 'Pancreatic necrosis associated with auricular fibrillation and flutter', American Heart Journal, **16**, 1938, p. 354.
37. Edgar Dittler, The Hippocratic Oath, New York: Liveright Publishing Company, 1938, jacket cover.
38. Ibid., pp. 179–80.
39. Ibid., p. 187.
40. Marc A. Rodwin, Medicine, Money, and Morals: Physicians' Conflicts of Interest, Oxford: Oxford University Press, 1993, p. 25.
41. Dittler, Oath (n. 37), p. 71.
42. 'Books: "The Hippocratic Oath"', New Yorker, 7 May 1938, p. 94.
43. 'The Hippocratic Oath', Journal of the American Medical Association, **113**, 1939, p. 1158.
44. Frank Luther Mott, A History of American Magazines, Cambridge, MA: Harvard University Press, 1968, Vol. 5, pp. 502–5.
45. 'Martin Arrowsmith: the scientist as hero', in Charles E. Rosenberg, No Other Gods: On Science and American Social Thought, Baltimore: Johns Hopkins University Press, 1976, pp. 123–32.
46. Sinclair Lewis, 'The Hippocratic Oath', Hearst's International-Cosmopolitan June 1935, p. 24.
47. Ibid., p. 161.
48. Lloyd C. Douglas's Green Light, Boston and New York: Houghton Mifflin, 1935,

was the best-selling novel of that year (using bookstore data); see Frank Luther Mott, *Golden Multitudes*, New York: MacMillan Company, 1947, p. 281. Mott characterised 1930s readers as 'weary of strident rebellion, and more tolerant of bolder comment on sex and criticism of entrenched ideas' (pp. 253–54).
49. It is more than a little surprising that given the vast popularity of Douglas' medical and religious fiction (he also published *The Robe* in 1942, which led the bestseller list for three years before becoming a successful film) that he has received so little critical attention. For biographical information, see Virginia Douglas Dawson and Betty Douglas Wilson, *The Shape of Sunday: An Intimate Biography of Lloyd C. Douglas*, Boston: Houghton Mifflin Co., 1952.
50. Douglas, *Green Light*, (n. 48) p. 24.
51. Apparently Douglas's prospective son-in-law, a mining engineer, suggested Rocky Mountain spotted fever for the 'spectacular scientific climax' needed for the book. Douglas read Paul de Kruif's *Men Against Death* for some of the details he used in the novel; see Dawson and Wilson, *The Shape of Sunday* (n. 49), pp. 266–67.
52. J.G. Avery, 'The oath of Hippocrates and its use at the present day', *Medical Journal of Australia*, 1, 1936, pp. 299–303 at p. 301.
53. See Henry Longan Stuart, 'House call', *New York Times*, 8 March 1925; Joanne Trautmann, 'Medical ethics in literature', in *Encyclopedia of Bioethics*, New York: Free Press, 1978, Vol. 3, pp. 1008–15 at p. 1012.

CHAPTER TWELVE

Hippocrates, Holism and Humanism in Interwar France

George Weisz

This essay explores the various meanings of Hippocratism in France and particularly the growing identification of that term with a certain kind of medical holism. As the various essays in this book collectively demonstrate, Hippocrates has, in the course of history, been identified with and made to represent a bewildering variety of medical values and ideologies. Much the same was true in France during the nineteenth century when many different readings and representations of Hippocrates coexisted easily, if not always peacefully. I will briefly illustrate this nineteenth-century pluralism of meanings before concentrating on the twentieth-century appropriation by French holists of the 'father of medicine'.

I began this project by creating a bibliography of all French-language works published between 1800 and 1959 that include the words 'Hippocrates' or 'Hippocratic' somewhere in their title or subtitle. By examining the holdings of many libraries[1] as well as citations and bibliographies in publications examined, I came up with 148 titles published in France (and, in one or two cases, Belgium) during this 150-year period.[2] There are many difficulties associated with a source of this type, starting with the fact that works dealing with Hippocrates do not necessarily announce this fact in their title. At best, such a bibliography is, like the visible part of an iceberg, a guide to material that is largely hidden.[3] Furthermore, entries in a library's catalogue can vary from an individual reprint of a journal article to periodicals appearing over an extended period and multivolume collections. Despite such disparities, I decided at the outset to simply count *entries* as they appeared in catalogues. (Different editions of a work were counted separately if the dates of publication differed.) The results, while not susceptible to multiple regression analysis, are remarkably clear and are summarised in Figure 12.1.

To briefly recapitulate: there was remarkable interest in the reputed father of medicine or in his ideas during the first 40 years of the nineteenth century. Publication fell off considerably in the 90 years after 1840, rebounding briefly and spectacularly during the 1930s. More striking than raw numbers is the nature of the works that were published in the different periods. During the first half of the nineteenth century, the predominant form of publication was the

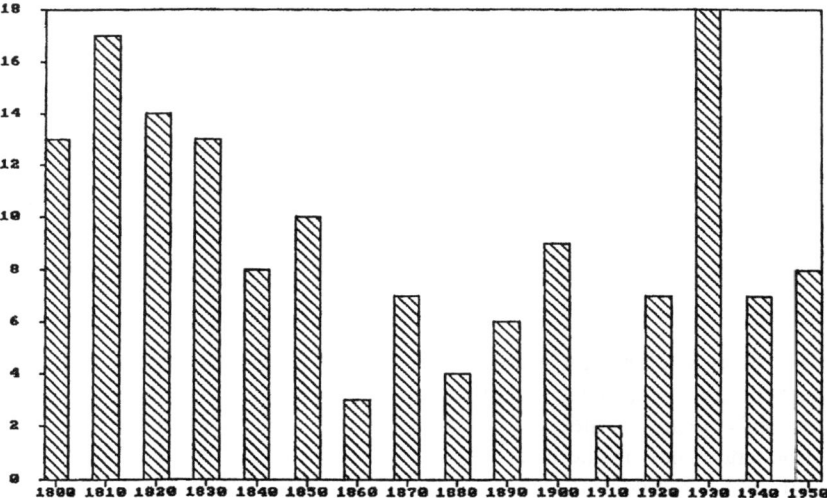

Figure 12.1   Hippocratic titles by decade

Hippocratic text, issued either singly or in various permutations and combinations. One reason for the falling off in the total number of publications after the mid-century was a decline in the number of such textual editions as a consequence of the gradual appearance of Émile Littré's definitive edition of the Hippocratic *Corpus* which came to dominate the publishing landscape.[4] Works published from 1850 to 1920 are very diverse including those defending specific medical doctrines and more scholarly literary and philosophical studies. But in the 1920s and especially the 1930s, entries referring to Hippocrates or his writings were predominantly ideological, reflecting the spread of a movement of holistic or 'synthetic' medicine that was rapidly gaining in popularity. In what follows, I shall briefly discuss writings on Hippocrates from 1800 to 1920 before delving more deeply into the meanings assigned to Hippocrates by the emerging holistic movement of the interwar period.

The long nineteenth century

Well over half the titles published before 1860 were entirely or largely composed of Hippocratic texts,[5] with editions of the *Aphorisms* being particularly numerous. Texts might or might not contain sections discussing and explicating Hippocratic ideas or doctrines. This pattern of publication undoubtedly reflects popular medical demand for classics that may well have been displayed rather than actually read. But at least some of the publications were stimulated by the medical education system. The Paris Faculty of Medicine was set up in 1794 with a course in Hippocratic medicine that was to be given by the dean of the faculty, Thouret. The course was never actually offered and the chair was abolished in 1811, but the leading translator of the period, François de Mercy, claims to have been encouraged by the government and by the faculty to undertake Hippocratic translations. While most of the 15 or so titles he produced were translations of this sort, several were pamphlets that sought unsuccessfully to convince the government that he deserved a chair in Hippocratic medicine or, at the very least, an annual stipend to continue his translation work.[6]

Discussions of Hippocratic ideas, whether appended to textual editions or standing alone, expressed the most varied perspectives. However, by and large, authors navigated between two stances. The first turned the father of medicine into an object of historical study and frequently involved some criticism of his work according to the standards of nineteenth-century medical science. A second stance was to consider Hippocratic ideas as either a still-valid body of knowledge or as a source of contemporary medical doctrines. The first position was more frequently expressed during the first half of the nineteenth century, as Hippocratic ideas lost much of their pertinence in the wake of the emergence of the Paris School which was based on pathological anatomy. However, many authors combined the two positions in nuanced ways.

René Laennec's famous MD thesis,[7] for instance, began with the premise that the universal popularity of the Hippocratic writings was due to the fact that they included so many indisputable observations and facts. But these observations and facts were widely misunderstood because they lacked any framework of systematic doctrine. Laennec saw his task as explicating this doctrine and determining which ideas were erroneous and which valid. While Hippocrates's *methods* of rigorous observation were universal and the basis of all medical science, his *doctrines* could be adopted or rejected.[8] In fact, Laennec went on to claim Hippocrates as a precursor of the anatomo-pathological method; in his nosological statements Hippocrates had occasionally tried to distinguish maladies on the basis of the kinds of organic lesion they produced; 'and this basis, when it exists ... is certainly the most solid one that can be chosen'.[9] But in matters of nosology, Laennec continued, the moderns were far superior.[10]

In contrast, for the leader of the Montpellier School of vitalism, P-J. Barthez, Hippocrates was the founder of 'the true Science of medicine ... it is only by adopting his general manner of seeing that one can add to the progress of this science ...'.[11] Far from having merely collected facts, he was the source of the 'fundamental dogmas' of medical science. In contrast, Galen had been a mere commentator of these essential dogmas which he had degraded and overloaded with systems.[12] Hippocrates was also a moral exemplar by virtue of his lack of interest in money and glory. Barthez did, however, express one serious reservation. Hippocrates had been too attached to natural methods and to the medical powers of nature. He did not realise that nature rarely provided spontaneous cures for serious maladies. Medicine thus had to impose movement on nature through methods that were 'either analytical or empirical'.[13]

During the Restoration such doctrinal disagreements heated up. De Mercy was probably being opportunistic when he justified the creation of a chair of Hippocratic medicine on the grounds that it would permit him 'to erect a barrier against the vices of systems' and sects.[14] But at least one frequently revised and reprinted work championing the most popular system of the day, Broussais' physiological medicine, clearly opposed Hippocratic doctrine.[15] And vitalists, for their part, certainly saw Hippocratic doctrine as a bulwark against anatomical localism which was becoming increasingly popular.[16] Representatives of the Paris School, in contrast, presented the 'father of medicine' as a precursor, an emblem of rigorous clinical observation and the experimental method, who had liberated medicine from religious explanation and philosophical systems.[17]

But the real thrust of the Paris School of medicine was not so much to appropriate Hippocrates as to historicise him. The work of Émile Littré was especially important in this connection, as was, to a lesser extent, the slightly later work of Charles Daremberg who began publishing his translations in the 1840s.[18] Littré's contribution was particularly rich and complex, not surprisingly given that his work on Hippocrates spanned more than 20 years. At one level, it has been noted, his Hippocrates was closely connected with French scientific expeditions and was used practically to develop a science of hygiene for hot countries based on geography and medical topography; Michael Osborne has thus emphasised Littré's attempt to 'dehistoricize' Hippocrates and make his work contemporary.[19] But at another and perhaps more profound level, Littré's translations, like those of Daremberg, deconstructed and historicised the traditional *Corpus*. Although both men rejected the extreme view that Hippocrates was not a real historical figure, they did demonstrate that most of the details of his life, as they were then known, were the stuff of legend. More importantly, they convincingly argued that the texts of the *Corpus* were of varied authorship. But the most important consequence of the work of these scholars was to turn Hippocrates into a historical subject who needed to be understood rather than glorified.[20] In Littré's wake, 'Hippocrates ceases to be a medical model to become an ancient author among the others'.[21] At the start of the project, the major medical justification for Littré's monumental work was that it would enable doctors to appreciate the changes which medicine had undergone since antiquity. This would 'fortify ... judgement', develop impartiality and teach respect for facts.[22] There was no question of imparting practical medical knowledge. It is thus not surprising that vitalists and other doctrinaire Hippocratists preferred the much older translation of Jean Baptiste Gardeil.[23]

From 1850 to the 1920s, works devoted to the father of medicine continued to appear, although they declined in number. Excluding sporadic textual editions, works were of several sorts. Hippocrates was a subject of scholarship not just for historians of medicine[24] but also for philosophers and literary scholars.[25] Although Hippocratic doctrines were no longer very relevant to mainstream medicine, some doctors combed the *Corpus* for examples of modern practices.[26] A few did more substantial historical research; J.C. Petrequin prepared a classic edition of Hippocratic texts on surgery.[27] The ethnic pride of Greeks living in France produced several works including a short-lived journal called *Hippocrate* focusing especially on works written by doctors who were Greek or of Greek origin.[28] Another French doctor of Greek origin wrote a book purporting to demonstrate that Hippocrates had been a precursor of the antiseptic method.[29] But a body of writing that is both quantitatively significant and particularly relevant to the later interwar period is that which sets up Hippocrates as an alternative to mainstream medicine.

Hippocratic doctrines, particularly the emphasis on the body's 'natural' tendency to heal itself, remained central to vitalists seeking to rally medical opinion to the doctrines of traditional medicine.[30] Inventors of new medical systems also rushed to align themselves with the father of medicine. One writer sought to make Hippocrates the initiator of the 'dosimetric method' which meant utilising 'defervescent' alkaloids as therapeutics for a wide variety of ills. Facing squarely the fact that Hippocrates had never spoken of this form of therapeutics and had in fact favoured expectant methods (allowing nature to take its course), the author responded simply that had he had the benefits of modern medical knowledge, Hippocrates *would have been* favourable to dosimetry. Quite ingenuously, he also expressed the attraction of Hippocratic patronage for alternative methods such as his:

> Dosimetry has been so often vilified by those who should bless it, that we have been obliged to place it under the protection of a great name. And we can [do this] because this is the doctrine of the father of medicine brought into relation with the means of modern science.[31]

Apart from vitalism, the most important doctrine which linked itself to Hippocrates was homoeopathy. By means of some selective reading, homoeopaths could find a variety of resources in the Hippocratic *Corpus*. Above all there was the law of similitude, and some authors were content to refer to it exclusively to justify homoeopathic practice (conveniently ignoring other references to the law of opposites).[32] Others, like Pierre Jousset, a leader of the eclectic branch of French homoeopathy developed more complex references to Hippocrates that reflected his more nuanced therapeutic position. In a book published in 1902 when the prestige of pasteurism was at its height,[33] Jousset linked together Hippocratic medicine, homoeopathy and pasteurism in a single tradition, distinct from, and in opposition to, the Galenic tradition. Galenism in this version was based on a single principle, the law of contraries, in which therapeutics aimed at suppressing an etiological agent. It was furthermore based on reasoning and dogmatism rather than observation. The Hippocratic tradition, by contrast, was based on observation and recognised *two* laws – the law of similars and the law of contraries. The former applied to maladies with internal causes; the latter suppressed symptoms. Homoeopathy and pasteurism were based on the same principles. While the latter utilised contraries for aseptic surgery it utilised similars to boost immunities in much the same way as homoeopathy – by treating an infectious malady with the microbe that caused it but using that microbe in an attenuated form.

The 1920s and 1930s

During the interwar period, various types of book about Hippocrates continued to be published. There was, for instance, a catalogue of Hippocratic texts held at the Bibliothèque Nationale,[34] as well as a few more or less scholarly discussions of Hippocratic texts[35] including a re-issue of Laennec's MD thesis. But the majority of works were ideological in nature, identifying Hippocrates with critiques of orthodox medicine and with various forms of alternative medicine. The especially large numbers of works published in the 1930s were predominantly of this sort.[36] To understand this phenomenon one must be aware that France, like many other nations during this period, was undergoing a holistic revival in medicine. I have presented my perspective on the French holistic movement of the interwar period in considerable detail elsewhere;[37] the outlines of my present analysis proceeds as follows.

I begin with a fundamental distinction between the *pragmatic* holism of those who saw themselves as functioning within the mainstream of medical science and practice and *doctrinaire* or ideological holism – the call to reject putatively dominant medical values in the name of a holistic approach that would rejuvenate medicine. Many domains or groups within late nineteenth- and early twentieth-century medicine were pragmatically holistic in the sense that individuals studied or treated specific problems systemically and contextually either because this was the traditional way in which to do things or because it seemed to be the best way to deal with specific problems. In some cases, such holistic views may have been shaped by larger social or ideological commitments but they nonetheless constituted relatively limited research strategies that must be distinguished from doctrines or ideologies about the state of medical knowledge in which holism became the *only* acceptable way to study the body and practise medicine.

By the early 1920s there was a growing body of scientific and medical activity that can be characterised as pragmatically holistic but that was not perceived as antagonistic to the principal currents of mainstream scientific medicine. The most significant of these were developments in such fields as endocrinology, the physiology of the central nervous system and immunology, all of which encouraged systemic orientations and shifted attention from causal agents of illness to the body's responses to such agents. Others were the widespread use of 'natural' therapies in various domains, particularly the tuberculosis sanatorium movement and the widespread use of mineral waters. The ideological holism that did exist was located primarily at the margins of the medical profession, particularly in the growing naturopathic and homoeopathic movements. I suggest that, during the second half of the 1920s, pragmatic and ideological forms of holism gradually moved closer together as ideological holists utilised the extensive body of research produced by pragmatic holists to justify and legitimate their views. At the same time, the therapeutic and theoretical disarray that reigned during this decade seems to have made many French doctors increasingly open to alternative therapies – particularly to homoeopathy which received enormous attention in the medical press. By the 1930s, in the context of professional, social and international crisis, ideological holism had spread widely within mainstream medicine. It brought together (literally) representatives of mainstream academic medicine with followers of alternative medical therapies – most notably homoeopathy which played a crucial mobilising role throughout this process.

In many respects, works on Hippocrates and Hippocratism simply reflect these developments. In these works, Hippocratism was synonymous with holistic ideas and advanced along with them, eventually receding with them as well. But I shall also suggest that ideas about Hippocratism were formative, helping to consolidate medical opinions and identities around several key concepts.[38]

One way of conceptualising these developments is to think of various sorts of consensus emerging around different holistic concepts. The notion of 'temperament' or, later, 'biotype' brought together representatives of many different medical tendencies interested in patterns of variation in individual susceptibility and resistance to disease. But it remained restricted to a relatively narrow circle of specialists interested in such matters. On the other hand, the concept of 'terrain', emphasising the individual body's primary role in disease processes and healing, as opposed to external etiological agents, attracted a very broad consensus within French medicine. Other notions such as 'nature' and 'synthesis' also attracted various degrees of assent. If one were to characterise the French holistic movement as a collection of partially overlapping notions generating partially overlapping consensuses and if one attempted to illustrate this spatially, the notions of 'Hippocratic', and especially 'neo-Hippocratic', medicine would be located close to the centre.

During the 1920s one finds relatively few works devoted to Hippocrates. Like holism more generally, interest in the father of medicine was located mainly at the margins of official medicine among Montpellier vitalists,[39] and naturopaths such as Paul Carton. Carton, a physician in the suburbs of Paris, was a remarkably prolific writer. He developed a 'synthetic' doctrine of healing centred on semi-vegetarian diets, but also including physical exercise and spiritual mental health. The mix was laced with a strong dose of the occult. In addition to writing countless books setting out and defending his views while belittling both orthodox medicine and the various vegetarian, nudist and naturopathic groups which he viewed as unworthy competitors, Carton directed a national society and a journal.[40]

Carton emphasised the Hippocratic roots of his ideas. In a book published in 1923, he featured excerpts from the Hippocratic writings that corresponded to his own views.[41] Significantly he did not use Littré's historicised translation but rather the older one by Gardeil, characterised as 'the more precise, the more alert, the more clairvoyant, the more naturopathic'.[42] His texts were in two sections, one centring on the unity of the cosmos and the second on the conditions for a healthy life. The meaning of Carton's Hippocratism is evident in his introductory essay. It was primarily a return to medical tradition and to 'antique virtues of clairvoyance [a word he was fond of] and simplicity'. Simplicity meant recourse to spiritual resources rather than material acquisitions, and to the rules of a simple hygienic life as opposed to an enormous therapeutic armamentarium. He maintained that the real causes of illnesses were violations of a healthy life, especially offences of diet and hygiene. Although he was willing to use modern medicine selectively, Carton, unlike most other French holists who were enamoured of immunology, opposed serums and vaccines on the grounds that they made it possible to ignore the rules of a healthy life and because 'natural immunities alone possess a real and durable value to preserve and heal'.[43]

During the 1930s interest in Hippocrates increased dramatically. Published works tell only a small part of the story. In the middle of this decade, the Academy of Medicine which, for over a century, had lacked any representation of Hippocrates (although it did contain a large statue of Asclepius) finally remedied the situation when a francophile Greek physician donated a large marble statue of the father of medicine that was placed in the main assembly hall amid much fanfare. It served as a reminder of the filiation between Hippocrates and the Academy 'his spiritual child and heir' and as a symbol of interwar Franco-Greek friendship (that was becoming increasingly important as war approached).[44] More significantly, perhaps, the Hippocratic oath, which had been required of graduating doctors only at the Montpellier Faculty of Medicine during the nineteenth century, was gradually introduced to other faculties of medicine. The motivation seems to have been the economic competition that resulted from a huge rise in the number of physicians practising in France; this created the perception of serious problems concerning unethical behaviour among physicians and pressure mounted for reintroducing the oath as a way of combating such medical misbehaviour. In 1935 the professorial council of the Paris Faculty of Medicine, citing the 'movement' in its favour and the examples of at least three other faculties, decided to reintroduce the oath at the graduation ceremony.[45]

However, most of the interest in Hippocrates was expressed in publications. Representatives of official medicine made some isolated efforts to claim Hippocrates as an intellectual precursor. The former dean of the Paris Faculty of Medicine, Henri Roger, wrote an introduction and commentaries for a new illustrated edition of Littré's translation of the Hippocratic *Corpus*.[46] Here and in an article directed at the medical profession, Roger presented a thoroughly historicised, multiple authored, *Corpus* whose writers had inveighed against inductive philosophers and called for rigorous observation. Hippocratic writers had, moreover, not accepted the Platonic duality of body and soul but had assumed a unity that was essentially materialistic – a concept that Roger found 'grandiose, fruitful in a different way from the metaphysics of spiritualists'.[47] Furthermore, they had recognised that the brain was the source of psychic manifestations, something many modern thinkers – Bergson in particular – had difficulty accepting.[48] The major authors not only rejected supernatural causation of disease but, in some works, expressed pantheistic views 'not too far removed from modern ideas on universal determinism'. And they recognised that 'the point of departure for illnesses must be placed outside of the sick organism' in such agents as miasmas and diet, even if the mechanisms of the disease involved internal factors such as humoral balance.[49] It would be difficult to find a figure more antithetic to the emerging holistic movement then was the Hippocrates presented by Roger. Despite such efforts, however, the physician of Cos was largely appropriated by holistic healers during this period.

The 1930s began with a remarkable 'biography' of Hippocrates by Gaston Baissette, a young doctor and novelist. Originally an MD thesis at the Paris Faculty of Medicine, it quickly found a publisher and commercial success.[50] Both thesis and book are remarkable for their effort to rid Hippocratic scholarship of a century of critical historical studies reflecting 'a permanent will toward diminution and disassociation' and which 'had revealed themselves to be sterile for the spirit'.[51] Baissette instead proposed 'by an act of love ... to approach the secret of such a genius ... an effort to eliminate all vain compilation'.[52] All the legends about his life denied by historians were accepted here as facts on the grounds that, even if not strictly true, they were inspired by truthful narratives which, in any case, had a place in a 'rational and necessary biography of Hippocrates'.[53] The biography itself, written in a purple prose that has defied my efforts at translation, is less important for our purposes than his conclusion that the work of Hippocrates possesses an absolute unity that attached medicine to all the sciences: 'It appears to us necessary in medicine to return to the Hippocratic spirit whose vast syncretism opens the way to all progress.'[54] The essence of this syncretism was an awareness that all manner of perspectives are correct and that differences could be reconciled: 'For Hippocrates there was identity in variety.'[55] This unity had been destroyed by

Cartesianism but even before that, by Galen: 'Galen seems to us to play the role of an evil genie, of a rancorous and ambiguous personage, who substituted a spirit of dogmatism for the spirit of investigation supported by facts, thus destroying this unity of science ... .'[56]

Baissette went on to borrow a vision of history from a book published the previous year by the homoeopath–psychoanalyst, René Allendy (best known today, perhaps, for being a lover and first analyst of Anaïs Nin). According to this view which would be widely repeated in the holistic literature, medical history was distinguished by the conflict between two opposing, indeed contradictory, 'poles' within medicine. One understood illness as the accidental product of an external agent that could be identified through 'analysis' and then combated directly. The other viewed illness as a product of internal processes linked to all the various conditions of life. It could be grasped only through 'synthesis'. One of these two tendencies was always dominant and, until recently, this had been 'analytical' medicine represented by Galen, most doctors of the modern period and, above all, pasteurism. The 'synthetic' tradition for Allendy included the medicines of China and India, Hermeticism, vitalism and homoeopathy, as well as Hippocrates. Baissette joined Allendy in viewing recent developments in medical science that emphasised the primacy of the 'terrain' in illness, as well as widespread medical experimentation with alternative therapies, as indicators that the tide was turning and that 'synthesis' would soon be in the ascendant.[57]

The most extraordinary thing about this self-consciously ahistorical work is that it was not denounced, or at least dismissed, by French historians of medicine. While Henry Sigerist, recently arrived in Baltimore, dismissed it with faint praise ('There is no harm in it as long as we are aware that we are reading fiction and not history'),[58] the professor of the history of medicine at the Paris Medical Faculty, the neuro-psychiatrist Maxime Laignel-Lavastine, chose Baissette to write the article on Hippocrates in the first volume of the lavishly illustrated, multi-authored history of medicine that he was organising.[59] The choice is less surprising in the light of Laignel-Lavastine's own introduction to the above work in which he declared that his primary aim was to discover the nature of medical humanism 'which with literary, scientific and religious humanism will come together in a happy synthesis, in the birth of a new humanism'.[60] The utility of this sort of history was essentially pedagogical. Consequently, although conventional erudition was important, he cited approvingly the example of Henri Berr's efforts to promote a more general 'synthetic' history and argued that 'one must know how to raise one's eyes, contemplate the entire landscape, look at the heavens and take a synthetic look at patient analytical elaboration'.[61]

Laignel-Lavastine was both consistent and indefatigable in pursuing this aim. From 1933 to 1939, he edited a journal called *Hippocrate*, which published a remarkably eclectic mixture of articles on medicine, medical history, physics and literature, among other subjects, in pursuit of an elusive medical humanism, which he identified with Hippocrates who had sought complete understanding of man.[62]

The various still rather inchoate, meanings of Hippocratism – syncretism, humanism, plus specific medical concepts like vitalism and the healing power of nature – were gradually coming together. In large measure this was due to foreigners who brought to France 'neo-Hippocratism', already established in Italy, Germany and Britain. In 1933 the Italian medical historian Arturo Castiglioni lectured at the Paris Academy of Medicine and repeated the conclusions of his well-known history of medicine that had recently appeared in French translation.[63] The modern orientation of medicine, he proclaimed, was becoming increasingly Hippocratic; by this he meant not just that it was moving closer to the work of the master or to Greek medicine but towards an older 'Mediterranean' medical tradition whose origins went back to Babylonian and Egyptian medicine, and especially the 'Italic' philosophical school associated with Heraclites. It thus combined many ancient medical ideas with the products of scientific progress, something made possible because the conceptions of 'the ancient Masters' were nothing but 'an intuitive vision of those truths of which modern science has furnished proofs'.[64] Castiglioni had little impact, partly because he addressed himself to an institution unlikely to be sympathetic and partly because his views were idiosyncratic.[65] Nonetheless, medical holism associated with Hippocrates continued to advance and soon afterwards two medical theses on the subject were successfully defended at the Paris Faculty of Medicine.[66]

Significantly one of the two theses was written by a homoeopath,[67] for homoeopaths, as mentioned earlier, had long identified themselves with Hippocratic medicine. Furthermore, they were among the prime beneficiaries of the growing popularity of holism and alternative medicines. There was extraordinary interest in homoeopathy in the medical press of the 1920s and 1930s.[68] According to one observer, many doctors saw 'the disciples of Hahnemann as kinds of precursors ... on the road to "the return to Hippocrates"'.[69] An institutionalised neo-Hippocratic movement was born in 1935 at the annual meeting of the progressive, eclectic wing of French homoeopathy associated with the Leopold-Bellan Hospital in Paris and the journal *L'Homéopathie moderne*. For some years this group, under the leadership of Fortier-Bernonville and Marcel Martiny, had been seeking to create a scientifically respectable form of homoeopathy more closely integrated with mainstream medicine. Among those invited to its Hahneman Days conference of 1935 were Laignel-Lavastine and a leader of British neo-Hippocratic medicine, Alexandre Cawadias. Cawadias was a Greek who had studied medicine in Paris before moving on to Britain where he became involved in efforts to bring together homoeopathy and mainstream medicine.[70] An excellent French speaker, he had recently published several articles in *L'Homéopathie moderne* on this theme.[71]

The presence of Laignel-Lavastine as an observer symbolised the growing friendliness of scattered parts of the medical establishment to homoeopathy. But Cawadias was there to sell neo-Hippocratism to French homoeopaths.

Cawadias's message was simple.[72] Neo-Hippocratism represented the growing convergence between scientific homoeopathy and expanding segments of official medicine. It was based on three general principles that both groups could agree on:

1. The primacy of the clinic. This did not exclude the results of the laboratory so long as the hierarchical primacy of clinical observation was clearly recognised.
2. A dynamic and individualised conception of illness that was based on a differential biology rooted in notions of temperament, constitution, and character. Individual reactions also had to be seen in terms of the influence of society and the cosmos.
3. Rational treatment meant natural treatment. Treatment sought to aid the body's own reactions to illness.[73]

Having himself moved increasingly toward homoeopathic practices which he now utilised for about 80 per cent of his patients, Cawadias could assure his listeners that his proposed synthesis with mainstream medicine included a significant and in no way subordinate role for homoeopathy. He was so convincing that, at the final banquet, Marcel Martiny proposed not only that an international neo-Hippocratic meeting be organised in Paris, but also that Laignel-Lavastine serve as president and that Cawadias serve as secretary general.[74] Subsequently in 1937, the First International Neo-Hippocratic Congress did indeed take place in Paris. Moreover, Laignel-Lavastine did indeed serve as president but Marcel Martiny, rather than Cawadias, filled the role of secretary-general. A year later a National Neo-Hippocratic Congress took place in Marseilles. As a result, an international neo-Hippocratic movement was set up with Laignel-Lavastine as president and Pierre Delore, who in 1936 had published the most influential statement of French medical holism,[75] as secretary-general. A national organisation was also founded under the presidency of Lucien Cornil, dean of the Marseilles Faculty of Medicine. The outbreak of war prevented the convening of a second international congress that was scheduled to take place on the island of Cos at the end of 1939.

Neo-Hippocratic medicine gave new prominence to homoeopathy (and, to a lesser extent, naturopathy) but its true significance in the French context was to bring together many of the holistic tendencies that had emerged during the previous decade. Within the movement there were, of course, prominent homoeopaths such as Fortier-Bernonville and Allendy, naturopaths such as the Marseilles hospital surgeon, Joseph Poucel, and medico-literary figures such as Paul Desfosses, the chief chronicler of holism in the prestigious journal, *La*

Presse médicale. Members of the Parisian medical elite – including faculty professors like Paul Carnot, Maurice Loeper and René Leriche of the Collège de France – were prominent as members of the committees of patronage but senior Parisian mandarins, with the exception of Laignel-Lavastine, rarely participated actively; this was left to younger men such as the Parisian hospital physicians, Guy Laroche and André Jacquelin. Provincial medical elites were somewhat more active; participants included Lucien Cornil, dean of the Marseilles Faculty of Medicine, J. Techoueyres, director of the medical school at Reims, and faculty professors Jules Guiart (Lyon) and Jean Fiolle (Marseilles). Pierre Delore would be named professor at the Lyon Faculty of Medicine in 1944.[76]

There were also some glaring absences. Alexis Carrel whose 1936 book, *L'Homme cet inconnu*, had received considerable attention in the French medical press, was apparently invited but declined to attend because he insisted that medicine should not be bound by doctrines like vitalism and pythagorianism, and that it required more, rather than less, laboratory experimentation and observation which was preferable to the history of medicine, 'a science of uncertain presumptions'.[77] In fact the muscular eugenic approach that he championed was conspicuously missing from the neo-hippocratic congresses. Elite Parisian 'terrain' theorists such as Jean Darier and Émile Sargent also did not take part. Although many participants spoke or wrote positively of religion and spirituality, the absence of representatives of Christian humanist medicine, such as René Biot, is also striking. Other absences are more easily explained. One of the inventors of cinematography, Auguste Lumière who for years had been proclaiming the revival of a new 'humoralism' not only did not attend but wrote a work criticising neo-Hippocratism for ignoring his theories of 'floculation'.[78] Léon Vannier, leader of the more intransigent wing of homoeopathy, attacked neo-Hippocratism as a snare that would weaken the true Hippocratic medicine, homeopathy.[79] Carrel, Biot, Lumière and Vannier contributed prominently to a collection of essays about alternative medicine published just before the end of the Second World War.[80] This included an essay on neo-Hippocratic medicine by Marcel Martiny and another on more traditional Hippocratic medicine but, overall, it presented a holism that was more eclectic, more Catholic and more hostile to official elite medicine than was neo-Hippocratism.

Reflections on neo-Hippocratism and holism

If I am correct in characterising holism as a collection of interconnected notions and metaphors each capable of attracting different but overlapping degrees of assent, the obvious question to ask is: what did appeals to Hippocrates and Hippocratic medicine add to holism that other popular terms such as vitalism, synthesis and nature did not? Or to put it another way, why did holists choose to identify themselves with the label 'neo-Hippocratism', a neologism that was, in Martiny's words, 'impoverished and shocking, but ... rich and traditionalist'.[81]

There are some fairly banal answers like the timeless need for the non-orthodox of all shades to enlist the patronage of universally respected authorities – a need well expressed by the founder of dosimetry in the late nineteenth century. (There was also a related need to create historical filiation for ideological opponents, as evidenced by the demonisation of Galen.) Furthermore, the vitalist tradition, of which many holistic currents were clearly an outgrowth, had long been identifying itself with Hippocrates. For the past century, many of the specific medical concepts utilised by holists had been associated with the Hippocratic *Corpus*. Moreover, the term 'Hippocratic' was almost a synonym for 'medical' and it was thus instantly recognisable unlike a term like 'neo-vitalist' which, although probably more accurate as a characterisation of the movement, had narrow, specialised associations.

Appeals to Hippocrates also enriched some of the other keywords and notions of holism. 'Synthesis' as a form of thought was perhaps the most fundamental concept of French holism. For a thinker like Pierre Delore it signalled the epistemological reconciliation of science and tradition, analysis and synthesis, terrain and external cause, body, mind and soul, cell, organism and cosmos, official medicine and all forms of alternative healing. Ultimately, I would argue, 'synthesis' also offered the promise of wider social reconciliation at a time when the European social order seemed to be disintegrating. Appeals to Hippocrates added to this abstract notion a purported model of 'synthesis' that had already been achieved and was recoverable. The textual inconsistencies and contradictions that scholars had explained as a consequence of multiple authorship could now be cast as visible manifestations of the ability to reconcile and synthesise multiple, even contradictory, points of view.

The notion that was probably most identified historically with Hippocratism was that of 'nature' or 'natural' healing.[82] Here, the common reference to Hippocrates served, in fact, to obscure disagreements about what constituted naturism – one of the few issues on which holists disagreed.[83] The common starting point for everyone was that Hippocrates had posited that illness was the method by which the body, directed by some sort of vital force, re-established its normal equilibrium. Illness thus needed to be guided to a positive conclusion rather than be suppressed. There was also widespread consensus that the healing power of nature did *not* mean that physicians should adopt a purely 'wait-and-see' stance. Medical intervention was required in order to stimulate and direct the body's recovery, and this intervention should be 'natural'. It was on the definition of 'natural' that disagreements commonly arose.

Paul Carton represented one extreme when insisting that this meant submission to the laws of nature and hygiene, especially through diet. At another extreme were those who understood 'natural' as anything which aimed not to suppress illness but to stimulate the healing response of the 'terrain'. Techniques for doing so could range from the gentle and subtle 'imponderables' prescribed by homoeopaths to various more invasive techniques including immunological serums and 'shock' provoked by the injection of foreign substances (and later by electricity). Jean Fiolle even postulated that one aspect of effective surgery was the general shock it inflicted on the organism.[84] (The significance of the notion of 'shock' during this period demands more systematic analysis.) An intermediary position was that therapies should, as much as possible, use therapeutic elements found in nature: sunshine, waters, air, electricity and, remarkably to us, radioactivity. The popularity of such physiotherapies has many explanations including a widespread revival of the notion that the cosmic environment was often the cause of imbalances in the body; therefore if it was properly manipulated, it could also promote equilibrium.[85] I suspect, too, that the fact such modalities were often based on the products of modern physics was also significant since, as I have argued elsewhere, the discipline of physics enjoyed enormous prestige and influence in holistic circles.[86]

Everyone, including Carton, recognised that, in certain cases, fairly dramatic procedures were required. But in fact, neo-Hippocratism offered even greater therapeutic flexibility because its declared aim was to combine the best of traditional and modern therapies. Its spokesmen made it clear that, while 'natural' and simple therapies were desirable, it was unthinkable not to use all modern therapies with proven efficacy.[87]

'Humanism' as a holistic term, referred generally to the need to focus on human beings rather than organs, bacteria or experimental animals. In its specifics it had a variety of connotations. There was a Christian humanism applied to medicine that had at its source recognition of the unique spirituality and divine quality of each individual.[88] By contrast, the humanistic Hippocratism of Laignel-Lavastine focused on setting medicine within a broader cultural context that could produce a more profound understanding of human beings. Traditionally, such culture had been the product of exposure to Greek and Latin literature but, since the turn of the century, classical languages had no longer been a prerequisite for medical studies. This seemed like a major misfortune to many French doctors who were usually at the forefront of sporadic efforts to reintroduce classical language requirements for entry to university programmes. One of the many advantages of the appeal to Hippocrates was that it renewed the connection to a classical heritage that, for many, remained the source of true culture. But the 'neo' in neo-Hippocratic meant that all forms of modern culture were also relevant to the cultural synthesis that was emerging. An enormous interest in oriental thought and practices was also justified by this perspective.[89]

In the final analysis, appeals to Hippocrates were explicitly and most fundamentally appeals to the past which expressed considerable discomfort with contemporary science and, more generally, with the world that science had created. It was not just the pasteurism, the 'analytical' orientation, or even the apparent intellectual disarray of medical science which was under scrutiny but the very status of science itself. During the interwar period a number of works critical of the excessive claims of science[90] were published, and the theme was taken up more briefly in many holistic writings. Such critiques were bolstered by recent work in physics that seemed to call into question traditional notions of objective knowledge.[91] If science was a necessary, but insufficient, form of knowledge, as was believed, with what other forms of knowing could it be supplemented? Intuition was one possibility made respectable by Henri Bergson. Spiritual authority or experience were popular alternatives. But while neo-Hippocratic spokesmen certainly invoked these forms of knowing, the movement basically rested on the historical authority of the past, understood as the collective experiences of mankind.

The claims of the past did not just apply to medical science. There is an unmistakable distaste in much holistic writing for contemporary civilisation which was widely perceived to be in crisis and on the verge of world conflagration. It is true that, although it grew out of the soil of interwar social dislocation and widespread contempt for liberal democracy, French medical holism, unlike German holism, remained — whether out of conviction or prudence — largely apolitical both in word and deed. But the movement nonetheless had a clear aura of conservatism and nostalgia for a simpler and better ordered social world that reflected a widespread mood (rather than a coherent ideology) among the French middle classes.

Neo-Hippocratic spokespeople emphasised that they were not advocating a simple return to the medicine of antiquity but a new sort of synthesis between medical tradition and science. This was the great appeal of the movement — it promised both the immutable truths of the past *and* the benefits of scientific progress. But if this promise attracted some, it also alienated many others. Despite his own growing nostalgia for mystical Catholicism, Alexis Carrel's negative response to neo-Hippocratism was clearly the expression of a belief that knowledge of healing, as well as of social organisation, could be based only on rigorous science. By the same token, the absence of representatives of the Christian humanist brands of holism may be a consequence of the fact that these had little need to appeal to *medical* traditions of the past; in their view, science needed to be supplemented by *Christian* truths applied to the social world.

Yet another aspect of Hippocratism concerned the philosophical imagination, the need to speculate and freely construct explanatory theories that explained the world in ways that rigorous scientific work ordinarily failed to do. This was especially critical in the crisis atmosphere of the interwar years when there were apparently few certainties. Among the attractions of modern physics for medical holists was its ability to 'explain' in relatively simple and elegant terms vast areas of reality and, at the same time, allow its practitioners to engage in metaphysical speculation. Hippocratic physicians wanted the same intellectual freedom and scope. Certainly, neo-Hippocratism was supposed to include both speculation *and* rigorous science – a claim that provoked Alexis Carrel's renewed wrath. Medicine, according to Carrel, certainly had to extend its perspectives but it had to refrain from confusing the domain of science with the domain of philosophy.[92]

> As a scientific discipline, medicine is independent of all doctrine. It has no more right to be vitalist than mechanist, materialist than spiritualist. It is not any more appropriate that it follows Hippocrates or Paracelsus, Freud or Mrs. Eddy. Observation and experience are the only sources of knowledge.[93]

Conclusion

For all its fundamental cultural strangeness, for the medical historian of the 2000s there is also a curiously familiar tone in much neo-Hippocratic literature. It is no accident that so many of those involved in the movement had institutional positions or a strong amateur interest in medical history. The problem, then as now, had to do with a perceived narrowness in the education and perspective of doctors that was at variance with the complexities of humane healing in the modern world. At a time when sociology, psychology or ethics had virtually no place in medical schools, it was left to history, which *did* have a modest place, to try singlehandedly to remedy the situation. In this context, yet another of the consequences of the appeal to Hippocrates was the valorisation of medical history.

Yet this was medical history of a particular sort; it was an appendage of clinical medicine, reflecting *medical* debates and concerns. At a time when historical understanding of the Hippocratic *Corpus* was changing dramatically due to the work of classicists such as Ludwig Edelstein and others in the German- and English-speaking worlds, one finds in the country of Littré and Daremberg, virtually no serious historical scholarship, or even awareness of recently published scholarship. In a review of the literature on Hippocrates published in 1934, Henry Sigerist cited only two twentieth-century works in French – Gaston Baissette's biography and Henri Roger's new edition of Littré's translation, both of which he summarily dismissed as works of scholarship.[94] A leading French classicist has more recently admitted that, after Littré, Hippocratic scholarship, a field once 'the privileged domain of French science becomes the domain of German erudition'.[95] This situation is a by-product of the inability of medical history in France to transform itself into an autonomous discipline with its own methods, problems and debates and its consequent status as a sinecure for retired, literary-minded clinicians. (This situation has begun to change in recent years but continues to a considerable degree.)

In the absence of real classical scholarship in France and the almost exclusively *clinical* concern with the subject, it becomes easier to understand the growing interwar identification of Hippocrates with holism. For there is an intrinsic inequality between proponents of mainstream medicine and holists in their need for, and identification with, Hippocrates. The former certainly wished to appropriate so prestigious a historical figure but they characteristically did so briefly, in passing, and in the company of numerous heroes and emblematic figures such as Laennec, Pasteur, Claude Bernard and many others whose work corresponded more closely to the values of twentieth-century medicine. Holists, on the other hand, had other precursors but no other heroes of comparable stature. This fundamental imbalance, as much as the growth of medical holism, accounts for the holistic appropriation of Hippocrates in interwar France.

Acknowledgements

Research for this essay was made possible by a grant from the Social Sciences and Humanities research Council of Canada.

Notes

1. Libraries consulted were: in Paris, the Bibliothèque Nationale, Bibliothèque de l'Académie de Médecine, Bibliothèque de la Faculté de Médecine de Paris, the British Library, The National Library of Medicine (Bethesda), the Health Sciences and Osler Libraries of McGill University, the Health Sciences and Arts and Sciences Libraries of the Université de Montréal.
2. Articles in journals or edited collections were not included unless a reprint was catalogued by one the libraries.
3. Some of what is hidden by this procedure is uncovered in Ann F. Laberge's essay in this volume (Chapter 9).
4. Emile Littré, *Oeuvres complètes d'Hippocrate: Traduction nouvelle ...*, 10 Vols, Paris: J.B. Baillière, 1839–61. The only real competitor to this collection was an older work, Jean Baptiste Gardeil, *Traduction des oeuvres médicales d'Hippocrate, sur le texte grec*, 4 Vols, Toulouse: Fages et Meilhac, 1801 and republished several times during the century.
5. The exact figure is 57 percent of the titles.
6. F.-C.-F. de Mercy, *Considérations sur la naissance des sectes ... et sur la nécessité de créer une chaire d'Hippocrate*, Paris: Eberhart, 1816; idem, *Demande à messieurs les Professeurs de la Faculté de Médecine de Paris du rétablissement d'une chaire d'Hippocrate*, Paris: de Vigor Renaudière, 1821. On Laennec's bid for this chair see Jacalyn Duffin, *To See With a Better Eye: A Life of R.T.H. Laennec*, Princeton, NJ, Princeton University Press, 1998, pp. 73–75.

7. René-Théophile-Hyacinthe Laennec, 'Propositions sur la doctrine d'Hippocrate, relativement à la médecine pratique, présentées et soutenues à l'Ecole de médecine de Paris, le 22 prairial an XII', Paris: Didot jeunne, an XII [1804]. This was republished in 1923 (Paris: Maurice Letusle).
8. Ibid., p. 9.
9. Ibid., p. 33.
10. Ibid., p. 37. On these matters, see also the essay by Ann F. La Berge in this volume (Chapter 9) and Jacalyn Duffin, *To See With a Better Eye* (n. 6).
11. Paul-Joseph Barthez, *Discours sur le génie d'Hippocrate, Inauguration du buste d'Hippocrate, faite à l'Ecole de Médecine de Montpellier*. Montpellier: l'Imprime de Tournal, an IX [1801], p. 3. The version I consulted was a reprint dated 1816.
12. Ibid., pp. 5–6.
13. Ibid., pp. 6, 21–22. For a more detailed examination of Barthez's views in the context of Montpellier vitalism see Elizabeth William's essay in this volume (Chapter 8).
14. De Mercy, *Considérations sur la naissance des sectes* (n. 6), p. 2.
15. M.S. Houdart, 'Quelques réflections sur Hippocrate', Thèse de médecine, Faculté de Médecine de Paris, 1821; *Etudes historiques et critiques sur la vie et la doctrine d'Hippocrate, etc.*, Paris: Baillière, 1836; 2nd revised and enlarged edn, Paris: Baillière, 1840; idem, *Examen critique de la vie d'Hippocrate* 4th rev. edn, Paris: Baillière, 1852; idem, *Réflexions sur Hippocrate*, Paris: Nogent le Rotrou, 1908.
16. Charles Alphonse Auguste Hardy Des Alleurs, *Du génie d'Hippocrate et de son influence sur l'art de guérir*. Paris: Bechet, 1824.
17. Jean Eugène Dezeimeris, *Résumé de la médecine hippocratique; ou, Aphorismes d'Hippocrate, classés dans un ordre systématique, et précédés d'une introduction historique*, Paris: Fortin et Masson, 1841, p. xxvii. For a discussion of different approaches to Hippocrates during this period see the essay by Ann La Berge, Chapter 9 in this volume.
18. Littré, *Oeuvres complètes* (n. 4); Charles V. Daremberg, *Le serment; La loi; De l'art Du medecin; ...*, Paris: Lefevre, 1843; idem, *Oeuvres choisies d'Hippocrate, traduites ... accompagnées d'arguments, de notes, et précédées d'une introduction par C. Daremberg ...*, 2nd rev. edn, Paris: Labe, 1855.
19. Michael A. Osborne, 'Resurrecting Hippocrates: hygienic sciences and the French scientific expeditions to Egypt, Morea and Algeria', in David Arnold (ed.), *Warm Climates and Western Medicine: The Emergence of Tropical Medicine, 1500–1900*, Amsterdam: Rodopi, 1996, pp. 84–86.
20. Daremberg, *Oeuvres choisies*, (n. 18), p. xlvii.
21. Jacques Jouanna, 'Littré, éditeur et traducteur d'Hippocrate', in *Actes du Colloque Émile Littré, 1801–1881: Paris 7–9 octobre 1981*, Paris: Albin Michel, 1983, p. 296.
22. Littré, *Oeuvres complètes*, (n. 4), Vol. 1, 1839, p. 477.
23. Gardeil, *Traduction des oeuvres médicales d'Hippocrate* (n. 4).
24. Charles Daremberg, *La médecine entre Homère et Hippocrate*, Paris: Librairie Académique, 1869. A more general history that uses Hippocrates as a starting point is J.M. Guardia, *Histoire de la médecine d' Hippocrate à Broussais et à ses amis*, Paris: Doin, 1884.
25. Emmanuel Chauvet, *Mémoire sur la philosophie d'Hippocrate*, Thèse Faculté de Lettres de Paris, 1856; Aimé Vingtrinier, *Un exemplaire d'Hippocrate annoté par Rabelais*, Lyon: Mougin-Rousand, 1887; Jean Psichari, *Sophocle et Hippocrate à*

propos du 'Philoctéte à Leemnos', extract from *Revue de philologie, de litérature et d'histoire anciennes*, Paris: C. Klincksieck, 1908; René Sturel, *Rabelais et Hippocrate (notes bibliographiques)*, Nogent-le-Rotrou: Imp. de Daupeley-Gouverneur, 1908.

26. Amédée Le Plé, *La chirurgie d'Hippocrate*, Rouen, 1878. René Briau, *Hippocrate et la lithotomie*, 2nd edn, Paris, 1879. Dr A. Courtade, *L'otologie dans Hippocrate*, extract from *Archives internationales de laryngologie*, January 1904; and *Recherche historiques la rhinologie dans Hippocrate*, extract from *Archives internationales de laryngologie, otologie et rhinologie*, Paris, nd.
27. J.C. Petrequin, *Chirurgie d'Hippocrate*, ed. E. Jullien, 2 Vols, Paris: Imprimerie nationale, 1877–78.
28. *Hippocrate: revue mensuelle illustrée, scientifique, historique, patriotique*, 1898–1901, p. 1. Not surprisingly it published many Hippocratic texts.
29. M. Sourlangas, *Étude sur l'Hippocrate: son oeuvre*, Paris: G. Steinheil, 1894.
30. Edouard Auber, *Institutions d'Hippocrate, un exposé philosophique des principes traditionnels de la médecine... Suivi d'un résumé du naturisme, du vitalisme et de l'organicisme et d'un essai sur la constitution de la médecine*, Paris: Baillière, 1864; idem, *De la fièvre puerpérale devant l'Académie de Médecine et des principes du vitalisme hippocratique appliqués à la solution de cette question*, Paris: Baillière, 1858.
31. Adolphe Pierre Burgraeve, *Etudes sur Hippocrate au point de vue de la méthode dosimétrique*, Paris: Chanteaud, 1881.
32. Dr Flasschoen, *Le triomphe de l'homéopathie: réforme médicale, néo-hippocratisme, doctrine dynamico-spécifiste*, Paris: L. Sauvaitre, 1908.
33. Pierre Jousset, *Hippocrate, Hahnemann, Pasteur*, Paris: Baillère, 1902.
34. *Catalogue des ouvrages d'Hippocrate conservés au département des Imprimés*; Extrait de tome 72 du *Catalogue général des livres imprimés de la Bibliothèque Nationale*, Paris: Imprimerie nationale, 1921.
35. Victor Magnien, *Les facultés de l'âme d'après Platon, Hippocrate et Homère*, extract from '*L'Acropole*', *Revue du Monde Hellénique*, October–December 1926, Le Puy: Imprimerie de la Haute-Loire, 1928,; Jean Dumortier, *Le vocabulaire médical d'Eschyle et les écrits hippocratiques: Collection d'études anciennes, publiée sous le patronage de l'Association Guillaume Bude*, Paris: Imprimerie A. Taffin-Lefort, 1935.
36. Of 18 works published during the 1930s, 67 per cent fall into this category.
37. George Weisz, 'A moment of synthesis: medical holism in France between the wars', in Christopher Lawrence and George Weisz (eds), *Greater than the Parts: Holism in Biomedicine, 1920–1950*, New York and Oxford: Oxford University Press, 1998, pp. 68–93.
38. In what follows I will concentrate on works in my Hippocratic bibliography but will occasionally bring into discussion periodical articles focussing on Hippocratism and medical holism more generally.
39. Dr Paul Négre, *Une vieille tradition dans une vieille faculté: La serment d'Hippocrate*, Montpellier: Imprimerie Firmin et Montane, 1923.
40. For Carton's own version of his story see Paul Carton, *L'apprentissage de la santé: histoire d'une création et d'une défense doctrinale*, Paris: Maloine, 1933. He was the founder and guiding light of the Société Naturiste Française and edited the *Revue naturiste*.
41. Paul Carton, *L'essentiel de la doctrine d'Hippocrate extrait de ses oeuvres*, Paris: Maloine, 1923. See idem, *Alimentation, hygiène et thérapeutique infantiles en exemples; méthode naturiste ou hippocratique*, Paris: Maloine, 1922.

42. Carton, *L'essentiel de la doctrine d'Hippocrate* (n. 41), p. 12. This preference for Gardeil's work was not uncommon among vitalists. See Auber, *Institutions d'Hippocrate* (n. 30), p. xiv.
43. Carton, *L'essentiel de la doctrine d'Hippocrate* (n. 41), p. 9.
44. Both points were made in the speeches celebrating the installation. See *Bulletin de l'Académie de Médecine*, **118**, 1937, pp. 390, 393.
45. Meeting of 7 November 1935 in Archives Nationales (Paris), AJ16 6294. Also see 'Le serment d'Hippocrate', *Presse thermale et climatique*, **76**, 1935, p. 787.
46. Hippocrate, *Oeuvres complètes*, preface and commentary by Georges Eugène Henri Roger, trans. Littré, Paris: Javal et Bourdeaux, 1932–34.
47. Henri Roger, 'La philosophie d'Hippocrate', *Presse médicale*, **41**, 1933, p. 521.
48. Ibid., p. 422.
49. Ibid., p. 722.
50. Raymond Gaston Baissette, 'Aux sources de la médecine: vie et doctrine d'Hippocrate', MD thesis, No. 335, Paris 1931; idem, *Hippocrate*, Paris: Grasset, 1931. This book was translated into German and Italian.
51. Baissette, 'Aux sources de la médecine' (n. 50), pp. 10, 11.
52. Ibid., p. 12.
53. Ibid., p. 263.
54. Ibid., p. 264.
55. Ibid., p. 231.
56. Ibid., p. 237.
57. Ibid., pp. 241–47. A more detailed discussion of Allendy's book *Orientations des idées médicales*, Paris: Au Sans-Pareil, 1929, can be found in Weisz, 'A Moment of Synthesis' (n. 37).
58. Henry E. Sigerist, 'Notes and comments: on Hippocrates', *Bulletin of the Institute of the History of Medicine*, **2**, 1934, p. 193.
59. Gaston Baissette, 'Hippocrate', in Maxime Laignel-Lavastine (ed.), *Histoire générale de la médecine, de la pharmacie, de l'art dentaire et de l'art vétérinaire*, Vol. 1, Paris: Albin Michel, 1936, pp. 233–77. By 1949 four volumes had appeared. The last included an essay on homoeopathy by Michel Martiny.
60. Maxime Laignel-Lavastine, 'Introduction', in *Histoire générale de la médecine*, (n. 59), p. 10.
61. Ibid., pp. 11–12.
62. 'Avant propos', *Hippocrate: revue d'humanisme médical*, **1**, 1933, p. 4.
63. A. Castiglioni, *Histoire de la médecine*, trans. J. Bertrand and F. Gidon, Paris: Payot, 1931.
64. G. [*sic*] Castiglioni, 'L'orientation de la pensée médicale contemporaine considérée du point de vue historique', *Bulletin de l'Académie de Médecine*, Series 3, **109**, 1933, pp. 429–36. The quote is on p. 436.
65. For instance, he saw neo-Hippocratism as a return to a biological orientation from a more purely clinical one whereas most French holists saw it as a return to clinical medicine. His emphasis on 'Mediterranean' traditions also had limited resonance in France. Writing in 1934, Henry Sigerist, 'On Hippocrates' (n. 58), pp. 212–13, cited no French texts in his discussion of neo-Hippocratism.
66. Alfred Walter Waddington, 'La tradition hippocratique et le renouveau actuel du vitalisme', MD thesis, No. 317, Paris, 1934; Léon Cottenceau, 'Le néo-hippocratisme', MD thesis, No. 314, Paris, 1935.
67. This was Cottançeau. Waddington was more influenced by Carton's naturopathy, but one of those he thanked in his acknowledgements was the homoeopath-psychoanalyst René Allendy.

68. See Weisz, 'A moment of synthesis' (n. 37).
69. René Dumesnil, *La renaissance de l'Hippocratisme*, Paris: np, 1938, p. 887. (This is reprinted from the *Revue de Paris*.)
70. Phillip A. Nicholls, *Homeopathy and the Medical Profession*, London and New York: Croom Helm, 1988, p. 234.
71. Alexandre Cawadias, 'La méthode néo-hippocratique', *L'Homéopathie moderne*, **2**, 1934, pp. 485–97; and idem, 'L'étude morphologique du malade et son importance clinique en médecine néo-hippocratique', *L'Homéopathie moderne*, **2**, 1934, pp. 728–40.
72. Alexandre Cawadias, 'Le néo-hippocratisme et l'homéopathie', *L'Homépathie moderne*, **4**, 1935, pp. 66–82.
73. Ibid., p. 67; M. Laignel-Lavastine, 'Le néo-hippocratisme', *Presse médicale*, **45**, 1937, pp. 1215–16.
74. *L'Homépathie moderne*, **4**, 1935, p. 108.
75. Pierre Delore, *Tendances de la médecine contemporaine*, Paris: Masson, 1936. This work is discussed in detail in Weisz, 'A moment of synthesis' (n. 37).
76. At the Second International Neo-Hippocratic Congress in 1953 the number of faculty professors who participated actively was larger.
77. As reported by B. Aschner, 'Hippocratisme pratique', in *Actes du Ie Congrès international de Médecine néo-hippocratique*, Paris: np, 1937, p. 36. Carrel briefly alluded to these views in Alexis Carrel, 'Le rôle futur de la médecine', in Alexis Carrel, Auguste Lumière et al., *Médecine officielle et médecine hérétique*, Paris: Plon, 1945, pp. 1–9.
78. August Lumière, 'A propos du Premier Congrès de Médecine Néo-hippocratique', in *Les slogans de la médecine*, Lyon: Sézanne, 1941, pp. 277–314.
79. Léon Vannier, *Néo-hippocratisme et homéopathie*, Paris: Doin, 1938.
80. *Médecine officielle* (see n. 77) appeared in 1945.
81. Marcel Martiny, 'Nouvel-hippocratisme', in Carrel et al., *Médecine officielle*, p. 141.
82. Littré's dictionary defined '*hippocratisme*' as 'the doctrine which attempts to imitate Hippocrates, giving to this imitation the particular sense of following nature, that is to say of studying the spontaneous effort that it makes and the crises that it produces'. See Emile Littré and Charles Robin, *Dictionnaire de médecine, de chirurgie, de pharmacie, des sciences accessoires et de l'art vétérinaire*, 12th edn, Paris: Baillière, 1865, p. 717.
83. Baissette, 'Hippocrate' (n. 59), is set up as a refutation of Carton's earlier presentation of a naturopathic Hippocrates.
84. Jean Fiolle, *Journal intime d'un chirurgien*, Paris: Amiot-Dumont, 1952, pp. 32–36.
85. Alfred Martinet, *Energétique clinique; physiopathologie thérapeutique*, Paris: Masson, 1925, p. 399.
86. Weisz, 'A moment of synthesis' (n. 37).
87. Martiny, 'Nouvel-hippocratisme' (n. 81), p. 145.
88. René Biot, *Au service de la personne humaine*, Joigny: Vulliez, 1934; idem, *Le Corps et l'âme*, Paris: Plon, 1938; Henri Bon, *Précis de médecine catholique*, Besançon: Alcan, 1936; A. Vincent, *Vers une médecine humaine*, Paris: Ed. Montaigne, 1937. Joseph Okinczyk, *Humanisme et médecine*, Paris: Labergerie, 1937; G. Regard, *Étude biologique et scientifique des grands problèmes religieux*, Lausanne: Payot, 1937.
89. See especially Jean Fiolle, *La crise de l'humanisme*, Paris: Mercure de France, 1937.

90. Jean Fiolle, *Scientisme et science*, 3rd edn, Paris: Mercure de France, 1936; Lecomte de Noüy, *L'homme devant la science*, Paris: Flammarion, 1939; Rémy Collin, *Message social de savant*, Paris: Albin Michel, 1941.
91. Delore, *Tendances de la médecine* (n. 75), pp. 6–7. While holism itself was generally ignored by leading spokesmen of official medicine, relativistic interpretations of physics hit closer to home and provoked responses. See Henri Roger, 'La crise du déterminisme', *Presse médicale*, **49**, 1941, pp. 129–32, 179–82; Gustave Roussy, 'L'avenir de la science', *Presse médicale*, **51**, 1943, pp. 582–83 and idem, 'Des brèches dans le mur', *Presse médicale*, **52**, 1944, pp. 286–87.
92. Carrel, 'Le rôle futur de la médecine' (n. 77), p. 3.
93. Ibid.
94. Sigerist, 'On Hippocrates' (n. 58), pp. 193, 198.
95. Jouanna, 'Littré' (n. 21), p. 299.

CHAPTER THIRTEEN

The Name and the Word: Neo-Hippocratism and Language in Interwar Britain

David Cantor

In the years after the First World War several commentators began to detect a revival of medical interest in Hippocrates and Hippocratic medicine. Hippocrates was invoked as the inspiration for constitutional, social, physical and psychological medicine, as well as homoeopathy and neo-humoralism.[1] While some traced the roots of this revival to the late nineteenth-century,[2] most accepted that it had gained particular impetus after the First World War, and the Italian historian Arturo Castiglioni claims to have coined the term neo-Hippocratism in 1925 to describe this interest.[3] Whatever the truth of such a claim, the label became increasingly popular in Britain in the 1920s and 1930s and the growing interest in Hippocrates was often portrayed as a broader reaction against certain aspects of nineteenth-century medicine. It was a 'revolt against the system, formalism, academics, professionalism, materialism, and analysis of the nineteenth century', as one physician put it in 1932[4] – a 'revolt in favour of vitalism, humanism, individualism, and synthesis, a return to [the] Hippocratic doctrine'.

For many British neo-Hippocratists this revolt was also against the ways in which language had come to be used in modern medicine. In their view, the growing influence of laboratory scientists, specialists, big business and state officials within medicine had resulted in a valuation and use of words that was inimical to clinical medicine. Neo-Hippocratists claimed that all these groups placed a reliance on words for transmitting knowledge that would work to undermine the effectiveness of medicine. In the bleak future controlled by these groups, they claimed, diagnosis would mean little more than matching patients to the definition of disease found in a book. The problem was that 'real' patients never fitted easily into such written categories, and neo-Hippocratists maintained that such a method could be disastrous in terms of treatment. For them such definitions were what they called 'fictions' – useful methods of classifying knowledge, perhaps, but never more than a prelude to practical diagnosis on real patients.

Words were quite problematic to neo-Hippocratists. Clinical practice, they claimed, could not be reduced to them. They were, at best, a highly imperfect vehicle for transmitting clinical knowledge: nothing substituted for practical experience gained at the patient's bedside, an 'incommunicable knowledge'.[5] Although words might help make sense of the real world by helping to organise knowledge, they were not to be confused with reality itself. They represented artificial categories of classification, fictions or fantasies. Their value in organising knowledge was always contingent. The problem for neo-Hippocratists was that, in modern medicine, the distinction between the artificial and the real seemed to blur. People increasingly treated words as if they were real things in themselves. Naming something prompted individuals to act as if that name was the reality itself rather than an attempt to make sense of reality. People's ideas were no longer grounded in experience of the real world. They derived their experience of 'reality' from books, and this secondhand 'reality' was increasingly taken to be authentic. As one physician put it, people were being 'hypnotised' by names.[6]

The recognition that words had the power to make the artificial seem real prompted neo-Hippocratists to define themselves in relation to the ways in which others employed words. On the one hand, they defined themselves against those who, they claimed, succumbed to such power, notably specialists, laboratory scientists, academic medicine, state officials and the general public, all of whom tended to treat words as if they were the things they represented. On the other hand, they also defined themselves against those who they suggested used words in ways that encouraged others to view abstractions as material objects, or at least to confuse the distinction between a word and its object. The same villains can be detected here – specialists, laboratory scientists and state officials who spread their own subordination to the word to others through medical textbooks, official memoranda and other means. More broadly, this group could also include demagogues, dictators and advertisers who caused the broader public to act as if nations, political parties and the brandnames of commercial products were real things. Concerns about language thus illustrate neo-Hippocratists' anxieties not only about changes in the organisation of medicine, but also about the broader social, economic and cultural problems of the inter-war years.

Alexander Cawadias and British neo-Hippocratism

Some of the characteristics of British neo-Hippocratism can be illuminated by a key figure in the movement, Alexander Cawadias, a Greek physician resident in London. Born in 1884, Cawadias was the son of Professor P. Kavvdias, General Director of Antiquities and Fine Arts, who had restored the ancient theatre at Epidaurus.[7] Cawadias studied at the Universities of Heidelberg, Bonn and Paris, graduating B. ès L. Paris (1900) and MD (1910), and returning to

Athens in 1912 on the outbreak of the Balkan Wars. A personal friend of the Greek royal family, in 1914 he was appointed chief of the Medical Clinic in the Evangelisomos Hospital, Athens on the nomination of Queen Olga. In 1926, two years after the declaration of the Greek republic, he followed the royal family into exile in London, and eventually took British citizenship. In later years, he would trace the origins of neo-Hippocratism to pre-war Athens, Genoa and Madrid and, perhaps with his own experience of exile in mind, concluded that 'political reasons disrupted this new Mediterranean Medicine'.[8]

After leaving Greece, Cawadias obtained his British medical qualifications at Durham and established a large consulting practice in the Harley Street area, particularly among expatriate Greeks.[9] He retained his friendship with the King of Greece, entertaining him at his Wimpole Street home, and developed, as far as his straitened circumstances allowed, the life and style of a cultured gentleman and scholar. According to his daughter, his study included a huge desk, cluttered with medical books, the Greek classics (Plato and Demosthenes) and a sprinkling of English paperback thrillers.[10] There was a giant round ashtray in the shape of a coiled snake which overflowed with cigarette ends, untidy bulging bookcases, a framed Hippocratic oath, and the busts of Socrates, Hippocrates and Napoleon. It may be that Cawadias' interest in the classics reflected his family and Greek origins, but it also reflected his aspiration to emulate English gentlemanly culture. A knowledge of Greek and ancient Greek culture was a distinguishing and self-defining mark of the social elite in interwar Britain, albeit probably not the mark it had been for their Victorian and Edwardian forebears.[11]

Although Cawadias had an unusual background for a British physician, he rapidly established himself as a key figure in the British neo-Hippocratic movement. Two years after arriving Britain, he gave a keynote speech to a 1928 conference on neo-Hippocratism held at the Linnean Society, perhaps the first neo-Hippocratic conference in the country.[12] He developed his ideas on neo-Hippocratism in his 1931 book *The Modern Therapeutics of Internal Diseases*,[13] and was involved in efforts to found the International Society of Neo-Hippocratic Medicine in the 1930s under Maxime Laignel-Lavastine (psychiatrist and professor of the history of medicine at the Paris Faculty of Medicine).[14] Cawadias evoked the common image of neo-Hippocratism as 'a reaction from the intense analytical work of the nineteenth-century',[15] giving numerous papers on the areas of medicine of interest to neo-Hippocratists – endocrinology, health education, physical medicine and constitutional medicine – and becoming involved in efforts in the early 1930s to heal the fractures between homoeopathy and orthodox medicine.[16] In 1937 he was elected president of the medical history section of the Royal Society of Medicine, and his presidential speech was on neo-Hippocratism. During the same year he spoke on the subject at the First International Congress on Neo-Hippocratism held in Paris.[17]

Cawadias thus highlights British neo-Hippocratism's close connections with continental – and especially French – neo-Hippocratic movements. But he also argued that there were particular reasons as to why the movement was so strong in England.[18] In his view, the work of English physiologists on the unity of the organism facilitated its reception, as did certain cultural and institutional features of English medicine. English doctors, he suggested, were particularly attracted to tradition and history; they were not allowed to forget Hippocrates. They were judged by both their character and their therapeutic success, and success, he claimed circuitously, was only possible with a Hippocratic perspective. All were facilitated by organisations such as the Royal College of Physicians and the medical history section of the Royal Society of Medicine.

Thus, for Cawadias, neo-Hippocratism was something that found particular support among the clinical elite to which he aspired. He singled out two Royal physicians, Lords Dawson and Horder,[19] as advocates of the neo-Hippocratic view. Both had accompanied him to Paris in 1937, as had another Royal physician, his friend the homoeopath Sir John Weir.[20] Cawadias also praised the general practitioner Sir James Mackenzie as 'probably the greatest clinical leader of neo-Hippocratism'.[21] He also lauded another physician, Francis Crookshank, who had developed an anti-realist, nominalist conception of disease.[22] He could also have listed many others who urged a return to Hippocrates in the 1920s and 1930s: the list of names is extensive, but includes Sir Robert Hutchison (Great Ormond Street and London Hospitals),[23] Sir Walter Langdon-Brown (Regius Professor of Physic Cambridge),[24] John Ryle (Guy's Hospital),[25] Alexander Gibson (Oxford),[26] Robert Moon (National Hospital for Diseases of the Heart),[27] Arthur Brock (Edinburgh),[28] as well as lesser known physicians such as Matthew Ray (London),[29] Reginald Hodder (Penge),[30] and the expatriate, Archibald Adam Warden (Cannes).[31]

As such names suggest, Hippocrates was particularly popular among those who aspired to what Christopher Lawrence has styled patrician values – clinicians who practised (or sought to practise) among the rich and influential and who offered charitable service in the voluntary hospitals.[32] Hippocrates, of course, provided the model personality for such physicians; his oath was a focus for the discussion of ethics.[33] But he also provided an opportunity for them to look back to an ancient world of supposed organic unity in which the ideas and practice of medicine were said to reflect the dynamic and synthetic nature of the social order. In such a society, these physicians believed, the body was seen as a fragile, integrated, self-regulating entity that existed in complex and constantly changing relation to the environment and mind. A disturbance in the internal workings of the body could lead to illness, as could changes in the environment or the person's mental state. For many commentators, such a view of the body provided a justification for bedside diagnostic skills focused on the individual patient, for a natural history of disease generated through bedside observation, and for an emphasis on the healing role of Nature, all of which characterised Hippocratic medicine according to these commentators. Hippocrates and Hippocratic medicine thus legitimated the authority of the generalist clinician over those whom they feared increasingly challenged their authority – the specialist, the laboratory practitioner and the medical bureaucrat, the very groups that, according to the neo-hippocratists, misused language.

Words and social disorder

But the turn to Hippocrates was about much more than internal medical politics. Hippocrates also provided a means of expressing anxieties about the social, economic and cultural upheavals of the First World War and the post-war world. To many of these physicians, the roots of these problems went back to the urban–industrial transformation of the nineteenth century. This transformation, they claimed, had created a world that was changing so rapidly that it was almost impossible to adapt to, and had led to a sense of anxiety and nerve strain.[34] It was also a world that was increasingly fragmented and mechanistic in outlook, often characterised by a 'herd mentality' that undermined higher qualities of individuality and reason. To neo-Hippocratists the war had exacerbated all these problems. While men had found comfort in the 'brotherhood of the trenches', this brotherhood had also promoted the confusion of the mass mind. As a consequence, neo-Hippocratists suggested the post-war period was characterised by delusion and sentimentality.

If the war had highlighted the problems of the mass mind, it also highlighted the thin dividing line between civilisation and barbarism. Its legacy was often characterised as a war after the war.[35] 'The post-war period has not brought us peace,' commented Arthur Brock in 1923.[36] 'It has brought us into a state halfway between that of actual war and that of the pre-war period – a kind of *status bellicosus*, a state of latent war, of *wardom*.' The 1920s and 1930s seemed increasingly polarised: nations divided against nations, labour against capital, communism against fascism, and countless other divisions besides, often working against each other. As Sir Walter Langdon-Brown put it: 'The building up of vertical walls between nations is being countered by horizontal lines of cleavage, which threaten to divide Europe into Fascists and Communists.'[37] Brock argued that the 'peace' was more a balance of opposing forces, than a harmony of mutually complementary groups and individuals: 'Everybody, every section of the community, every country, is "up against" something or somebody.'[38]

Language played a central role in neo-Hippocratists' accounts of the divisions of the inter-war years. The 'fire-eating' speeches[39] of dictators and demagogues and the sensationalism of the press barons and advertisers all demonstrated the power of language to inflame otherwise stable individuals.

Words seemed to have the ability to make individuals behave as if nations, empires, labour and capital were real entities. As Brock put it:

> Nations were all looked upon as absolutely separate things. ... Yet, of course, the absolute idea of nationality is a bit of pure political specialism, and is, as such, in perpetual conflict with facts. What is and what is not a country has been determined on the most arbitrary principles.[40]

To Brock and other neo-Hippocratists, such 'entities' were actually abstractions or fictions. While such fictions could usefully help organise social life, what concerned neo-Hippocratists was the extremity of loyalty to such entities. Such loyalty had brought the world to war in 1914 and ensured that peace would never be more than a balance of opposites. Put another way, words seemed to have the ability to create group loyalties, be it to nation or party, and it was not simply a matter of how such words were expressed. The sensationalist language of demagogues and advertisers might create group loyalties, but so too might the colder language of science. To neo-Hippocratists the analytical language of science served to subdivide things off from one another: the roots of the problem were in the 'fragmented' minds that thought this way. What was increasingly apparent to neo-Hippocratists was that this tendency towards fragmentation was also present in medicine. And the very groups that challenged the authority of the general clinician – the laboratory scientist, the specialist and the bureaucrat – seemed to be the principal offenders.

The links between concerns about language, social fragmentation, medicine and the First World War can be illuminated by the Scottish physician, sociologist and classicist, Arthur Brock, a specialist in the treatment of nervous diseases and the translator of Galen for the Loeb classics series. To Brock the origins of the problem went back to before the war. 'The pre-war public mind was fragmented, and the fragments did not cohere',[41] he claimed; it was 'broken up, disparate, thinking in compartments'.[42] Brock claimed that the pre-war mind was best described in terms of 'dissociation', 'disintegration' and 'split personality'.[43] The extreme form of this mentality, according to Brock, was neurasthenia. Doctors, he claimed, saw increasing numbers of neurasthenics before the war, the characteristic feature of which was the very lack of solidarity – the segregation of parts – that also characterised the broader pre-war mind.[44] The wartime epidemic of shell-shock was evidence of much the same pathology. 'The essential element of shell-shock was fragmentation or "dissociation" of the mind,' he stated.[45] To Brock such fragmented minds subdivided the world into artificial compartments which took on a seemingly independent existence and which names only served to make concrete.

For Brock, pre-war Germany, with its highly specialised education system, powerful state bureaucrats, and mechanistic or separatist explanations of biological, psychological and social phenomena, was the principal example of a society that encouraged such mental compartmentalisation. Such fragmentation was at the root of German aggression: the specialised nature of German education, he claimed, had led to the 'moral enfeeblement' that led to the First World War, 'for how else can we explain the Docility or mass-hypnotism that lead these hapless millions into war?'.[46] Brock portrayed a pre-war world divided along lines of nationalism, race, gender and class, all encouraged by increasingly powerful state officials whose own minds were almost pathologically compartmentalised. In such a world individuals began to lose their moral strength and their will, people *'were allowing themselves to become weak'*.[47] They were workshy and they avoided trouble and pain through drugs, alcohol, food, sentimentality, sex and spectacle – '[t]he dope and the dream', as Brock put it.[48] Increasingly, people ceased to think for themselves, aiming to do as others did, to be told what to do. In short, '[i]ndividuals disappeared in the crowd'.[49] For Brock, as for many other commentators, crowds were credulous, mindlessly willing to be led and to imitate, and vulnerable to mass hypnosis.[50]

For Brock, neo-Hippocratism was thus constructed as a revolt against Germany. It was in Germany that such a crowd mentality had been most apparent, German pharmaceutical companies had provided the 'dope' and German music (especially Wagner) had provided the 'dream' that allowed individuals to escape from life and into what Brock called 'an other worldly region'.[51] And what concerned him was the impact of such German influences on Britain. German drugs had flooded the British market, and were close to controlling 'our philosophy of life'.[52] Furthermore, British medicine imitated German infatuations with state and laboratory medicine, specialisation and abstract thinking. It was here that Brock's anti-German sentiments blurred into anti-Semitism. German medicine's propensity for abstractedness, he speculated, might be due to the large number of Jews in German medicine:

> This race was for so long precluded by selfish convention and laws from sharing in European culture that the minds of its thinkers had been practically forced away from the concrete totality of life into materialistic or metaphysical by-ways.[53]

Brock himself wanted British medicine to reject much that he conceived of as particularly German or Jewish in British medicine: specialisation, laboratory medicine and the growing importance of the state. Other neo-Hippocratists echoed his point.[54] 'We in England have ... worshipped too long and too blindly the false gods set up in the Teutonic laboratories by exclusively *à posteriori* investigators,'[55] commented F.G. Crookshank in 1919. ' "This England" of ours is a quaintly individualist country,' noted Lord Horder in the 1930s, echoing Brock's concern about the influence of the mass mind in medicine. 'A good many things which in other countries are left to a central bureau are done here by the people themselves as a result of their own initiative.'[56]

If British neo-Hippocratists rejected the institutional structures of German medicine, they also tended to reject its mechanistic, reductive and solidistic outlook. As Cawadias put it, 'Britain never submitted to the dictature of Virchow' – the man Cawadias and many neo-Hippocratists blamed for much of modern medicine's reductive tendency – 'and biological thought here has always tended towards unity'.[57] For Cawadias, British physiologists and biologists had demonstrated the neo-Hippocratic principle of the 'unity of the organism'. He praised the work of Bayliss and Starling on the endocrines' role in chemical integration, the work of Gaskell and Langley on the integrating action of the vegetative nervous system, and that of Charles Sherrington on the integrating role of the cerebral cortex. Thus neo-Hippocratism was not a rejection of the laboratory, but a rejection of certain allegedly German tendencies towards reductionism and mechanism they saw as within it. As Cawadias noted, the 'word *Neohippocratism* indicates that our contemporary doctrine is an adaptation to modern scientific research of the doctrine of Hippocrates'.[58] Indeed, Robert Hutchison argued that the development of biochemistry, endocrinology and medical psychology had themselves 'brought about a change of doctrine which is variously described as "Neo-Hippocratism", "individual" or "constitutional" medicine'.[59] To neo-Hippocratists, these sciences demonstrated the need to treat the body as a whole. In other words, their work demonstrated the primacy of the general clinician in diagnosing and treating disease. Only a general clinician could hope to understand all the factors that went to make up a disease, and to evaluate the results of the laboratory.

Finally, British neo-Hippocratists also rejected what they regarded as German medicine's materialist or realist tendency to reify disease categories, 'to believe that there actually exist in Nature objects or things, known as "special diseases," that attack people physically as do Bolshevicks or Huns', as Crookshank put it.[60] For Crookshank, diseases were 'fictions', as they also were to Cawadias, although they disagreed on the philosophical basis of this claim.[61]

For Cawadias this claim was based on '[t]he nominalistic principle [which] is opposed to the realistic ... according to which diseases have a substantial reality'.[62] According to nominalists, Cawadias argued, diseases were 'mere names, artificial categories of classification of the morbid phenomena. They do not correspond to reality',[63] and the only choice was whether they should be abandoned altogether or kept as an aid to diagnosis. Nominalism thus rejected any connection between words and material reality, but its place as a key philosophical tenet of neo-Hippocratism was challenged by a rival conceptualist principle. According to Cawadias, conceptualism was a weaker version of realism, in which diseases were 'concepts existing in our minds and express real similarity in things themselves'[64] and one its chief advocates was Crookshank.

Crookshank's objection to nominalism was that it would result in physicians doing little more than sticking a label on a patient that signified nothing but *flatus vocis* – literally, the breath of the voice, a phrase used to describe the ultra-nominalist opinion that universals have no substantial or conceptual existence, but consist in nothing more than the mere sound of their names. (Even Cawadias seems to have acknowledged the futility of the ultra-nominalist position, arguing that diseases were essential to understanding the patient.) For Crookshank conceptualism allowed the practitioner to put 'in due relation the THING, the THOUGHT and the NAME'.[65]

Limited minds

What concerned neo-Hippocratists about the ability of words to make the abstract seem real was what it said about those who succumbed to them. For neo-Hippocratists such individuals were profoundly limited: they lacked imagination and ideas. And often in neo-Hippocratic discourse, limitation blurred into confinement. Those who succumbed to the word had inflexible, narrow, compartmentalised minds; they were unwittingly confined by their own limitations and unable to rise above them. They were slaves to system, fettered by facts as well as bound by words. Thus Crookshank urged his readers not to regard 'our universals, our laws, our generalizations and our hypotheses ... [as] immutable, and insusceptible of modification', to fall into what he called the 'bonds of academic slavery'. It was academics who regarded such systems as unchangeable, a fact that, for Crookshank, derived from their own subordination to the word:

> For the Academic, in the end, bows down and worships, not the ideal God whom he symbolizes verbally but the very symbol itself – the NAME or WORD which comes to be his Idol and so no longer the symbol which indicates the convenient Idea that resumes his experiences or perceptions.[66]

If Crookshank saw academic medicine as subordinated to words, Brock saw state medicine as much the same. Although Hippocrates was invoked by George Newman and John Ryle to justify an expanded role for the state in medicine after the war, Brock took a very different view.[67] For Brock the state could never be a solution to medicine's problems, since it was part of the problem itself and the state official was one of the central villains. Along with specialists, Brock claimed that state officials tended towards neo-scholasticism, a sophistical tendency to speak of mere words as if they were real things. They did this because they were trapped by their own psychology. He continued:

> ... it must never be forgotten that the official himself has a psychology, and that, however well he may begin, and however high his original qualifications may be, the further he gets away from real patients of flesh and blood, the more does his own psychological state tend to partake of the pathological. An excessive devotion to [disease] 'entities' is among the milder symptoms of this neurosis, which, in its best-known forms, has been christened 'departmentality'.[68]

The prospect of what Brock regarded as such stunted intellectuals determining treatment caused him to despair for medicine's future if the state took over. The individual state official blurred too easily into the mass, to become one of so many cogs within an inanimate organisation: 'The State is lifeless; it is only a machine. We must regain sanity by our own individual efforts.'[69]

Specialists also exhibited intellectual limitations that they were unable to rise above, and which were linked to their fascination with words. Brock and Horder referred to the 'myopia'[70] and James Mackenzie to the 'limited experience' and 'limited outlook'[71] of the specialist, while Cawadias labelled it the 'narrow specialistic outlook'.[72] For Cawadias, such a narrow outlook could have disastrous results in practice. Such a specialist, he claimed:

> ... will overrate certain symptoms, those included in his special horizon, and underrate others. It will be impossible for him to *see* the whole individual patient. He will run after the shadow of the local or fictional disease, and thus let the reality, the condition of the diseased individual, escape him.[73]

Such 'reality' was not, however, something that was grounded in words; it was rooted in experience of medical practice. Thus, Cawadias was at pains to dissociate words from practical therapeutic success. Such a specialist, he noted, might 'become a great writer, a powerful terminologist, skilled in technical details of exploration, but he will be unable to cure a single individual'.[74] For example, a heart specialist could not cure someone labelled as suffering from a disease of the heart, because 'diseases of the heart do not exist'.[75] The imagination that conjured up such fictions was poor indeed.

Pessimism about the intellectual life of specialists betrayed uncertainties about the future. Neo-Hippocratists often portrayed themselves fighting a rearguard action against the relentless onslaught of the specialist and laboratory scientist. 'We may agree with Sir Arthur Keith that specialism is inevitable as medical science evolves,' commented Hutchison, 'but none the less we may be permitted to regret it. For specialism, however favourable to the accumulation of facts, is bad for the philosophy of knowledge.'[76] Skilled terminologists they might be, but it was unclear to Hutchison whether specialists even understood each others' words, for 'the terminology of the different specialties is now become so esoteric that other workers cannot understand it if they would'.[77] He speculated that all laboratories should close for five years to allow time to digest the already huge accumulation of knowledge and think out new lines of advance.[78] A.J. Brock agreed:

> Is not Dr Hutchison's complaint against the 'medical organism' in effect just this, that from a defective sense of humour it has failed to digest its material, to assimilate what is good in it, and to reject the irrelevant *perittomata*, with the result that these latter are now menacing its further advance?[79]

Faced with what Hutchison regarded as the inevitability of specialism, neo-Hippocratists disagreed on what the solution might be. Hutchison wanted bridge-makers to bridge the gap between the laboratory and the clinic, but Brock feared that this would only bring about a new group of officials, presumably exhibiting the scholasticism of existing state bureaucrats: 'Surely the link which he [Hutchison] desiderates is already existent in the mental constitution of the average general practitioner[?]'[80] To others, however, it was quite unclear whether the division between specialism and generalism could be maintained absolutely. Cawadias who, in his early articles, argued that 'specialisation in diagnosis [is] impossible'[81] (diagnosis being the central part of internal medicine for him), subsequently permitted an element of specialisation even within general medicine. 'There is a tendency nowadays even among ardent Neohippocratists, to maintain these specialties', he wrote in 1937 of neurology, cardiology, endocrinology, gastroenterology, and dermatology, 'but to introduce into their practice the constitutional outlook.'[82]

What was particularly disturbing to these physicians was the way in which the narrow outlook of unreformed specialists and laboratory scientists prompted them to lump individual patients together as a mass. Such specialists seemed unable to view patients as individuals, preferring to slot them into prefixed categories. In other words neo-Hippocratists saw specialists as grouping individuals according to whether they shared some organic lesion or cellular disruption: the individual patient did not exist except as a member of a group which shared certain common characteristics, so the whole 'patient' began to fade away to become, for instance, a case of high-blood pressure as defined by the words in a medical textbook. Thus Crookshank castigated the practitioner who 'diligently making a diagnosis in strict accordance with differential tables and tests, searches his text-books in confusion for the treatment appropriate to the disease he suspects'.[83] No 'real' patient could be found in such books, as the phrase 'in confusion' suggests. Cawadias makes the point:

> The physician who is advised – as I [Cawadias] read in the advertisement of one of these works – to have such books on his table for rapid reference, while examining his patient, will be enabled to determine a fictional label, but that fiction will simply make him lose contact with reality, with the suffering individual who has entrusted himself to his care.[84]

Indeed, Cawadias feared that the constitutional outlook might be subverted by such a perspective and urged his readers not to reify the biotype: the biotype was:

> ... also a fictional construction made for purposes of classification. To say that a patient has an arthritic or a pyknic constitution is as fictional as to say that he has 'pneumonia', or 'typhoid fever'.[85]

Repeatedly, neo-Hippocratists called for a return to the individual patient, and by extension a return to a broader mentality able to take on board all the complexities of human life. Brock urged '[A]bove all, let our slogan be: "Back to the individual patient and the individual practitioner"'.[86] Hutchison called neo-Hippocratism 'the science of the individual'.[87] Cawadias argued that '[t]he clinician must pass on from the diagnosis of the disease to the diagnosis of the diseased individual. ... The whole of the individual, psychical as well as physical.'[88] Neo-Hippocratists saw 'official' medicine's representation of the body as fragmented because it treated the components of the body – cells, organs or tissues, for example – as independent of each other and of the rest of the organism; the body as separate from its environment; the action of a microbe as separate from the response of the body on which it acted; and the disease as quite separate from the body. All this was encouraged by a realist attitude to language. Such was the grip of words on the realist's mind that those who subscribed to a fragmented vision of the body confused their partial vision with the 'whole' thing. They saw diseases as real entities, attacking the body from without or located in particular lesions within the body. By emphasising the fictional nature of such 'entities', neo-Hippocratists hoped to loosen the grip of such words on the mind. They seized on the 1918 influenza outbreak as evidence of the limitations of reductive bacteriology.[89]

Neo-Hippocratists' response

Neo-Hippocratists responded in a number of ways to those groups and individuals who, in Crookshank's phrase, idolised the word. In the first place, they argued that words were quite insufficient to fully develop clinical practice. In part, it was a problem of translation: specialist terminology was often incomprehensible to clinicians, if not, as Hutchison noted, to other specialists. Another issue was, as Cawadias suggested, that the skills of the terminologist had little to do with therapeutic success and could be positively detrimental. Words could never entirely capture the nature of clinical practice: recall the confusion of Crookshank and Cawadias' imaginary physicians searching textbooks for a suspect disease. In contrast, neo-Hippocratic diagnosticians might experience difficulty in putting a diagnosis into the conventional language of medical textbooks. As Crookshank put it, 'The elderly practitioner who, remote from libraries and from laboratories but near to Nature, is hesitant when asked for verbal diagnosis in terms of recent convention'[90] – conventions, that is, found in books and emanating from laboratories. The world of practice and the world of words were incommensurable.

In contrast to the word-bound world of academic medicine, neo-Hippocratists often construed themselves as cultivating 'natural' gifts, easily harmed by specialists and laboratory scientists. For example, Cawadias noted how early specialisation destroyed the 'natural gift'[91] of intuition so necessary to clinical practice. Such intuition, he claimed, could only be developed by all-round clinical education involving early and permanent contact with patients. Hutchison agreed on the importance of intuition, 'so often disparaged by the experimentalist'.[92] On a broader canvas, Brock claimed that it was man's 'natural instincts, his intuitions' that would save civilisation by healing the divisions of the post-war years. But, for Brock, it was not the specialist that possessed such 'natural faculties',[93] only what he called the 'plain man' trying to shape his environment. This environment included the 'verbalistic', 'that part of our surroundings which consists of *words*', he explained.[94] And, playing on the phrase found in popular health manuals, he urged 'we must become every man his own philologist and learn carefully to scrutinise our environing words.'[95]

In Brock's imagination, neo-Hippocratic physicians were the equivalent of this 'plain man'; they were generalists healing the divisions in medicine, as the 'plain man' healed divisions in society. Both shared a closeness to nature, an opposition to specialist terminologists and a complex identity as physicians to the body politic. For Brock – the plain thinking man was the *vis medicatrix naturae* of the societal body: 'man at length becomes his own healer',[96] he noted. The generalist played a similar role in healing the illness in a medical organism, including its verbal environment. Thus, Langdon-Brown literally played the role of nature when, in a speech to Edinburgh medical students, he attempted to rescue the word 'disease' from Thomas Lewis's revival of the notion of diseases as entities:

> But on the whole, the present tendency is to regard disease, as the name implies, as the sum total of the uncomfortable reactions of an individual to some perturbation in his external or internal environment, possibly in both.[97]

By now it should be clear that, although neo-Hippocratists saw no particular connection between words and things, words nevertheless formed a means of asserting distinction. When neo-Hippocratists argued that words had no material reality, they created a distinction between those who maintained a separation between words and their objects (neo-Hippocratists) and those who believed that words had a material existence or who tried to persuade others of this fact (often specialists, laboratory scientists, bureaucrats and others whom neo-Hippocratists mistrusted). Yet neo-Hippocratists did not see neo-Hippocratism as something purely for those who were verbally skilled. Like many other gentlemen of the inter-war years, they imagined themselves as part of an extended grouping of 'practical' or 'plain men' allied against the evils of modernity.[98] In their view the return to Hippocrates was something that united a broad range of practitioners, from Harley Street to the humblest general practitioner. Ironically, this alliance meant that a knowledge of Hippocrates was unnecessary to the practice of Hippocratic medicine. Brock's 'plain man' and Crookshank's elderly practitioner did not have to know of Hippocrates. For Hippocratic medicine was 'in fact now being practised successfully by not a few who are guiltless of any acquaintance with the Hippocratic Collection'.[99]

Such an image of a broad-based movement provided neo-Hippocratists with another means of asserting their own significance. In their imagination their movement extended far beyond the elite, with roots in an older world unimpressed by the lesser innovations of the present. It was a world that extolled wisdom and refused to confuse it with knowledge – one that looked to the timeless virtues of nature and countryfolk, refusing to abandon tradition in the midst of change. It was often an inarticulate world, but was eloquent all the same. It valued experience more than book-learning, practice more than the word – values that scholarly neo-Hippocratists were also coming to recognise. Here in the plain or practical man were the vestiges of a 'primitive' world with lessons for the present – an authentic England or Britain ignored at its peril by modern civilisation. The plain man, like Hippocrates, was instinctively opposed to modern tendencies towards analysis and fragmentation. He was without ambition or adornment, anchored in a practical world that crossed class barriers. Throughout the nineteenth century it had been plain men who had held faith with the holistic vision of the ancients, intuitively mistrusting the modern tendencies towards reductivism, mechanisation, standardisation and mass medicine. They might have known nothing of the Hippocratic *Corpus*, but they were often far more Hippocratic that those who invoked the name of the father of medicine – or so the leaders of neo-Hippocratism claimed.

The turn to the plain man thus illustrates a general point of this essay, that neo-Hippocratism was a response to what its followers regarded as the problems of modernity: the increasing fragmentation of society, its anonymity, its narrowing of vision, and the confusion between fact and fantasy that seemed to characterise it. Even the ancient world seemed in danger of misrepresentation. Fewer and fewer doctors appeared able to read Greek, and neo-Hippocratists repeatedly criticised the ways in which the language was constantly misused. Cawadias feared 'that the limitation of the action of the physician to the placing on the patient of a Greek or Latin label provokes many ironical comments on the part of non-medical thinkers'.[100] And Brock chided state bureaucrats for the tendency to reduce patients not only to diseases but, even worse, to 'entire abstractions, ciphers, [and] Greek names'.[101]

In retrospect, neo-Hippocratic concerns about the misuse of Greek – and the repeated attempts to recapture something of the original meaning of Greek words[102] – can also be seen as part of a longer-term process in which the classical world was marginalised in British culture. Elite physicians had long complained about the ignorance of Greek and Latin, especially among grammar school entrants to medical training.[103] But since the late nineteenth century such complaints had coincided with attempts to distinguish between language and the culture it carried. Some classicists urged an abandonment of compulsory Greek and the promotion of Greek culture: Greece, not Greek, as the classicist Gilbert Murray put it, attacking the use of the language as a class badge, much as neo-Hippocratists attacked it as a false badge of learning.[104] Both agreed that the language of liberty should not be foisted on individuals. Was not the modern tendency to slot people into pre-existing disease categories conjured out of Greek names precisely such an imposition? It is no coincidence that neo-Hippocratism emerged only shortly after compulsory Greek was abandoned at Oxford and Cambridge.[105]

By the 1940s neo-Hippocratism had begun to lose its momentum. Not only had Greek declined as a mark of the social elite, so had the elite itself and, with it, both the faith in Greece and the fantasy of a union of 'plain men'. Neo-Hippocratism – originally anti-specialist – was increasingly absorbed (as Cawadias seems have recognised above) into the outlook of new specialities such as constitutional, psychological, social and physical medicine. There are some signs of a brief revival in the mid-1940s,[106] a response perhaps to the threat of a state medical service, but, increasingly, physicians looked back to an earlier flourishing of the movement. As one commentator put it in 1944: 'There is much to be said for a "return to Hippocrates" warmly advocated a few years ago by those who saw danger in the present-day trend of medicine.'[107]

Acknowledgements

I am very grateful to the College of Physicians of Philadelphia for supporting the research on which this essay is based, and to Monique Bourque for excellent research assistance. An earlier version was given at a conference on holism in Montreal in May 1995.

Notes

1. On constitutional medicine see Sarah Tracy, 'George Draper and American constitutional medicine, 1916–1946: reinventing the sick man', *Bulletin of the History of Medicine*, **66**, 1992, pp. 53–89. On social medicine see Dorothy Porter, 'John Ryle: doctor of revolution?', in Dorothy Porter and Roy Porter, *Doctors, Politics and Society: Historical Essays*, Amsterdam and Atlanta: Rodopi, 1993, pp. 247–74. On holistic neurology and psychology see Anne Harrington, 'Other "ways of knowing": the politics of knowledge in interwar German brain science', in Anne Harrington (ed.), *So Human a Brain. Knowledge and Values in the Neurosciences*, Boston: Birkhäuses, 1992, pp. 229–44; also idem, *Reenchanted Science: Holism in German Culture from Wilhelm II to Hitler*, Princeton, NJ: Princeton University Press, 1996. On neo-humoralism and neo-Hippocratism see David Cantor, 'Cortisone and the politics of empire: Imperialism and British medicine, 1918–1955', *Bulletin of the History of Medicine*, **67**, 1993, pp. 463–93 esp. pp. 475–77; also idem, 'The contradictions of specialization. Rheumatism

and the decline of the spa in inter-war Britain', *Medical History (Supplement)* (10), 1990, pp. 127–44 esp. pp. 140–42. On homoeopathy in Britain see Phillip A. Nicholls, *Homeopathy and the Medical Profession*, London: Croom Helm, 1988, especially p. 234. where he highlights the connections between the thawing of relations between homoeopathic and orthodox medicine in the early 1930s and the neo-Hippocratic movement. See also Christopher Lawrence and George Weisz, *Greater than the Parts. Holism in Biomedicine, 1920–1950*, New York and London: Oxford University Press, 1998; and Stephen Cross and William R. Albury, 'Walter B. Cannon, L.J. Henderson, and the organic analogy', *Osiris*, 3, 1987, pp. 165–92.
2. Sir William Hamer's history of epidemiology described a return to Hippocratic methods from the 1890s, suggesting that it was Creighton's multivolume *History of Epidemics in Britain* that was instrumental in bringing a return to Hippocratic methods. See Sir William Hamer, *Epidemiology Old and New*, London: Kegan Paul, Trench, Trubner & Co. Ltd, 1928, p. ix. On Creighton as a Hippocratist pioneer of the psychotherapy movement see F.G. Crookshank, 'Introduction to the English edition', in Hans Prinzhorn, *Psychotherapy. Its Nature – Its Assumptions – Its Limitations. A Search For Essentials*, trans. and ed. Arnold Eiloart, London: Jonathan Cape, 1932, pp. 15–25, esp. p. 16.
3. Arturo Castiglioni, *A History of Medicine*, 2nd edn, New York: Alfred A. Knopf, 1947, p. 1143; also idem, 'Neo-hippocratic tendency of contemporary medical thought', *Medical Life*, **41**, 1934, pp. 115–46 where he suggests that he coined the term in 1926. See also Bernard Aschner, *The Art of the Healer*, New York: Dial, 1942; and Bernard Aschner, 'Neo-hippocratism in everyday practice', *Bulletin of the History of Medicine*, **10**, 1941, pp. 260–71.
4. F.G. Crookshank, 'The new psychology and the health of the people', *Purpose*, July–September 1932, pp. 122–27 at p. 123.
5. Christopher Lawrence, 'Incommunicable knowledge: science, technology and the clinical art in Britain 1850–1914', *Journal of Contemporary History*, **20**, 1985, pp. 503–20.
6. Arthur J. Brock, *Health and Conduct*, London: Williams and Norgate, 1923, p. 180 (note); and Arthur J. Brock, *Greek Medicine Being Extracts Illustrative of Medical Writers From Hippocrates to Galen*, London and Toronto: J.M. Dent & Sons, 1929, p. 1.
7. 'Dr. A. Cawadias. Exponent of neo-hippocratism', *Times*, 23 November 1971; A.W.F., 'Cawadias, Alexander Polycleitos', in Gordon Wolstenholme (ed.), *Lives of the Fellows of the Royal College of Physicians of London Continued to 1975*, London: Royal College of Physicians, 1982, pp. 95–96. Alexander Cawadias himself drew on his father's work in 'From Epidauros to Galenos. The principle currents of Greek medical thought', *Annals of Medical History* (NS) 3, 1931, pp. 501–14 at p. 503. See also Mary Henderson, *Xenia – A Memoir. Greece 1919–1949*, London: Weidenfeld and Nicolson, 1988. I am grateful to Lady Henderson, the daughter of Alexander Cawadias for telling me about her father in interview, June 1994.
8. A.P. Cawadias, *Clinical Endocrinology and Constitutional Medicine*, London: Frederick Muller, 1947, p. 360.
9. He was also physician to the St John Clinic and Institute of Physical Medicine in London.
10. Henderson, *Xenia* (n. 7), pp. xvii–xviii. Compare this with the portrayal of gentlemanly or patrician medical culture in the lives of Horder and Langdon Brown in Christopher Lawrence, 'A tale of two sciences: Bedside and bench in

twentieth-century Britain', *Medical History*, **43**, 1999, pp. 421–49, esp. pp. 421–25.
11. Christopher Stray, *Classics Transformed. Schools, Universities, and Society in England, 1830–1960*, Oxford: Clarendon Press, 1998. For the importance of classical Greece to the Victorians see Frank M. Turner, *The Greek Heritage in Victorian Britain*, New Haven and London: Yale University Press, 1981; Richard Jenkyns, *The Victorians and Ancient Greece*, Cambridge MA, Harvard University Press, 1980; G.W. Clarke (ed.), *Rediscovering Hellenism. The Hellenic Inheritance and the English Imagination*, Cambridge: Cambridge University Press, 1989.
12. A.P. Cawadias, 'The neo-hippocratic theory as a basis of medical thought and practice', *Archives of Medical Hydrology*, **7**, 1929, pp. 148–52.
13. A.P. Cawadias, *The Modern Therapeutics of Internal Diseases: An Introduction to Medical Practice*, London: Bailière, Tindall and Cox, 1931.
14. Cawadias, *Clinical Endocrinology* (n. 8), p. 360.
15. A.P. Cawadias, 'Neohippocratism', *Proceedings of the Royal Society of Medicine*, **31**, 1937, pp. 27–38 at p. 38.
16. Nicholls, *Homeopathy* (n. 1), pp. 234. As George Weisz argues in this volume, Cawadias was keen to promote neo-Hippocratism among homoeopaths. See also Cawadias, 'La méthode néo-hippocratique', *L'Homéopathie Moderne*, **2**, 1934, pp. 485–97. Alexandre Cawadias, 'L'étude morphologique du malade et son importance clinique en médecine néo-hippocratique', *L'Homéopathie Moderne*, **2**, 1934, pp. 728–40. Alexandre Cawadias, 'Le néo-hippocratisme et l'homéopathie', *L'Homépathie Moderne*, **4**, 1935, pp. 66–82.
17. Cawadias, 'Neo-Hippocratism' (n. 15), pp. 27–38. A.P. Cawadias, 'Les étapes historiques du neo-hippocratisme', in Ier Congrès International De Médecine Néo-Hippocratique, *Les Actes*, 1937, pp. 17–34.
18. Cawadias, 'Les étapes' (n. 17), p. 19.
19. On Horder see Lawrence, 'Tale of two sciences' (n. 10). See also Mervyn Horder, *The Little Genius. A Memoir of the First Lord Horder*, London: Duckworth, 1966. On Dawson see Francis Watson, *Dawson of Penn*, London: Chatto and Windus, 1950; Charles Webster, 'The metamorphosis of Dawson of Penn', in Porter and Porter, *Doctors, Politics and Society* (n. 1), pp. 212–28.
20. Weir discusses the relations between homoeopathy and Hippocratism in John Weir, 'Samuel Hahnemann and his influence on medical thought', *Proceedings of the Royal Society of Medicine*, **26**, 1933, pp. 668–76.
21. Cawadias, *Modern Therapeutics*, (n. 13) p. 4. On Mackenzie see Alex Mair, *Sir James Mackenzie MD 1853–1925. General Practitioner*, London: Royal College of General Practitioners, 1986. Mackenzie himself seems to have referred to Hippocrates only rarely.
22. Cawadias, 'Neo-Hippocratism' (n. 15), p. 29. On Crookshank see Douglas Robb, 'Individual psychology and the work of F.G. Crookshank', *New Zealand Medical Journal*, **33**, 1934, pp. 221–27. For an example of Crookshank's interest in Hippocrates see F.G. Crookshank, 'Airs, waters, and places', *Proceedings of the Royal Society of Medicine (Section of Balneology)*, **19**, 1925–26, pp. 17–22.
23. Robert Hutchison, 'Harvey: the man, his method and his message for us to-day', *British Medical Journal*, 24 October 1931, pp. 733–39. On Hutchison see Alan Moncrieff, 'Sir Robert Hutchison, Bart. (1871–1960)', *Journal of Pediatrics*, **58**, 1961, pp. 137–39. Alan Moncrieff, 'Hutchison, Sir Robert', in E.T. Williams and Helen M. Palmer (eds), *Dictionary of National Biography, 1951–1960*, Oxford: Oxford University Press, 1971, p. 526; Anon, 'Hutchison, Sir Robert', in Richard

R. Trail, *Lives of the Fellows of the Royal College of Physicians of London Continued to 1965*, London: Royal College of Physicians, 1968, pp. 208–9; Anon, J.R.B. Dixey, S. Leonard Simpson and Frank Rigall, 'Sir Robert Hutchison', *British Medical Journal*, 20 February 1960, pp. 571–73; 27 February 1960, pp. 655–56; 5 March 1960, pp. 735–36; 26 March 1960, p. 973. Kenneth H. Tallerman, 'Sir Robert Hutchison, Bt., M.D., F.R.C.P.. I. At the Hospital for Sick Children, Great Ormond Street, London', *Archives of Disease in Childhood*, **26**, 1951, pp. 365–67; Arthur G. Maitland-Jones, 'Sir Robert Hutchison, Bt., M.D., F.R.C.P.. II. At the London Hospital', *Archives of Disease in Childhood*, **26**, pp. 367–68; Langley Porter, 'Robert Hutchison at the London Hospital circa 1900: reminiscences of a clinical clerk', *Archives of Disease in Childhood*, **26**, 1951, pp. 369–72; Donald Hunter, 'The sayings of Robert Hutchison', *Archives of Disease in Childhood*, **26**, 1951, pp. 467–68; Alfred White Franklin, 'A handlist of the writings of Sir Robert Hutchison', *Archives of Disease in Childhood*, **26**, 1951, pp. 469–75.

24. Sir Walter Langdon-Brown, 'Art and fashion in medicine', *British Medical Journal* (Supplement), 16 March 1935, pp. 93–98. On Brown see Lawrence, 'Tale of two sciences' (n. 10).

25. John A. Ryle, 'The Hippocratic ideal', *Lancet*, 8 December 1934, pp. 1263–68. On Ryle see Porter, 'John Ryle' (n. 1); Dorothy Porter, 'Changing disciplines: John Ryle and the making of social medicine in Britain in the 1940s', *History of Science*, **30**, 1992, pp. 137–64.

26. Alexander George Gibson, *The Physician's Art. An Attempt to Expand John Locke's Fragment De Arte Medica*, Oxford: Clarendon Press, 1933, pp. 51–52; 'Gibson, Alexander George', *Lives of the Fellows of the Royal College of Physicians 1826–1925*, compiled by G.H. Brown, London: Royal College of Physicians, 1955, p. 530.

27. R.O. Moon, *Hippocrates and His Successors in Relation to the Philosophy of Their Time*, London: Longman, Green and Co., 1923, p. vii. On Moon see Anon and Arthur MacNalty, 'R.O. Moon' *British Medical Journal*, 8 August 1953, pp. 343–44; Anon, 'Robert Oswald Moon', *Lancet*, 8 August 1953, p. 303; Anon, 'Moon, Robert Oswald', in, *Lives* (n. 26), pp. 503–4.

28. Arthur J. Brock, 'Neo-hippocratism and state control of medicine', *British Medical Journal*, 28 November 1931, pp. 1012–13. See also Arthur J. Brock, 'Child guidance clinics and neo-hippocratism', *British Medical Journal*, 16 January 1932, pp. 122–23. On Brock see David Cantor, 'Arthur John Brock and humanism in early twentieth-century British medicine', precirculated paper for the 'Humanism Conference', Wellcome Institute for the History of Medicine, London, 16 February 1996; Dominic Hibbert, 'A sociological cure for shellshock: Dr. Brock and Wilfred Owen', *The Sociological Review (NS)*, **25**, 1977, pp. 377–86.

29. Matthew B. Ray, 'Historical sketch', *Archives of Medical Hydrology*, **7**, 1929, pp. 143–45; Matthew B. Ray, 'The Hippocratic tradition', *Post-Graduate Medical Journal*, **10**, 1934, pp. 27–31, 67–74, 116–22. Matthew B. Ray, 'Concepts of disease', *Archives of Medical Hydrology*, **5**, 1927, pp. 227–28. Matthew Ray is discussed in David Cantor, *Medicine, Philanthropy, and the Rheumatic Diseases in Britain, 1920–1970*, forthcoming. See also F.B., 'Matthew Burrow Ray', *British Journal of Physical Medicine*, **13**, 1950, p. 240; C.B. Heald, 'Matthew Burrow Ray', *Annals of the Rheumatic Diseases*, **9**, 1950, p. 280.

30. Reginald Hodder, 'Neo-hippocratism', *British Medical Journal*, 19 December 1931, p. 1160.

31. A.A. Warden, 'Neo-hippocratism', *British Medical Journal*, 28 November 1931, pp. 1011–12. See also Archibald Adam Warden, *English Handbook to the Paris Medical School, with Prefatory Letters by Lord Lister and W.W. Keen*, London: Churchill, 1903 (second edition 1910). Warden was a former consultant physician to the American and British Hospitals in Paris.
32. Christopher Lawrence, 'Still incommunicable: clinical holists and medical knowledge in interwar Britain', in Lawrence and Weisz, *Greater Than the Parts* (n. 1), pp. 94–111. For an alternative view of Hippocratism see Steve Sturdy, 'Hippocrates and state medicine: George Newman outlines the founding policy of the Ministry of Health', in ibid., pp. 112–34.
33. For Hippocrates as the model physician see Charles Singer, 'Medicine', in R.W. Livingstone (ed.), *The Legacy of Greece*, Oxford: Clarendon Press, 1923, pp. 201–48 at p. 212. For a reference to his *Oath* see F.G. Crookshank, 'The medico-legal relations of venereal disease', in L.W. Harrison, *The Diagnosis and Treatment of Venereal Diseases in General Practice. The Routine Management of Syphilis and Gonorrhoea Employed in the St. Thomas's Hospital Venereal Diseases Department*, London: Humphrey Milford/Oxford University Press, 1931, pp. 452–506 at p. 470.
34. Lord Horder, 'The strain of modern civilization', *Nature*, 26 September 1936, pp. 529–31.
35. Paul Fussell, *The Great War and Modern Memory*, New York and London: Oxford University Press, 1975. Modris Eksteins, *Rites of Spring: The Great War and the Birth of the Modern Age*, New York and London: Anchor Books, 1990. Samuel Hynes, *A War Imagined: The First World War and English Culture*, London: Bodley Head, 1990.
36. Brock, *Health and Conduct* (n. 6), p. 235.
37. Sir Walter Langdon-Brown, 'The seventeenth Maudsley Lecture: The biology of social life', *Journal of Mental Science*, **83**, 1937, pp. 1–14 at p. 5.
38. Brock, *Health and Conduct* (n. 6), p. 2.
39. Horder, 'Strain of modern civilization' (n. 34), p. 530.
40. Brock, *Health and Conduct* (n. 6), pp. 24–25.
41. Ibid., p. 26.
42. Ibid., p. 24.
43. Ibid.
44. Ibid., pp. 4 and 26. For other suggestions that neurasthenia and functional diseases of the nervous system were on the rise see Horder, 'Strain of modern civilization' (n. 34), p. 529.
45. Brock, *Health and Conduct* (n. 6), p. xviii.
46. Ibid., p. 86.
47. Ibid., p. 28 (emphasis in original).
48. Ibid., p. 29.
49. Ibid., p. 31.
50. D.L. LeMahieu, *A Culture for Democracy. Mass Communication and the Cultivated Mind in Britain Between the Wars*, Oxford: Clarendon Press, 1988; John Carey, *The Intellectuals and the Masses. Pride and Prejudice Among the Literary Intelligentsia, 1880–1939*, London: Faber and Faber, 1992.
51. Brock, *Health and Conduct* (n. 6), p. 30.
52. Ibid.
53. Ibid., p. 91.
54. On American graduates studying in Germany, see also James Mackenzie in 'The Special British Mission to America', *New York Medical Journal*, **108**, 1918, pp.

112–17, at p. 115.
55. F.G. Crookshank, 'The importance of symptoms', *West London Medical Journal*, **24**, 1919, pp. 50–60 at p. 54.
56. Lord Horder, 'Heat, health and happiness', *Gas World*, 29 April 1939, pp. 385–86 at p. 385.
57. Cawadias, 'Neohippocratism' (n. 15), p. 30. See also Cawadias, 'Les étapes' (n. 17). For other attacks on Virchow see Castiglioni, 'Neo-hippocratic tendency' (n. 3); and Hutchison, 'Harvey' (n. 23), p. 737.
58. Cawadias, 'Neohippocratism' (n. 15), p. 28.
59. Robert Hutchison, 'Medical progress 1936–37', *Practitioner*, **139**, 1937, pp. 313–18 at p. 317.
60. Crookshank, 'Importance of symptoms' (n. 55), p. 53.
61. Cawadias, 'Neo-hippocratic theory' (n. 12), p. 149. F.G. Crookshank, 'Types of personality, with special reference to individual psychology', *Lancet*, 8 March 1930, pp. 546–48 at p. 546. Cawadias, *Modern Therapeutics* (n. 13), pp. 39–45.
62. Cawadias, 'Neohippocratism' (n. 15), p. 28.
63. Ibid.
64. Ibid.
65. F.G. Crookshank, 'The relation of history and philosophy to medicine: introductory essay', in Charles Greene Cumston, *An Introduction to the History of Medicine From the Time of the Pharaohs to the End of the XVIIIth Century*, London: Kegan, Paul Trench Trubner, 1926, pp. xv–xxxii at p. xxx. For Crookshank's attitude to language see also his essay in C.K. Ogden and I.A. Richards, with supplementary essays by B. Malinowski and F. G. Crookshank, *The Meaning of Meaning: A Study of the Influence of Language Upon Thought and of the Science of Symbolism*, London: K. Paul, Trench, Trubner, 1923. On Ogden see W. Terrence Gordon, *C.K. Ogden: A Bio-bibliographic Study*, Metuchen, NJ: Scarecrow Press, 1990; P. Sargant Florence and J. R. L. Anderson (eds), *C. K. Ogden: A Collective Memoir*, London: Elek, Pemberton, 1977.
66. Crookshank, 'Introductory essay' (n. 65), pp. xxix–xxx.
67. Sturdy, 'Hippocrates and state medicine' (n. 32); Porter, 'John Ryle' (n. 1).
68. Brock, 'Neo-hippocratism' (n. 28), p. 1012.
69. Brock, 'Child guidance clinics' (n. 28), p. 123.
70. Brock, *Health and Conduct* (n. 6), p. 88; Lord Horder, 'Clinical medicine', *St. Bartholomew's Hospital Journal*, **43**, 1936, pp. 73–77 at p. 75; idem, 'The clinician's function in medicine', *New York State Journal of Medicine*, **36**, 1936, pp. 843–48 at p. 846.
71. James Mackenzie, 'A plea for a clinical physiology', *British Medical Journal*, 28 June 1924, pp. 1122–25 at p. 1124. See also his comments on the narrow conception of research in 'Clinical research', *British Medical Journal*, 24 January 1920, pp. 105–11 at p. 105. More generally, see James Mackenzie, *The Future of Medicine*, London: The Joint Committee of Henry Frowde and Hodder & Stoughton, 1919.
72. Cawadias, *Modern Therapeutics* (n. 13), p. 59.
73. Ibid.
74. Ibid., pp. 59–60.
75. Ibid., p. 60.
76. Hutchison, 'Harvey' (n. 23), pp. 735–36.
77. Ibid., p. 736.
78. Ibid.
79. Brock, 'Neo-hippocratism' (n. 28), p. 1013.

80. Ibid.
81. Cawadias, 'Neo-hippocratic theory' (n. 12), p. 150.
82. Cawadias, 'Neohippocratism' (n. 15), p. 38.
83. F.G. Crookshank, 'Bradshaw Lecture on the theory of diagnosis', *Lancet*, 6 November 1926, pp. 939–42 and 13 November 1926, pp. 995–99, at p. 942. (A correction to the quotation on p. 939 can be found at *Lancet* 4 December 1926, p. 1202.)
84. Cawadias, *Modern Therapeutics* (n. 13), p. 52.
85. Ibid., p. 46.
86. Brock, 'Neo-hippocratism' (n. 28), p. 1013.
87. Hutchison, 'Harvey' (n. 23), p. 737.
88. Cawadias, 'Neo-hippocratic theory' (n. 12), p. 149. See also Crookshank, 'Importance of symptoms' (n. 55), p. 56.
89. F.G. Crookshank, 'Science and Health', in F.S. Marvin (ed.), *Science and Civilization*, London: Humphrey Milford/Oxford University Press, 1923, pp. 247–78 at p. 259; F.G. Crookshank (ed.), *Influenza. Essays By Several Authors*, London: William Heinemann, 1922.
90. Crookshank, 'Theory of Diagnosis' (n. 83), p. 942.
91. Cawadias, 'Neo-hippocratic theory' (n. 12), p. 150.
92. Hutchison, 'Harvey' (n. 23), p. 738.
93. Brock, *Health and Conduct* (n. 6), p. 251.
94. Ibid., p. 255 (emphasis in original).
95. Ibid., p. 256.
96. Ibid., p. 251.
97. Sir Walter Langdon-Brown, 'Changing conceptions of disease', *Edinburgh Medical Journal*, 43, 1936, pp. 13–28 at pp. 15–16.
98. A image of the 'plain man' can be found in the novels of John Buchan. On Buchan's concerns about civilisation see Juanita Kruse, *John Buchan (1875–1940) and the Idea of Empire*, Lewiston: Edwin Mellen Press, 1989. For a recent account of the relations between science, medicine, modernity and Englishness that appeared after this volume was in press, see Christopher Lawrence and Anna K. Mayer, *Regenerating England. Science, Medicine and Culture in Inter-war Britain*, Amsterdam and Atlanta: Rodopi, 2000.
99. Crookshank, 'Introductory essay' (n. 65), p. xxx.
100. Cawadias, *Modern Therapeutics* (n. 13), p. 52.
101. Brock, 'Neo-hippocratism' (n. 28), p. 1012.
102. See, for example, Cawadias' attempt to define words and phrases such as 'philosophy of medicine', 'doctrine' and 'theory' by reference to the ancient Greek in Cawadias, 'Neohippocratism' (n. 15), p. 29.
103. See, for example, the debates over dead languages in Professor Grant, 'University of London. Address on the study of medicine, delivered at the opening of the medical school, October 1st, 1833', *Lancet*, 5 October 1833, pp. 41–50 at pp. 42–43. A.T. Thomson, 'Report of the address delivered at the commencement of the medical session of 1836–37, at London University', *Lancet*, 8 October 1836, pp. 75–82 at pp. 78–79. See also the comments of the professor of greek in the University of Edinburgh, J.S. Blackie, 'In the Medical Department of Our University, justly celebrated as it is, who knows or expounds Hippocrates? Who cares for Greek?', *On the Advancement of Learning in Scotland*, Edinburgh: Sutherland and Knox, 1855, p. 17.
104. Stray, *Classics Transformed* (n. 11), p. 222.
105. Ibid., especially chapter 9.

106. Hippocratic methods, Douglas Guthrie claimed in 1945, had been revived by Sydenham and Boerhaave, 'and to-day it is again engaging the attention of some of the best minds in medicine'. See Douglas Guthrie, *A History of Medicine*, London: Nelson, 1945, p. 60.
107. Douglas Guthrie, 'Reform in Medical Education', *British Medical Journal*, 25 March 1944, p. 432.

CHAPTER FOURTEEN

A Model for the New Physician: Hippocrates in Interwar Germany

Carsten Timmermann

'How could they do it?' is probably the most common question asked about German doctors in the twentieth century. How could doctors play such a major part in the killing machinery of Auschwitz? How could they do it, in view of their Hippocratic oath? Robert Jay Lifton has suggested that Nazi doctors perverted medical ethics by valuing the health of the *Volk* over that of the individual. This 'ultimate absurdity', he argues, turned healers into killers. He quotes the witness at the Nuremberg trials against Nazi doctors, the physician Werner Leibbrandt, who referred to the Nazi embrace of Hippocrates as 'an ironical joke of world history'.[1] Leibbrandt assumed – as does Lifton – that there was something quintessential and self-evident about Hippocrates.[2] The Nazis are said to have abused and violated the true Hippocrates but, in this essay I shall argue that the story was more complicated, and that the boundaries between good and evil were less clear. I will attempt to show that the reception of the Hippocrates myth in parts of the medical community before 1933 invited its appropriation by Nazi officials.

Hippocrates today is associated with humane medicine, with a strong emphasis on the individual patient (as opposed to depersonalised, large-scale hospital medicine), with organicist, even vitalist, connotations. But can we assume that Hippocratism did not carry different meanings when Nazi physicians underwent their training? As in Britain and France, a holist, neo-Hippocratic movement emerged in Germany among physicians and alternative practitioners in the mid-1920s.[3] Worries about specialisation and the role of the laboratory, about state and mass medicine and the commercialisation of healing, along with the experience of economic and intellectual crisis, led many to proclaim a 'crisis in medicine'.[4] Hippocratism was seen as a solution to this crisis. In Britain, interwar neo-Hippocratism was mainly concerned with the individual. In Germany, however, in the wake of losing the First World War and in face of economic hardship, parts of the educated élite began to value the survival of the collective, the *Volk*, more highly than that of the single individual.[5] Along with fellow intellectuals, German Hippocratists were not only concerned with individual patients, but also with the *Volk*.

Was Hippocrates a carer for the individual or the guardian of public health?

The variety of meanings associated with Hippocrates in different national and historical contexts indicates that medical ethics are more malleable than we are often led to assume. Perceptions of role models and ethical codes are shaped by the contexts in which they are received as much as by their historical origins.[6] Current debates over ethical issues, for example, draw massively on the atrocities committed by Nazi doctors and are reinterpreted in the light of the democratisation and civil rights movements of the 1960s.[7] The purpose of this study is to unwrap some of the meanings read into the figures of Hippocrates, and increasingly also that of Paracelsus, in the context of the social and economic situation of the medical profession in interwar Germany. I will argue in this essay that physicians used Hippocrates in the crisis-ridden interwar years in order to lend an air of timelessness and ascribe a higher meaning to a professional ideology that was in fact highly interest-driven. I prefer the term 'ideology' to 'culture' or 'mentality' here because it does not have the deterministic connotations of the latter two. Ideology according to Karl Mannheim is an ambiguous concept. It allows for the conscious use of a set of ideas and values, which are nevertheless determined, to a certain degree, by an individual's socialisation in a distinct group or culture.[8]

Part of the ideology embraced by most German academics in the early twentieth century was the claim to be unpolitical. One way of sustaining this claim was by exploring political issues, as the Hippocratists did, through analogies drawn from the ancient world, referring to underlying higher values. Out of bourgeois élitism and frustration over their role in the welfare state, many of them developed sympathies for the political right. Increasingly they chose a 'fundamentalist' approach to problems arising from the modernisation of medicine and responded to a complicated, highly differentiated social reality by embracing a world-view based on symbols and myths. 'Myth' in this context does not imply the opposite of a 'fact' but rather a unifying legend born out of the desire to assign meaning to a fragmented reality.[9] The concept of fundamentalism is commonly used to analyse religious movements but it may serve here as a suitable analytical category.[10] 'Fundamentalists fight with a particularly chosen repository of resources which one might think of as weapons,' state Martin E. Marty and R. Scott Appleby in the introduction to the first volume of their monumental *Fundamentalism Observed*, '... they reached back to real or presumed pasts, to actual or imagined ideal original conditions and concepts, and selected what they regarded as fundamental.'[11] The myth of and the various qualities assigned to Hippocrates served as such weapons – tools in what I shall call in this essay an ideological toolkit, a miscellaneous collection of beliefs and ideas associated with the ideal doctor.

'Return to Hippocrates'

The myth of Hippocrates, paradoxically, became very popular just after all the medical schools in Germany had abandoned the ritual of oath-taking.[12] Hippocratism was partly a response to what many portrayed as a crisis in medicine and, indeed, in society after the First World War.[13] As is well known, the cause of crisis was most prominently set out by Oswald Spengler in his popular account of the 'Decline of the West'.[14] Following Spengler many intellectuals blamed Western 'civilisation' (as opposed to German 'culture') for the defeat of the Germans in the war. In the shape of *fin de siècle* decadence, 'civilisation' had weakened Germany's defences, just as American-style modernisation had strengthened her enemies. Many intellectuals felt humiliated by the Versailles Treaty and threatened by the 1918 revolution that turned Germany into a republic. War and inflation led to a national crisis of a scale previously unknown. The economic crisis could be easily interpreted as a symptom of decline.[15] German society was receptive to myths, torn between fascination for the great modernisation plans, such as the welfare state, and visions of a romantic past.[16] In medicine, the conflict between 'culture' and 'civilisation' found its expression in the ideals of the rural family doctor and the urban medical expert.[17] Medical authors constructed the 'crisis in medicine' in response to pressure for modernisation in the health and welfare system.

The political commitments of the Hippocratists involved in the crisis debate were diverse. Take, for example, the editorial board of the journal *Hippocrates*. In 1927 a group of doctors and supporters of alternative healing practices founded *Hippokrates*, led by the psychiatrist and head of the internal women's ward of the Stuttgart homoeopathic Robert Bosch Hospital, Heinrich Meng, and financially backed by the industrialist Robert Bosch.[18] The internist and medical historian at the University of Gießen, Georg Honigmann, was appointed editor-in-chief and the organisers succeeded in winning the support of an impressive list of co-editors, amongst them Henry E. Sigerist.[19] Sigerist was a left-leaning liberal and Heinrich Meng, the founder of the journal *Hippokrates*, had emerged from the war as a pacifist and had socialist sympathies.[20] Another popular and influential member of the board, however, the Danzig surgeon Erwin Liek, was a right-winger.[21]

Not all writings on Hippocrates and Paracelsus were overtly designed as contributions to the crisis debate. Publications dealing with, and alluding to, the two historical figures can be grouped into three overlapping genres. Essays on professional and general politics and reflections on the philosophy and theory of medicine constituted the largest group. Often rather cursory in style, they could be found in the general interest [*Feuilleton*] and professional politics [*Standespolitik*] sections of the journals.[22] Texts in this genre usually dealt with the 'crisis', taking up tropes and issues associated with the debate. Central to many of these publications was the assumption that physicians were part of an eternal, natural élite who could not realise their beneficial potential for humankind, due to the 'materialism' embodied in the expanding welfare state and the 'mechanistic attitude' associated with nineteenth-century medical science.

Practical guidelines for physicians, especially for general practitioners, constituted the second genre.[23] They contained recommendations and case studies on how to implement 'Hippocratic' medicine in everyday practice, often in order to overcome the 'crisis' and bring medicine back on to 'its historical main path'. Usually this implied calls to 'treat the whole patient and not only single organs'. Like those writing in the first genre, these authors saw their recommendations as remedies against fragmentation and the 'one-sidedness of modern medicine'.[24]

Studies in classical philology and the history of medicine constituted the third genre. Covering a wide range from scholarly to popular writings, they dealt directly with the lives and works of Hippocrates and Paracelsus.[25] The scholarly studies profited considerably from the increased interest in Hippocrates and Paracelsus. History of medicine as a discipline, medical historians suggested, had the potential to contribute valuable solutions to the 'crisis of medicine'. Henry E. Sigerist declared in 1930 that medicine had entered a new stage after the war, signified by medical practitioners developing an increasing interest in the history of medicine as they lost faith in the promises of nineteenth-century science:

> As in the romantic age one felt the urge to do justice to the fundamentals of healing, to assemble isolated findings into a whole, the urge for a philosophy of medicine. ... The structure of society had changed fundamentally. The physician had not found his place yet in the new society. A new physician ideal was emerging.[26]

Despite their diverse political affiliations, all Hippocratists believed that they were standing for a common cause: the renewal of medicine. In the following two sections I shall use the examples of two outspoken academic Hippocratists to illustrate how Hippocratism legitimated an élitist medical ideology which was later appropriated by Nazi officials.

The natural élite

August Bier (1861–1949) was the doyen, the grand old man, of German interwar Hippocratism. Professor of surgery and head of the famous *Ziegelstrasse* clinic of Berlin University since 1907, he did not restrict his activities to surgery but attempted to make this clinic the centre of a medical microcosm of various specialists, including such unorthodox and controversial practices as homoeopathy and the methods of 'natural healing.'[27] Bier's small medical empire was a material expression of his attempts to develop a unifying theory for all of medicine. He held his lectures and demonstrations in front of large audiences who loved his sarcastic remarks and admired his surgical skills. Occasionally he swapped the modern instruments for carpenters' tools to demonstrate his contempt for those surgeons who relied on modern technology rather than traditional manual skills.[28] A fine surgeon in a famous clinic, Bier was consulted by celebrities from both Germany and abroad.

Bier became a patron of unorthodox practitioners. He argued for a scientific engagement with homoeopathy, following the theories of the pharmacology professor Hugo Schulz, a former colleague at the University of Greifswald at an earlier stage of Bier's career. Bier published articles on homoeopathy and, in 1926, he sent one of his assistants to Stuttgart to work at the homoeopathic hospital funded by the industrialist Robert Bosch.[29] To the outrage of many academic colleagues, he supported an initiative of the Prussian national assembly in 1919 to set up teaching positions for homoeopaths and natural healers in the country's universities.[30] He was also instrumental in the establishment of the Berlin Institute for the History of Medicine.[31] Bier based his theories of medicine on his readings of Heraclitus and Hippocrates, as well as on the speculative theories of the eighteenth-century Scottish physician John Brown. He published his ideas in a long series of articles in the *Münchener Medizinische Wochenschrift*.[32]

Bier's clinic was temporarily closed down in 1931 due to an acute cash shortage as well as administrative errors on the part of both the Prussian government and the university. The right-wing press used the opportunity to blame the Weimar system, and Bier retired to his countryside manor house. There he wrote books on 'Life' and 'The Soul' and looked after his private forest, which he saw as a great Heraclitian experiment. Bier's political allegiances were with the right. A staunch patriot, he is credited with the design of the new German army helmet in 1915, allegedly modelled on ancient Greek helmets. He was also a member of the right-wing bourgeois German National People's Party and, in 1932, signed an appeal of right-wing organisations to vote for Adolf Hitler in the presidential elections.[33]

The Hamburg immunology professor, Hans Much (1880–1932) liked to present himself as a polymath and true Renaissance man, a scientist and artist, philosopher and poet.[34] Apart from being a 'man of will,' he prided himself in possessing various other characteristics of the 'Nordic race'.[35] Starting his career as an assistant to the bacteriologist Emil von Behring, he was made head of the small Serological Institute at the Eppendorf Hospital in Hamburg in 1907. Besides medical and biological issues, Much published books and articles on philosophy, North German Gothic buildings and art, Buddhist thought, ancient Egypt and the Middle East, as well as novels and a drama.[36] Much's 1926 book, *Hippocrates the Great*, is by no means a historical study of Hippocrates.[37] Nevertheless, this did not prevent contemporary reviewers in the medical press from seeing the book as a valuable contribution to the ongoing debates over the future of medicine.[38]

'To talk about Hippocrates', Much opened his book, 'means to talk about the essence of medicine.'[39] He went about this by presenting his views on the world in the form of an impressionistic survey, grouped around a few quotes from Hippocratic writings but mainly drawing on his various fields of interest. Much's book leans towards a Spenglerian approach to history. Several ancient high cultures culminated in Hippocrates, he claimed. The Hippocratic writings, he argued, were not primarily manifestations of Greek culture, but of the older empires of ancient Egypt and of India.[40] Egypt had been a truly high culture, he claimed, and the Egyptians had been a 'truly beautiful people' of high race who incidentally also, like the modern ideologues of the Nordic race, 'recognised the long skull as the noblest form of skull'. The Greeks, in contrast, had 'faces without soul'.[41] Ancient Greece, in Much's view, was already more of a 'civilisation' than a high 'culture', and on the verge of decline.

Bier was not impressed with Much's attitude towards the Greeks. 'I thought,' he wrote, 'that the ... fashion of denying the Greeks any original culture and turning them into students of the oriental people had been overcome.' Much's book, he argued, could be viewed 'at best as a historical novel' and, even then, it was not a particularly good one. In Bier's view, Much had chosen the easy, but flawed, option of addressing the *Corpus Hippocraticum* 'with "genius and intuition" where only diligence, thoroughness and knowledge could meet the goal'.[42] Bier's reflections on the Hippocratic texts were part of a long-term project: 'I have used the services of two young philologists, the Messrs. W. Sauter and K. Levy, who were recommended to me as being exceptionally competent.'[43] He felt obliged to object to Much's ways of 'making [up] history'.

To Bier, Hippocrates represented what was great in Greek culture; to Much he represented the heritage of the Orient. Amidst all differences, however, there were striking similarities between Much's and Bier's approaches to Hippocrates. Both found it appropriate to present their personal views as resulting from the dialogue with an ancient culture – as a modern version of the dominant world-view of that culture. Both wanted to see these allegedly timeless values applied to modern medicine. And both attacked the same enemies. To Bier, the Greeks:

> ... had the wonderful gift, which scientists have almost lost today, to combine clear thinking, level-headed observation, sharp analysis – which we admire as great today and in which most of us see the [sole] goal of science – with that generalising and artistic ability, and thus [they created] the harmony of the whole, which today is lacking everywhere in the sciences, not only in medicine. This [lack of harmony] is the great disease of our times.[44]

It comes as little surprise that Bier used the Greeks to highlight the 'disease of our times' – 'naturalism', 'causalism' and 'mechanism'.[45] The rationalist nineteenth century had brought great progress to medicine, had freed the art of healing from the speculations of 'Naturphilosophie', but it was now time for a humanist turn, to bring back spirit into medicine.

On the surface, Bier and Much were talking about a theoretical problem, internal to medicine: the conflict between healing and medical science. Both stressed that it was an illusion to believe – as their opponents allegedly did – that medicine could ever be merely applied science. This illusion was behind the 'disease of our time' and the 'crisis of medicine'. Both talked about 'rules' of nature as opposed to natural 'laws'.[46] Believing in laws would imply that the body was merely a machine. In opposing this mechanistic simplification, Much's, as well as Bier's, line of argument followed a fairly popular Kantian line: we would never be able to understand life in all its fine details; we would only ever understand little bits. This was, however, a problem of 'pure reason'. Doctors had to apply 'practical reason'. Medicine to Bier was a very practical form of knowledge. Even without understanding every detail, doctors could act according to the rules of life.[47] They had to use 'intuition'. This meant that doctors had to be artists where science did not provide answers. To both Bier and Much, the importance of the right balance of empirical science and artistic intuition and skill was the central message of Hippocrates.

What might look to us like esoteric, theoretical elaborations was connected with rather profane, social claims. To both Bier and Much the medical profession, or the 'estate of physicians' [*Ärztestand*] as it was commonly called, constituted a social élite. 'Medical art', Much quotes Hippocrates on the frontispiece of his book, 'is of all arts the noblest.' The physician Elfriede Paul remembers from Bier's lectures that:

> Bier told us bluntly about his opinion that under the Greek doctors of the Classic age even stomach and head wounds healed after surgery without complications because those doctors were recruited from the aristocracy and the highest estates, and because unlike today not any 'plebeian' could become a physician.[48]

Medicine could not simply be studied; one had to be 'born' a physician and one's art could only be accomplished by apprenticeship and years of bedside experience. Physicians stylised themselves as a middle-class aristocracy, justifying their claims with their exclusive knowledge about life and death, which seemed to be in high demand in a society increasingly obsessed with biological explanations for social processes.[49] Much and Bier presented the ideal physician as a philosopher and priest, rather than as an expert of health management.[50] If the health system was controlled by the right priest–physicians, Much claimed, even increasing specialisation would not be a problem. Specialisation only led to 'cultural bankruptcy' if the specialists were not acting as servants of a greater whole, controlled by those who were 'spiritually more highly gifted'.[51] Much and Bier opposed the secularisation process which medicine seemed to undergo in modern society.[52] Against it, they promoted idealist visions of nature, worshipping the power of the soul and the will.

This peculiar combination of élitism, declinism and idealist ideology was not an uncommon attitude in the educated middle classes since the *fin de siècle*.[53] Members of the old bourgeoisie embraced it to distinguish themselves from the commercial and industrial élites and the 'new middle class' of white-collar workers who made their living in the expanding administrative bodies of companies and the modern state machinery. In the case of the medical profession, however, this élitist attitude also indicated a more specific problem: what was going to be the role and authority of the doctors in the expanding welfare state?[54] Doctors increasingly found their autonomy restricted by the growing sickness insurance funds,[55] whose elected administrative bodies were largely dominated by representatives of the trade unions.[56] Insurance fund doctors became employees of the funds and there is good evidence that, economically, they profited from this situation as the funds gave them access to large groups of the population which otherwise would have rarely consulted a doctor.[57]

The problem, however, became one of power and of sustaining their traditional middle-class status. It was a violation of the doctors' *Standesehre*, the 'honour of their estate', to be controlled by workers. In the Weimar Republic a further rise of the income thresholds for compulsory and voluntary sickness insurance worried many doctors. Large parts of the 'new middle class' joined the insurance membership. Furthermore, the funds claimed a say in health policy-making. What they could not claim, however, was that exclusive priestly knowledge, the membership in the Hippocratic club. The promotion of Hippocratic values against what the editor of the *Deutsche Medizinische Wochenschrift* called the 'materialistic – mechanising and spiritually stultifying – worldview of Social Democracy' can be understood partly as a reaction to the expansion of the insurance funds, which many doctors feared to be the first step towards the 'socialisation' of the medical profession.[58] In this context Hippocrates served right-wing and liberal doctors as a symbol of old-style individualistic practice and of opposition against socialist health reform plans.

Self-declared spokesmen for the medical profession, such as the Danzig surgeon Erwin Liek, presented the expansion of the insurance funds as part of an inherent socialist threat not only to middle-class values but also to the health of the nation.[59] This attitude, along with its close ties to Spenglerian declinism, resonates with what is known as '*Konservative Revolution*', a movement of middle-class intellectuals in the interwar years, harbouring blood-and-soil traditionalist, holistic and anti-urban tendencies.[60] Along with these 'Conservative Revolutionaries', Hippocratists such as Much and Bier called for a revolution against civilisation and the positivist outlook of late nineteenth century science – namely its effects on medicine. They embraced instead a world-view based on selectively chosen ancient and allegedly timeless ideas of wholeness and harmony. The programmes of the Hippocratists had distinctly fundamentalist character. They attempted to counter the differentiation evident in the increasingly complex and heterogeneous character of modern medicine and a growing fear of personal instability by embracing myths and symbols which promised a return to the stability they imagined had existed earlier.

New ethics

'Hippocratic medicine,' Much claimed, 'was ethics in the first place.'[61] While Hippocratic doctrines supported the élitist claims of the medical profession it also served to support a particular form of ethics. 'Preservation of a human life is obviously something marvellous,' Much declared. But Hippocrates had also recognised our dependence on the higher power of 'fate':

> We must lift this problem completely out of the realm of ethics... because the exaggerated, empty phrases of inferior centuries obstruct us here. Take an ideal State like the Platonic one, which was modelled on Sparta and which alone has any legitimacy, and we can address this question more easily. Of what use can it be to preserve the life of a cripple? Whoever sees an art in this rids himself of the right to talk about art at all. In the end there is never art at work in these institutions where the useless are nursed, just a wrong understanding of sympathy.[62]

The line Much takes with respect to 'useless cripples' is that of the retired law professor, Karl Binding, and the professor of psychiatry, Alfred Hoche, who in 1920 published a book on *The Permission to Destroy Life Unworthy of Life*.[63] In their controversial book they argued for an ethical and legal basis for the medical 'mercy' killing of what they called the 'mentally dead' – psychiatric patients with no or little prospect of improvement. These 'empty shells of human beings' were a burden on society, Binding and Hoche argued, and putting them to death could not be equated with other types of killing: it was permissible and useful. The book expressed the feelings of large sectors of the population after the First World War: why should the incurably sick and deranged be fed and nurtured while the bravest of the nation's young men had sacrificed their lives in the trenches for the *Volk*, and while mentally sane children were dying of starvation? Medical ethics would not be violated by this form of 'euthanasia'. The *Volk* was an organism, too, and had rights above that of the individual. Paul Weindling has suggested that, for Binding and Hoche, 'the war destroyed the value attached to individual life, shifting the emphasis to collective national survival'.[64]

Much apparently saw little problem in reconciling his favourable attitude towards the Binding and Hoche argument with his calls for the artist–doctor:

No, it is not man as such, as person, so pathetic and easily replaceable as part of a mass ... who makes medicine the noblest of all arts. It is the higher idea, here as in all other arts, the whole, the general, the great and fundamental which makes art an art. Not man but life is what makes medicine a first class art, the artistic handling of life as such in its highest form.[65]

Like Much, Bier was also concerned with the threat of 'inferiority' to the German *Volk*. In 1925 he complained that 'today the cult of the inferior is in power. For the healthy and stout they have no more sympathy. The inferior, however, is nurtured.'[66] Bier believed that physical education, modelled on ancient Greek gymnastics, was a suitable means to fight the decline of the race. He was a co-founder of the 'German College of Physical Education' (*Deutsche Hochschule für Leibesübungen*) in 1920, and its director until 1932. Compulsory exercise, he believed, should compensate for the missing army service. 'Nude exercise', the direct translation of the Greek for 'gymnastics', would be the best means of preventing tuberculosis.[67] The so-called 'life reform' (*Lebensreform*) movement had promoted fresh air, nudism and exposure to the sun as remedies against the evils of civilisation since the late nineteenth century.[68] Bier took up these ideas and incorporated them into his medical microcosm.

Much believed that the physician always had to be primarily an artist, a born genius whose creativity and use of intuition should not be restricted by bureaucracy. He also followed this creed with respect to experimental medical science: the experimenter was always to be governed by concern for the greater whole, otherwise he would descend into shallow specialism. Central to medical research was the insight into the impossibility of exactitude when dealing with biological phenomena. How could one expect animal models to behave exactly like human beings? In a paper on the common cold which he presented to the North-Western German Society of Laryngologists in 1926, Much tackled the problem of infection: was it mainly caused by bacteria or mainly by environmental influences, such as exposure to cold air or water?[69] In his view, both factors had an effect on the human 'constitution', which in turn led to the disease. The constitution was, in accordance with the principles he laid out in his Hippocrates book, the balance of substances in the body. The infection was therefore the disturbance of this peculiar balance, affected by bacteria and exposure to cold. Experiments with guinea pigs could not tell researchers anything reliable about the human constitution.[70] The best way to solve the problem, he suggested, was to get in touch with 'a reasonable asylum or prison director. ... One should expose a number of feebleminded persons or prisoners, who live under the same [standardised] conditions, with their consent to various "endemic causes" '.[71] The whole experiment, he claimed, was 'the opposite of inhumanity. It contributes to the battle [against the disease], and in this way the infinitely or temporarily useless help their fellow human beings and risk a cold at worst.' Such experiments on asylum inmates or prisoners, however artistic, would soon be illegal. In 1930 the Imperial Health Council (*Reichsgesundheitsrat*) issued new guidelines for experiments on humans.[72] In a letter to prison service officials in July 1931, the Prussian minister of justice stressed that according to these guidelines, experiments on prisoners were not permissible, even with the inmates' consent.[73]

The German Hippocrates

If, to men like Bier and Much, Hippocratism was reconcilable with eugenic ideas and musings over experiments on prisoners, what happened to Hippocrates after Hitler's rise to power in 1933? Not surprisingly, Third Reich medical officials took up the popular 'Back to Hippocrates' calls of the Weimar years.[74] According to the Nazi reading, central to Hippocratism was its opposition to the Weimar 'system', to mechanism and materialism which the Nazis related to Marxist and Jewish influences. Hippocrates turned into a patron of their 'national revolution'. The first volume of a series of books on 'The Doctor's Eternal Mission' (*Ewiges Arzttum*) contained a collection of Hippocratic texts. The series was edited by Ernst Robert von Grawitz, chief physician of the SS.[75] The leader of the SS and of the German police forces in the Third Reich, Heinrich Himmler, wrote the introduction to the volume. He praised 'the great Greek doctor Hippocrates' and his 'unity of character and accomplishment' which 'proclaims a morality, the strengths of which are still undiminished today and shall continue to determine medical action and thought in the future'.[76]

Paracelsus, the other great mythical doctor, was increasingly presented as the symbol of physicians' responsibility towards the German *Volk*.[77] To rightwing ideologues, Paracelsus had the advantage of being born on 'German' soil. However, authors often used the same phrases in describing the qualities of both Paracelsus and Hippocrates. Paracelsus was, as it were, the German Hippocrates. For example, Hans Hartmann, in his book on 'Paracelsus: A German Vision', wrote in 1941: 'The Hippocratic Oath and this vow [of Paracelsus to love the sick person more than himself] are in their deepest essence one and the same. Paracelsus says it just more simply and is carried by German feeling.'[78] According to Hartmann, Paracelsus, like Hippocrates, had recognised that there were aspects to the world which humans would never understand: 'The more he searches, the more he knows how much he does not know.' Like Hippocrates, Paracelsus was as much a philosopher as a physician, and that was what the modern German doctor should be – a 'philosopher of German kind' who can 'above all distinguish the core of things from the superficial and the appendages'.[79] Hartmann emphasised Paracelsus' attempts to overcome the division between physicians and surgeons in order to lead medicine back to its united Hippocratic roots. In this he was an example for the modern German doctor:

> There are questions which have arisen from the passage of centuries, and which exactly equal the questions of Paracelsus. These are all those questions dealing with the conflict between orthodox medicine and folk medicine.[80]

Like Hippocrates, Paracelsus was presented as a symbol of unity in medicine and of the Third Reich project of setting up a 'New German Art of Healing'.[81]

Paul Diepgen, who in 1928 in connection with the launch of the journal *Hippokrates*, had argued that his fellow historians of medicine should keep a professional distance from questions of daily politics, apparently changed his mind after 1933.[82] In 1934 he announced the dawn of a 'new ethics' for the Third Reich and offered the services of medical historians to the new government:[83]

> The patient in the new State will more than ever before be seen by the doctor as part of the whole of the *Volk*. Health counselling of the individual will always be shaped by his considering [the patient in the first place as] member of the *völkisch* community, the carrier of genetic material which serves the whole. ... A new ethics is announcing itself. There is no better help to finding one's way into what is new than to study the history of the medical profession.[84]

Diepgen's student, Karl Rothschuh, saw potential for 'tough conflicts' between 'the role of the doctor as trustee of the community' and 'his traditional role as trustee of individual well-being', as it was 'embodied for thousands of years in the Oath of Hippocrates'.[85] However:

> With good reason, our time values the health of the community higher than that of the individual. The physician will under certain circumstances be forced to harm an individual's body and soul if this individual represents a threat to the social body [*Volkskörper*].[86]

Diepgen attempted to bridge the apparent contradictions between the responsibilities of the physician towards the individual and the *Volk* by proposing a division of labour. In a speech to practitioners in the town of Cottbus in 1936 under the title 'Hippocrates or Paracelsus?', he suggested that embracing both role models would solve the problem:

> I think that the physician does best today who says: Hippocrates as well as Paracelsus shall be my example; because rationalism as well as intuition, scepticism as well as optimism, critique strictly adjusted to the individual case as well as breadth of thought, nationalism as well as understanding for the interests of the other peoples of the earth, youth as well as old age constitute together the true physician. [87]

Conclusion: the legacy of Hippocratism

In this essay I have attempted to analyse the use of Hippocrates as a rhetorical weapon and part of an ideological toolkit of German physicians in the 1920s and 1930s. Some of the defendants in the 1947 Nuremberg medical trials drew on the same ideological toolkit in their statements, using the same phrases as Much and Bier in the 1920s. I have argued that the Hippocratic professional identity promoted in medical schools and by parts of the medical press did not rule out experiments on prisoners or asylum inmates. They were considered inferior human beings, and the experiments allegedly served the good of the greater whole.

The physician Fritz Fischer, who had performed experiments on inmates of the Ravensbrück concentration camp, remembered having considered the ethical implications of human experiments in medical school and occasionally reflected on the topic 'by way of rounding up my complete picture. But I had utterly forgotten it later and never dreamed that it ever could constitute an actual problem for me.'[88]

> I knew that some people and doctors considered themselves, as free individuals, to regard such tests [upon human subjects] as necessary even in normal times ... and I knew that when one believes that medicine should be subdivided in some way and is not very keen on the clinical side, which in the last analysis derives from the ancient priest–doctor, and does no more than observe the invalid and his symptoms at the bedside ... such doctors who, entirely on their own initiative, in normal times, choose to experiment on human beings, are those who turn to the domain of natural science, feel themselves morally justified in doing so and are regarded by humanity as so justified, because ... in the view of a natural science applied to human biology the ultimate and decisive proof of a theory can only obtained by observation of a human subject.[89]

Fischer's statement combined, in a confused way, Much's notion of an ideal state with priest–doctors in leading functions and the Kantian argument of the limits of human understanding: the situation in which the concentration camp doctor found himself was 'beyond the grasp of one mind, on the level, that is, of the State'.[90] Gerhard Rose, professor of tropical medicine of the Berlin Robert Koch Institute who had commissioned typhus experiments on prisoners at Buchenwald, went further in his compliance with the demands of the state:

> Speaking as a doctor, I may stress the fact that in a certain clearly defined category of experiments ..., medical men in general and I myself would consider it immoral to employ voluntary subjects. For the psychological strain then borne by the physician in charge would be unacceptable. He has no right to acquiesce in an offer of suicide. Such experiments are in my view only admissible when the sovereign power of the State nominates subjects who have forfeited their lives by committing crimes against the community.[91]

Fischer and Rose used rhetorical figures from the same ideological toolkit as Much and Bier but applied them to rather different conditions. Much and Bier employed them against a political 'system' that they despised. The existing state powers of the Weimar Republic, as it were, stood between the doctors and an idealised state, where they would function as the omnipotent priests of biology. Hitler's regime allowed some doctors to move into such positions. The professional ethical codes constructed around representations of Hippocrates and Paracelsus did not prepare physicians for resistance. They did, however, prepare them for the *völkisch* ideals of the Nazi hierarchy and the élitist structures of the SS.[92]

Physicians and their ideologies were part of the bigger picture of Hitler's rise to power. The ideology many physicians embraced under the banner of Hippocratism scarcely prevented them from becoming involved in racist and discriminatory policies. It presented the doctor as a leader and member of a detached élite with the 'natural' right to make arbitrary decisions 'at a glance' without being accountable to anyone. The Hippocratism championed by such men as Bier, Much and Liek would not induce resistance but rather compliance with Nazi 'biological politics' and SS élitism. Declaring doctors to be priests of biology proved to be too successful for the profession's own good.

The problem of physicians' compliance with the Nazi authorities is far too complex to be dealt with in this essay.[93] It would seem, however, that resistance against the role these authorities assigned to the medical profession in many cases did not originate primarily in medical ethics, but in personal ties with other belief and value systems – for example, the Christian faith.[94] It seems, for example, that the criticism of 'the termination of so-called life not worth living' in a much hailed speech of the Freiburg pathologist Franz Büchner at Freiburg University, on 'The Oath of Hippocrates. The Fundamental Laws of Medical Ethics' in 1941 grew in the first place out of his Christian beliefs.[95] Büchner was known as 'the holy Franz' after the First World War. However, even his Christian faith does not seem to have prevented him, as head of the Freiburg Institute of Aeronautical Pathology, from taking part in the planning and evaluation of *Wehrmacht* experiments on prisoners in the Dachau concentration camp.[96]

Other stories could be told about German doctors and medical ethics than the one I have told here. I have hinted above at the diverse political backgrounds of the *Hippokrates* editors. There was also a distinctly non-Hippocratist tradition of concern with the ethics of medical research in Prussia. Albert Moll, an eminent psychiatrist and sexologist in Berlin, published a book on medical ethics in 1902, in which he rejected experiments on human subjects.[97] He wrote this book in the wake of the highly controversial 'Neisser case': in 1898 the Breslau dermatologist Albert Neisser published his experiments on eight young women who he had injected with an experimental syphilis serum in 1892. Four of them contracted the disease.[98] Moll was appalled by the reactions of his medical colleagues to the case, accusing them of hushing it up. He was a positivist and his line of argument was pragmatic: the foundation of medical ethics should be practice, not moral theories. His criticism was that most writings on medical ethics focused on questions of the 'medical estate' and of etiquette. Doctors should not, he thought, set up special professional ethical codes; they should rather reconcile their special professional duties with general ethical concerns.

Julius Moses, a physician, supporter of the naturopathy movement and socialist member of parliament, also campaigned against experiments on human subjects. Like other socialist doctors he did not use Hippocratic arguments. He did, however, draw extensively on Moll's book.[99] In 1930, when in the city of Lübeck more than 80 children died after vaccinations with a controversial tuberculosis vaccine, Moses suggested that they had been victims of an experiment.[100]

Why were Moll's and Moses' warnings not more successful with the large majority of doctors? Certainly, Moses' sympathies with the socialists and the alternative healing movement made him suspect to many of his colleagues. Moses himself blamed the profession's preoccupation with the 'honour of the estate' (*Standesehre*). He wrote:

> The dangers of experimenting, for the people's health and for medical science, are unfortunately not recognised by many doctors. ... This has to do, on the one hand with the strange attitude of physicians towards criticism, and on the other with the hypocritical arrogance ... and the wrong sense of solidarity, the fear about their prestige, which makes medics deaf and blind for the wrongs in their own realm.[101]

After the war, Alexander Mitscherlich and Fred Mielke published the officially commissioned documentation of the Nuremberg doctors' trials.[102] Mielke died soon afterwards and Mitscherlich was subsequently ostracised by the profession. Medical officials showed little interest in shedding light on the activities of some of their colleagues in the Third Reich,[103] and only the changed climate of the 1960s brought Mitscherlich recognition. Michael Kater has recently argued that a continuity of old *Standesehre* concepts is still evident in the practices of professional organisations today, despite all the changes the Auschwitz experience might have introduced to perceptions of medical ethics.[104] In face of a public which, since the 1960s, has demanded its 'patient rights', it seems that maintaining élitist claims and realising economic interests remained more attractive to representatives of the profession than accepting concrete criticism, and promoting transparency and ultimately accountability. The myth of Hippocrates has served this purpose well by disguising politics and lending an air of timelessness to the claims of the profession. Unaffected by his use in setting up Third Reich medicine and sanitised by post-war amnesia in Germany and elsewhere, Hippocrates still serves this function, ready to be appropriated and reinterpreted in correspondence with the medical ideals of an era.

Acknowledgements

I am grateful to Jon Harwood, Roger Cooter and John Pickstone for comments on earlier drafts of this paper. I am also indebted to a seminar audience at the Oxford Wellcome Unit for the History of Medicine and especially to the editor of this volume, David Cantor, for their useful criticism. The research leading to this chapter was generously supported by a Wellcome Trust PhD studentship.

Notes

1. Robert Jay Lifton, *The Nazi Doctors: A Study in the Psychology of Evil*, London: Macmillan, 1986, p. 32. What the Hippocratic code meant for experimental medicine was at the centre of a controversy between the prosecution and the defence at the Nuremburg Medical Trial. See Paul Weindling, 'The origins of informed consent: the International Scientific Commission on Medical War Crimes, and the Nuremburg Code', *Bulletin of the History of Medicine*, 75, 2001, pp. 37–71, esp. pp. 57–58. The body of literature on medicine and the Third Reich is substantial. See, for example, Michael H. Kater, *Doctors under Hitler*, Chapel Hill and London: University of North Carolina Press, 1989; Paul Weindling, *Health, Race, and German Politics between National Unification and Nazism, 1870–1945*, Cambridge: Cambridge University Press, 1989; Robert N. Proctor, *Racial Hygiene: Medicine under the Nazis*, Cambridge, MA and London: Harvard University Press, 1988; Fridolf Kudlien, *Ärzte im Nationalsozialismus*, Cologne: Kiepenheuer & Witsch, 1985; Walter Wuttke-Groneberg (ed.), *Medizin im Nationalsozialismus: Ein Arbeitsbuch*, Tübingen: Schwäbische Verlagsgesellschaft, 1980; Ernst Klee, *Auschwitz, die NS-Medizin und ihre Opfer*, Frankfurt-am-Main: S. Fischer, 1997.
2. So does, for example, Karl-Heinz Leven, 'Hippokrates im 20. Jahrhundert: Ärztliches Selbstbild, Idealbild und Zerrbild', in Karl-Heinz Leven and Cay-Rüdiger Prüll (eds), *Selbstbilder des Arztes im 20. Jahrhundert: Medizinhistorische und medizinethische Aspekte*, Freiburg-im-Bremen: H.F. Schulz, 1994, pp. 39–96 at pp. 75–80.
3. See Christopher Lawrence and George Weisz (eds), *Greater than the Parts. Holism in Biomedicine 1920–1950*, New York and Oxford: Oxford University Press, 1998.
4. Cf. Eva-Maria Klasen, 'Die Diskussion über eine "Krise" der Medizin in Deutschland zwischen 1925 und 1935', MD dissertation, Mainz; J.-Gutenberg University, 1984; Carsten Timmermann, 'Constitutional medicine, neoromanticisim and the politics of anti-mechanism in interwar Germany', *Bulletin for the History of Medicine*, forthcoming.
5. Cf. Detlev J. K. Peukert, 'The genesis of the "Final Solution" from the spirit of science', in David F. Crew (ed.), *Nazism and German Society 1933–1945*, London: Routledge, 1994, pp. 274–99.
6. Cf. Thomas Rütten, 'Receptions of the Hippocratic oath in the Renaissance: the prohibition of abortion as a case study in reception', *Journal of the History of Medicine and Allied Sciences*, 51, 1996, pp. 456–83 at p. 471.; Karl Deichgräber, 'Die ärztliche Standesethik des hippokratischen Eides', *Quellen und Studien zur Geschichte der Naturwissenschaften und der Medizin*, 3, 1932, pp. 29–49. See

also Ivan Waddington, 'The development of medical ethics – a sociological analysis', *Medical History*, **19**, 1975, pp. 36–51; Robert Baker, Dorothy Porter and Roy Porter (eds), *The Codification of Medical Morality: Historical and Philosophical Studies of the Formalization of Western Medical Morality in the Eighteenth and Nineteenth Centuries*, 2 vols, Dordrecht: Kluwer, 1993 and 1994.

7. See, for example, George J. Annas and Michael A. Grodin (eds), *The Nazi Doctors and the Nuremberg Code: Human Rights in Human Experimentation*, New York and Oxford: Oxford University Press, 1992; Rolf Winau, 'Medizin und Menschenversuch. Zur Geschichte des "informed consent" ', and Paul Weindling, 'Ärzte als Richter: Internationale Reaktionen auf die Medizinverbrechen des Nationalsozialismus während des Nürnberger Ärzteprozesses in den Jahren 1946–1947', both in Claudia Wiesemann and Andreas Frewer (eds), *Medizin und Ethik im Zeichen von Auschwitz. 50 Jahre Nürnberger Ärzteprozess*, Erlangen and Jena: Palm & Enke, 1996, pp. 13–29, 31–44; Ruth R. Faden, Tom L. Beauchamp and Nancy M.P. King, *A History and Theory of Informed Consent*, New York and Oxford: Oxford University Press, 1986.

8. Cf. Karl Mannheim, *Ideology and Utopia: An Introduction to the Sociology of Knowledge*, London: Routledge & Kegan Paul, 1936, esp. pp. 49–53.

9. Cf. Christoph Jamme, *Einführung in die Philosophie des Mythos*, Vol. 2: *Neuzeit und Gegenwart*, Darmstadt: Wissenschafliche Buchgesellschaft, 1991.

10. There is a substantial body of literature on fundamentalism, most of the works with a few exceptions on religious fundamentalisms. See, for example, Martin E. Marty and R. Scott Appleby (eds), *Fundamentalisms Observed*, The American Academy of Arts and Sciences, The Fundamentalism Project Vol. 1, Chicago and London: University of Chicago Press, 1991. Stefan Breuer has applied the fundamentalism concept to the secular cult around the German poet Stefan George; see Stefan Breuer, *Ästhetischer Fundamentalismus: Stefan George und der deutsche Antimodernismus*, Darmstadt: Primus Verlag, 1996.

11. Marty and Appleby, *Fundamentalisms Observed* (n. 10), p. ix.

12. Cf. Wilfried Nolte, 'Der Hippokratische Eid und die Abschlußeide der frühen und jetzigen deutschsprachigen Hochschulen – mit ergänzender Betrachtung ausländischer Eide', MD dissertation, Bochum: Ruhr University, 1981.

13. Cf. Klasen, *Diskussion über eine 'Krise'* (n. 4). See also Adolf Meyer, 'Die gegenwärtige Krise der Wissenschaften und die Aufgabe der Philosophie bei ihrer Beseitigung', *Hippokrates, Zeitschrift für Einheitsbestrebungen der Gegenwartsmedizin*, 3, 1931, pp. 393–416; Kurt Riezler, 'Die Krise der "Wirklichkeit" ', *Die Naturwissenschaften*, **16**, 1928, pp. 705–12.

14. Oswald Spengler, *Der Untergang des Abendlandes: Umrisse einer Morphologie der Weltgeschichte*. Vol. I.: *Gestalt und Wirklichkeit* (1918), 33rd–47th edn, Munich: C.H. Beck, 1923. Vol. II: *Welthistorische Perspektiven*, 1st–15th edn, Munich: C.H. Beck, 1922.

15. Gerald D. Feldman, *The Great Disorder: Politics, Economics, and Society in the German Inflation, 1914–1924*, Oxford: Oxford University Press, 1993. Fritz Stern, *The Politics of Cultural Despair: A Study in the Rise of Germanic Ideology*, Berkeley: University of California Press, 1961; Michael H. Kater, 'Hitler's early doctors: Nazi physicians in predepression Germany', *Journal of Modern History*, **59**, 1987, pp. 25–52.

16. Detlev J.K. Peukert, *The Weimar Republic. The Crisis of Classical Modernity*, London: Allen Lane, The Penguin Press, 1991.

17. Michael Hubenstorf, ' "Deutsche Landärzte an die Front!" Ärztliche Standespolitik zwischen Liberalismus und Nationalsozialismus', in Christian Pross, Götz

Aly and Ärztekammer Berlin (eds), *Der Wert des Menschen: Medizin in Deutschland 1918–1945*, Berlin: Edition Hentrich, 1989, pp. 200–23.

18. Heinrich Meng, 'Aus meinem Leben', *Hippokrates*, 33, 1962, pp. 305–10; Detlef Bothe, *Neue Deutsche Heilkunde 1933–1945. Dargestellt anhand der Zeitschrift 'Hippokrates' und der Entwicklung der volksheilkundlichen Laienbewegung*, Husum: Matthiesen, 1991.

19. The other editors were Bernhard Aschner, Louis R. Grote, Miroslav Mikulicic, Eugen Bircher, Walter Gerlach, Diedrich Kulenkampff, Erwin Liek, Max Hirsch, Adolf Buschke, Erich Langer, Arnold Friedländer, Karl Landauer, Heinrich Meng, Walter Riese, Paul Schilder, Erich Stern, Rudolf Tischner, Otto Leeser, Hans Graaz, Ferdinand Hueppe, Georg Lutz, Hans Much, Friedrich Wolter. Cf. Bothe, *Neue Deutsche Heilkunde* (n. 18), pp. 51–54.

20. Cf. Elizabeth Fee and Theodore M. Brown (eds), *Making Medical History: The Life and Times of Henry E. Sigerist*, Baltimore and London: Johns Hopkins University Press, 1997; Meng, 'Aus meinem Leben', and Bothe, *Neue Deutsche Heilkunde* (n. 18).

21. Hans-Peter Schmiedebach, 'Zur Standesideologie in der Weimarer Republik am Beispiel Erwin Liek', in Pross *et al.*, *Der Wert des Menschen* (n. 17), pp. 26–35.

22. See, for example, several articles in *Moderne Medizin*, special issue of *Süddeutsche Monatshefte*, 25, 1928, pp. 546–614; also Peter Schmidt, 'Krise der Medizin?', *Der Querschnitt*, 9, 1929, pp. 318–20; Wilhelm His, 'Die Krise in der Medizin', *Die Woche*, 1930, pp. 789–90; Hans Much, *Hippokrates der Grosse*, Stuttgart: Hippokrates Verlag, 1926; August Bier, 'Gedanken eines Arztes über die Medizin', *Münchener Medizinische Wochenschrift*, 73, 1926, pp. 723–26, 782–86, 1161–64; **74**, 1927, pp. 1141–47, 1186–88; **75**, 1928, pp. 265–68; idem, 'Beiträge zur Heilkunde aus der chirurgischen Universitätsklinik Berlin' *Münchener Medizinische Wochenschrift*, 77, 1930, pp. 569–74, 2112–14, **78**, 1931, pp. 113–16, 154–57, 408–11, 482–85, 540–43, 919–21, 961–63; idem, 'Hippokratische Studien', *Quellen und Studien zur Geschichte der Naturwissenschaften und der Medizin*, 3, 1932, pp. 1–28; Curt Elze, Louis R. Grote, Theodor Brugsch, Erwin Liek und Willy Meyer-Gross, *Grundlagen und Ziele der Medizin der Gegenwart*, Leipzig: Thieme, 1928; Eberhard Zeller, *Paracelsus. Der Beginner des deutschen Arztuums*, Burg Giebigstein: Werkstätten der Stadt Halle, 1936; Hans Hartmann, *Paracelsus. Eine deutsche Vision*, Berlin and Vienna: Verlag Neues Volk, 1941. Critical remarks on this use of Hippocrates and Paracelsus can be found in Henry E. Sigerist, 'Das Bild des Menschen in der modernen Medizin', *Neue Blätter für den Sozialismus*, 1, 1930, pp. 97–106 at p. 99. See also Udo Benzenhöfer, 'Zum Paracelsusbild im Nationalsozialismus', in Christoph Meinel and Peter Voswinckel (eds), *Medizin, Naturwissenschaft, Technik und Nationalsozialismus*, Stuttgart: Verlag für Geschichte der Naturwissenschaften und der Technik, 1994, pp. 265–73.

23. Bernhard Aschner, 'Was können wir aus dem Studium der Werke des Paracelsus und der Geschichte der Medizin überhaupt für die heutige ärztliche Praxis lernen?', *Wiener Medizinische Wochenschrift*, 76, 1926, pp. 1471–73; idem, *Die Krise der Medizin. Konstitutionstherapie als Ausweg*, Stuttgart, Leipzig, Zürich: Hippokrates Verlag, 1928; idem, 'Paracelsische Krebsbehandlung', *Biologische Heilkunde*, 13, 1932, p. 308; idem, 'Praktischer Hippokratismus. I. Die historische Methode als unentbehrliches Forschungsprinzip', *Wiener Medizinische Wochenschrift*, 86, 1936, pp. 314, 345–49, 402–6; idem, 'Neo-Hippocratism in Everyday Practice', *Bulletin of the History of Medicine*, 10, 1941, pp. 260–71; idem, *The Art of the Healer*, New York: Dial, 1942. August

Bier, *Über die Berechtigung des teleologischen Denkens in der praktischen Medizin*, Berlin: August Hirschwald, 1910; idem, 'Die Behandlung lokaler Infektionen mit dem Glüheisen', *Münchener Medizinische Wochenschrift*, **77**, 1930, pp. 1359–62.
24. The popular Vienna gynaecologist Bernhard Aschner claimed to have coined the term 'crisis of medicine'. See Sibylle Brunk-Loch, 'Bernhard Aschner (1883–1960): Sein Weg von der Endokrinologie zur Konstitutionstherapie, MD dissertation, Mainz: J.-Gutenberg University, 1995. Along with the Berlin homoeopath, Bastanier, Aschner was one of the vice presidents of the 1937 *Premier Congrès International de Médecine Neo-Hippocratique* in Paris. See *Premier Congrès International de Médecine Neo-Hippocratique, Les Actes*, 1937, pp. 35–55.
25. For example, Richard Koch, 'Medizin und Philosophie', *Münchener Medizinische Wochenschrift*, **76**, 1929, pp. 10–12; idem, 'Warum kamen die hippokratischen Aphorismen zu klassischer Bedeutung?', *Münchener Medizinische Wochenschrift*, **80**, 1933, pp. 189–91; Paul Diepgen, *Hippokrates oder Paracelsus?*, Stuttgart: Hippokrates Verlag, 1937; Franz Spunda, *Paracelsus*, Wien and Leipzig: König, 1925; Henry Ernest Sigerist, *Grosse Ärzte. Eine Geschichte der Heilkunde in Lebensbildern*, 3rd edn, Munich: J.F. Lehmann, 1954; Bodo Sartorius von Waltershausen, *Paracelsus am Eingang der deutschen Bildungsgeschichte*, Leipzig: Meiner, 1936; Will-Erich Peuckert, *Theophrastus Paracelsus*, Stuttgart and Berlin: Kohlhammer, 1944.
26. Henry Ernest Sigerist, 'Forschungsinstitute für Geschichte der Medizin und der Naturwissenschaften', in Ludolph Brauer, Albrecht Mendelssohn Bartoldy and Adolf Meyer (eds), *Forschungsinstitute. Ihre Geschichte, Organisation und Ziele*, Hamburg: Paul Hartung, 1930, Vol. 1, pp. 391–405 at pp. 396–97.
27. August Bier, 'Beiträge zur Heilkunde aus der chirurgischen Universitätsklinik Berlin. I. Abhandlung: Vorbemerkungen', *Münchener Medizinische Wochenschrift*, **77**, 1930, pp. 569–74. Cf. Hans-Uwe Lammel, 'Chirurgie und Nationalsozialismus am Beispiel der Berliner Chirurgischen Universitätsklinik in der Ziegelstraße', in Wolfram Fischer et al. (eds), *Exodus von Wissenschaften aus Berlin. Fragestellungen – Ergebnisse – Desiderate. Entwicklungen vor und nach 1933*, Berlin and New York: de Gruyter, 1994; Rolf Winau, 'August Bier', in Wilhelm Treue and Rolf Winau (eds), *Berlinische Lebensbilder: Mediziner*, Berlin: Colloquium Verlag, 1987, pp. 287–301; Karl Theodor Vogeler, *August Bier, Leben und Werk*, Munich: J.F. Lehmann, 1942.
28. Lammel, 'Chirurgie und Nationalsozialismus' (n. 27).
29. Geheimes Staatsarchiv Preußischer Kulturbesitz (GStA), Rep 76 Va, Section 1, Tit. VII, No. 24, 'Das Studium der homöopathischen Heilmethoden auf den hiesigen Universitäten', Typescript, Arnold Zimmer, Berlin-Zehlendorf, 4 January 1927: An den ärztlichen Direktor der chirurgischen Universitätsklinik Berlin, 'Bericht über meine Studienzeit am homöopathischen Krankenhaus in Stuttgart'.
30. Cf. GStA Rep 76 Va, Section 1, Tit. VII, No. 24, 'Das Studium der homöopathischen Heilmethoden auf den hiesigen Universitäten', *passim*; Universitätsarchiv der Humboldt-Universität Berlin, Medizinische Fakultät, No. 41, pp. 195–96. See also Petra Werner, 'Zu den Auseinandersetzungen um die Institutionalisierung von Naturheilkunde und Homöopathie an der Friedrich-Wilhelms-Universität zu Berlin zwischen 1919 und 1933', *Medizin, Gesellschaft und Geschichte*, **12**, 1994, pp. 205–19.
31. Universitätsarchiv der Humboldt-Universität Berlin (UA-HUB), Medizinische

Fakultät, No. 41, pp. 63, 206. See also Gabriele Bruchelt, 'Gründung und Aufbau des Berliner Institutes für Geschichte der Medizin und der Naturwissenschaften', MD dissertation, Berlin: Humboldt University, 1978, pp. 11–12.
32. Bier, 'Gedanken eines Arztes' and 'Beiträge zur Heilkunde' (n. 22). For John Brown and the reception of his theories see Guenter B. Risse, 'The History of John Brown's Medical System in Germany During the Years 1790–1806', PhD dissertation, Chicago: University of Chicago, 1971; Thomas H. Broman. *The Transformation of German Academic Medicine, 1750–1820*, Cambridge: Cambridge University Press, 1996, pp. 128–58.
33. Lammel, 'Chirurgie und Nationalsozialismus' (n. 27), p. 576.
34. Hans Much, 'Hans Much', in L.R. Grote (ed), *Die Medizin der Gegenwart in Selbstdarstellungen*, Leipzig: Felix Meiner, 1924, Vol. 4, pp. 188–226. On Much, see also Renate Schulze-Rath, 'Hans Much (1880–1932), Bakteriologe und Schriftsteller', MD dissertation, Mainz, J. Gutenberg University, 1993; Rainer Wirtz, *Leben und Werk des Hamburger Arztes, Forschers und Schriftstellers Hans Much (1880–1932) unter besonderer Berücksichtigung seiner medizintheoretischen Schriften*, Herzogenrath: Verlag Murken-Altrogge, 1991; Gabriele Winkler, 'Hans Much (1880–1932) als schöngeistiger Schriftsteller, dargestellt am Beispiel seines "Meister Ekkehart"', MD dissertation, Munich, Ludwig-Maximilians University, 1989.
35. Much, 'Hans Much' (n. 34), p. 191.
36. A.A. Friedländer, 'Hans Much', *Münchener Medizinische Wochenschrift*, 80, 1933, pp. 23–24; Hans Much, *Das ewige Ägypten*, Dachau: Einhorn-Verlag, 1927; idem, *Die Welt des Buddha*, Dachau: Einhorn-Verlag, 1924. For a recent study on orientalism and philhellenism in German cultural and educational politics, see Suzanne L. Marchand, *Down from Olympus: Archaeology and Philhellenism in Germany, 1750–1970*, Princeton, NJ: Princeton University Press, 1996.
37. Much, *Hippokrates der Grosse* (n. 22).
38. Reviews by [Henry E.] Sigerist, *Deutsche Medizinische Wochenschrift*, 53, 1927, p. 1151; [Wilhelm] His, *Klinische Wochenschrift*, 6, 1927, pp. 513–14; Max Nassauer, *Münchener Medizinische Wochenschrift*, 74, 1927, p. 248.
39. Much, *Hippokrates der Grosse* (n. 22), p. 8.
40. Ibid., pp. 206–8.
41. Ibid., p. 37.
42. August Bier, 'Beiträge zur Heilkunde aus der chirurgischen Universitaetsklinik Berlin. VIII. Abhandlung: Wesen und Grundlagen der Heilkunde. 2. Teil: Hippokratismus. 1.Abschnitt: Einleitung', *Münchener Medizinische Wochenschrift*, 77, 1930, pp. 2193–95 at p. 2194.
43. Ibid.
44. Quoted in Vogeler, *August Bier* (n. 27), p. 270.
45. For Much, see *Hippokrates der Grosse* (n. 22), p. 69.
46. For Bier see 'Beiträge zur Heilkunde' (n. 27), 569–74.
47. August Bier, 'Beiträge zur Heilkunde aus der chirurgischen Universitätsklinik Berlin. VIII. Abhandlung: Wesen und Grundlagen der Heilkunde. 1. Teil: Naturalismus', *Münchener Medizinische Wochenschrift*, 77, 1930, pp. 2112–14. Much, *Hippokrates der Grosse* (n. 22), pp. 11–14, 65–67, 111–12.
48. Elfriede Paul, 'Wegbegleiter auf unebener Strasse', in Günther Albrecht and Wolfgang Hartwig (eds), *Ärzte: Erinnerungen, Erlebnisse, Bekenntnisse*, Berlin: Der Morgen, 1972, p. 132, quoted after Lammel, 'Chirurgie und Nationalsozialismus' (n. 27), p. 570.

49. Cf. Weindling, *Health, Race, and German Politics* (n. 1).
50. Much, *Hippokrates der Grosse* (n. 22), p. 25.
51. Ibid., p. 29.
52. See also Paul Diepgen, 'Die Profanierung des ärztlichen Berufes', *Ärztliche Mitteilungen*, **27**, 1926, pp. 690–91.
53. Fritz K. Ringer, *The Decline of the German Mandarins: The German Academic Community, 1880–1933*, Cambridge, MA: Harvard University Press, 1969.
54. Cf. Paul Weindling, 'Bourgois Values, Doctors and the State: The Professionalization of Medicine in Germany 1848–1933', in David Blackbourne and Richard J. Evans (eds), *The German Bourgoisie. Essays on the Social History of the German Middle Class from the Late Eighteenth to the Early Twentieth Century*, London & New York: Routledge, 1991, pp. 198–223.
55. Alfons Labisch, 'From Traditional Individualism to Collective Professionalism: State, Patient, Compulsory Health Insurance, and the Panel Doctor Question in Germany, 1883–1931', in Manfred Berg and Geoffrey Cocks (eds), *Medicine and Modernity: Public Health and Medical Care in Nineteenth- and Twentieth-Century Germany*, Cambridge: Cambridge University Press, 1997, pp. 35–54. Claudia Huerkamp. *Der Aufstieg der Ärzte im 19. Jahrhundert. Vom gelehrten Stand zum professionellen Experten: Das Beispiel Preußens*, Göttingen: Vandenhoeck & Ruprecht, 1985.
56. Florian Tennstedt, *Soziale Selbstverwaltung. Geschichte der Selbstverwaltung in der Krankenversicherung*, Bonn: Verlag der Ortskrankenkassen, 1977.
57. Reinhard Spree, *Soziale Ungleichheit vor Krankheit und Tod*, Göttingen: Vandenhoeck & Ruprecht, 1981; Claudia Huerkamp. *Der Aufstieg der Ärzte*, (n. 55).
58. Julius Schwalbe, 'Bemerkungen zu dem vorstehenden Aufsatz', *Deutsche Medizinische Wochenschrift*, **45**, 1919, p. 78.
59. Erwin Liek, *The Doctor's Mission: Reflections, Reminiscences, and Revelations of a Medical Man*, London: J. Murray, 1930. Cf. Timmermann, 'Constitutional medicine', (n. 4).
60. Cf. Stefan Breuer, *Anatomie der Konservativen Revolution*, Darmstadt: Wissenschaftliche Buchgesellschaft, 1993; Rolf Peter Sieferle, *Die Konservative Revolution*, Frankfurt: Fischer, 1995.
61. Much, *Hippokrates der Grosse* (n. 22), p. 55.
62. Ibid., p. 130–31.
63. Karl Binding and Alfred Hoche, *Die Freigabe der Vernichtung lebensunwerten Lebens: Ihr Mass und ihre Form*, Leipzig, F. Meiner, 1920. Cf. Karl Heinz Hafner, and Rolf Winau, '"Die Freigabe der Vernichtung lebensunwerten Lebens". Eine Untersuchung zu der Schrift von Karl Binding und Alfred Hoche', *Medizinhistorisches Journal*, **9**, 1974, pp. 227–54; Lifton, *The Nazi Doctors* (n. 1), pp. 46–48, Peukert, 'The Genesis of the "Final Solution"' (n. 5); Weindling, *Health, Race and German Politics* (n. 1), pp. 394–97.
64. Weindling, *Health, Race and German Politics* (n. 1), p. 394.
65. Much, *Hippokrates der Grosse* (n. 22), p. 131.
66. Vogeler, *August Bier* (n. 27), p. 105.
67. August Bier, 'Gymnastik als Vorbeugungs- und Heilmittel', *Münchener Medizinische Wochenschrift*, **69**, 1922, pp. 993–98.
68. See, for example, Claudia Huerkamp, 'Medizinische Lebensreform im späten 19. Jahrhundert. Die Naturheilbewegung in Deutschland als Protest gegen die wissenschaftliche Universitätsmedizin', *Vierteljahresschrift für Sozial- und Wirtschaftsgeschichte*, **73**, 1986, pp. 158–82. Wolfgang R. Krabbe, *Gesellschaftsveränderung durch Lebensreform. Strukturmerkmale einer sozialreformerischen*

Bewegung im Deutschland der Industrialisierungsperiode, Göttingen: Vandenhoeck and Ruprecht, 1974.
69. Hans Much, 'Erkältung', *Münchener Medizinische Wochenschrift*, **73**, 1926, pp. 684–86.
70. Cf. Timmermann, 'Constitutional medicine', (n. 4).
71. Much, 'Erkältung' (n. 69), p. 685.
72. Cf. 'Kleine Mitteilungen', *Deutsche Medizinische Wochenschrift*, **56**, 1930, p. 591; 'Tagesgeschichtliche Notizen', *Münchener Medizinische Wochenschrift*, **77**, 1930, p. 615.
73. Bundesarchiv Berlin, R 1501: Reichsministerium des Inneren, No. 26226: 'Mißbräuchliche medizinische Eingriffe', p. 296.
74. Cf. Lifton, *The Nazi Doctors* (n. 1), p. 32.
75. B.J. Gottlieb. *Hippokrates. Gedanken über ärztliche Ethik aus dem Corpus Hippocraticum*, 2nd edn, Ewiges Arzttum 1, Prague, 1942. Cf. Leven, 'Hippokrates im 20. Jahrhundert' (n. 2), pp. 75–80.
76. Quoted from Lifton, *The Nazi Doctors* (n. 1), p. 32.
77. Cf. Benzenhöfer, 'Zum Paracelsusbild im Nationalsozialismus' (n. 22).
78. Hartmann, *Paracelsus* (n. 22), p. 162.
79. Ibid., p. 170.
80. Ibid., p. 159–6.
81. Bothe, *Neue Deutsche Heilkunde* (n. 18); Alfred Haug, 'Die "Synthese" von Schulmedizin und Naturheilkunde im Nationalsozialismus. Ein kritischer Rückblick', in Manfred Brinkmann and Michael Franz (eds), *Nachtschatten im weißen Land. Betrachtungen zu alten und neuen Heilsystemen*, Berlin: Verlagsgesellschaft Gesundheit, 1982, pp. 115–25.
82. Paul Diepgen, 'Einheitsbestrebungen der Gegenwartsmedizin und Medizingeschichte', *Klinische Wochenschrift*, **7**, 1928, pp. 855–56; Friedrich Kümmel, 'Im Dienst "nationalpolitischer Erziehung"? Die Medizingeschichte im Dritten Reich', in Meinel and Voswinckel (eds), *Medizin, Naturwissenschaft, Technik und Nationalsozialismus* (n. 22), pp. 295–319.
83. Paul Diepgen, 'Aufgaben und Bedeutung der Medizingeschichte', *Geistige Arbeit*, **1** (14), 1934, pp. 1–2.
84. Ibid., p. 1.
85. Karl Eduard Rothschuh, 'Theoretische Medizin. Begründung ihrer Notwendigkeit in der Gegenwart und eine Umreißung des Gebietes,' *Klinische Wochenschrift*, **14**, 1935, pp. 1401–5 at p. 1403.
86. Ibid., p. 1404.
87. Diepgen, *Hippokrates oder Paracelsus?* (n. 25), p. 30.
88. Alexander Mitscherlich and Fred Mielke, *The Death Doctors*, London: Elek, 1962, p. 186.
89. Ibid., p. 186.
90. Ibid., p. 189.
91. Ibid., p. 141.
92. See Kater, *Doctors under Hitler* (n. 1), pp. 70–73; also Lifton, *Nazi Doctors* (n. 1), pp. 447–51.
93. For some detailed studies, see publications cited in note 1.
94. Another group who resisted were the few socialist and communist doctors. Cf. Kater, *Doctors under Hitler* (n. 1), pp. 74–84.
95. Franz Büchner, *Der Eid des Hippokrates. Die Grundgesetze der ärztlichen Ethik*, Freiburg im Breisgau: Herder, 1945. Cf. Leven, 'Hippokrates im 20. Jahrhundert', (n. 2), pp. 65–74.

96. Klee, *Auschwitz* (n. 1), pp. 193–243, esp. 241–42.
97. Albert Moll, *Ärztliche Ethik*, Stuttgart: Enke, 1902; Julius Henri Schultz, *Albert Molls ärztliche Ethik*, Zürich: Juris, 1986.
98. Cf. Barbara Elkeles, 'Medizinische Menschenversuche gegen Ende des 19. Jahrhunderts und der Fall Neisser', *Medizinhistorisches Journal*, **20**, 1985, pp. 135–48; Winau, 'Medizin und Menschenversuch' (n. 7), pp. 21–24.
99. Cf. Julius Moses, *Der Kampf um die Kurierfreiheit*, Radebeul and Dresden: Madaus, 1930, pp. 72–75, 79–80; Daniel S. Nadav, *Julius Moses (1868–1942) und die Politik der Sozialhygiene in Deutschland*, Gerlingen: Bleicher, 1985; Susanne Hahn, 'Revolution der Heilkunst – Ausweg aus der Krise? Julius Moses (1868–1942) zur Rolle der Medizin in der Gesundheitspolitik der Weimarer Republik', in Pross *et al.*, *Der Wert des Menschen* (n. 17), pp. 71–85; Kurt Nemitz, 'Julius Moses – Nachlass und Bibliographie', *Internationale wissenschaftliche Korrespondenz zur Geschichte der deutschen Arbeiterbewegung*, **10**, 1974, pp. 219–41.
100. Julius Moses, *Der Totentanz von Lübeck*, Radebeul and Dresden: Madaus, 1930. See also Alberto Ascoli, 'Die Calmettesche Schutzimpfung und die Säuglingserkrankungen in Lübeck', *Deutsche Medizinische Wochenschrift*, **56**, 1930, pp. 1160–62.
101. Moses, *Der Kampf um die Kurierfreiheit* (n. 99), pp. 80–81.
102. Mitscherlich and Mielke, *The Death Doctors* (n. 88).
103. Christian Pross, 'Nazi doctors, German medicine, and historical truth', in Annas and Grodin, *The Nazi Doctors and the Nuremberg Code* (n. 7), pp. 32–52 at pp. 40–41.
104. Michael H. Kater, 'The Sewering scandal of 1993 and the German medical establishment', in Berg and Cocks, *Medicine and Modernity* (n. 55), pp. 213–34; idem, *Doctors under Hitler* (n. 1), pp. 1–11.

Index

Aberdeen, University of 93, 96
Abortion 245–8
Academic medicine 281, 288, 291
Academics, British Neo-Hippocratists' anxiety about 280, 288
Academy of Medicine, Paris 178, 190, 193, 194
Ackerknecht, Erwin 172 n.3, 185, 186, 187, 188, 193, 209
   Medicine at the Paris Hospital (1967) 188
Adam 67
Adams, Francis 10
Advertisers 281, 284
Albany Medical College 209
Albury, Randall 243
Alchemist(s) 61–2, 65, 82 n.25
Alcohol distillation 57 n.69
Alexandria 25
Allendy, René 266, 268
Alternative medicine 23 *see also* Homeopathy, Naturopathy, Hydropathy
Amerbach, Bonifacius 56 n.66
America *see also* Hippocratism/Neo-Hippocratism
   And French medicine 200–36 *passim*
   Identities of American Physicians 200–36 *passim*, 239–45
   Material culture 241–5
   Popular culture 1930s 245–53
   Reform of medicine (Nineteenth-Century) 204, 213
   Southern nationalism/identity 223–7
Analytical
   Medicine 266, 272
   Method 169
Anatomy 38, 102, 117–31, 189
Anatomy of a Humbug (1837) 218
Ancient
   Greek culture, to Americans 227
   Greek culture, to Britons 282
   Greek culture, to Germans 307–8
   Medicine 184, 188, 190, 192, 194
   Method of induction 191
   Physicians 193
   Spirit 187, 188, 189
   Theology 62
   World, images of 283, 293, 303
Ancients 180, 186
Andral, Gabriel 192, 194, 212, 219
   Pathological Hematology (1843) 192
Anthropological medicine 181
Anti-Semitism in Britain 286
Anxiety 284
Aphorisms 190, 192 *see also* Hippocratic writings
Apollo 23, 24, 26, 39, 81 n.16
   As father of medicine, 25
Appleby, R. Scott 303
   Fundamentalism Observed (1991) 303
Arabic physicians 59, 63, 164
Arbuthnot, John 137, 145, 146, 147, 148, 149
   An Essay concerning the Effectors of Air on Human Bodies (1733) 145–6
Archeus 66, 86 n.92, 98, 99, 120, 122
Aristotelian(ism) 61, 70, 84 n.49
Aristotle 8, 29, 30, 38, 72–3, 77, 86 n.77, 117, 123, 180, 191
Arrizabalaga, John 5
Artaxerxes 9, 18 n.44, 25, 28, 32, 244
Ärztestand 308
Asclepiads 8, 201
Asclepius 8, 22, 23, 24, 25
   Temple of 109
Aslakssøn, Kort 88 n.126
Astra (stars) 76–7
Astrology 46
Astronomy 62, 64, 81 n.15, 87 n.112
Astrum (astral body) 76, 87 n.106
Asulanus, Franciscus 57 n.68
Athens 25, 282
   Plague of 8
Atkinson, Brooks 246
Auber 194
   Traité de la science médicale (1853) 194
Augustine, Saint 44, 65, 83 n.33
Augustus 28
Auschwitz 302, 316
Auscultation 184, 185, 188
Avery, J.G. 253

Avicenna 39

Babylonian medicine 267
Bacon, Francis 27, 30, 45, 62, 91, 103, 104, 107, 138, 139, 140, 181, 191, 206, 211
   Advancement of Learning (1605) 138
   New Atlantis (1626) 119
   The Masculine Birth of Time (1603) 27
Baconianism 12, 205 *see also* Bacon, Francis
Bacteriology 291
Baissette, Gaston 10, 265–6, 273
Balfour, Sir Andrew 94
Balkan wars 282
Balzac, Honoré de 18 n.44, 98
Barbarism 284
Barbeyrac, Charles 159, 174 n.15
Barchusen, Johann Conrad 48
Barnum, P.T. 214
Baron d'Holbach 167
Barthez, Paul-Joseph 158, 167–70, 181, 186, 194, 259
   Cours de thérapeutique (1821) 170
   Nouveaux élémens de la science d l'homme (1858) 167, 194
Bartlett, Elisha 210–11, 218–19, 220
   A Discourse on the Times, Character and Writings of Hippocrates (1852) 212, 217
   A Philosophy of Medical Science (1844) 210, 211, 212, 220
   History, Diagnosis and Treatment of the Fevers of the United States (1847) 224
Basel 39, 79
Bathhurst, Ralph 125
Bauhin, Casper 117
Bayle, Gaspart-Laurent 182, 185, 189, 190
Bayliss Sir William Maddock 287
Bayly, Edward 143
Béarne 160, 171
Beastmaker Mountain 1
Beclard 206
Begbie, James Warburton 10
Bellvue Hospital (New York) 246
Bergson, Henri 265, 272
Berlin University 305
Bernard, Claude 274

Berr, Henri 266
Beverwijk, Johann 48
Bibliothèque Nationale 262
Bichat, Xavier 189, 193, 206
Bier, August 305–12
Big business 280
Bills of Mortality 98, 144, 145
Binding, Karl 310
   The Permission to Destroy Life Unworthy of Life (1920) 310
Biochemistry 287
Biot, René 269
Biotype 263, 290
Blackmore, Richard 91
Blood 192–3
Boerhaave, Hermann 105, 138, 140, 142, 159–60, 165, 186
Bologna 40
Bonaparte, Napoleon 157, 168, 182, 282
Books, Neo-Hippocratists' concerns about 281
Bosch, Robert 304
Botanical metaphors 121
Bouillaud, Jean-Baptiste 186, 188, 189, 190, 191, 192, 194
   Essai sur la philosophie médicale (1836) 188
Bowditch, Henry Ingersoll 222
Boyle, Robert 60, 80 n.9, 99, 104, 117, 123, 148
Brahe, Tycho 62, 81 n.15, 87 n.94 & n.109, 88 n.126
Brand names 281
Bridge-makers between laboratory and clinic 290
Britain *see* England, Scotland, Hippocratism/Neo-Hippocratism
Brock, Arthur John 283, 284–6, 288–9, 291, 292
Broman, Thomas 6
Brotherhood of the trenches 284
Broussais, François 185, 186, 187, 188, 189, 192, 194, 206, 221, 260
   Examination of Systems of Nosology (1816) 186, 189
   The History of Chronic Inflammations (1808) 186
Broussaisism 211, 221
Brown, John 306
Brownism 208, 211
Brunfels, Otto 56 n.68

INDEX 327

Buchenwald concentration camp 314
Büchner, Franz 315
Buddhism, in the writings of Hans Much 306
Burckhard, Peter 56 n.65, n.68
Bureaucrat(s) 284, 285
Burleigh, Walter 56 n.68
Burnet, Dr Thomas 95
   Hippocrates Contractus (1685) 95
   Treasury of Practical Medicine (1673) 95

Cabanis, Pierre-Jean-Georges 179, 182, 183, 185, 209
   On the relations between the Physical and Moral Aspects of Man (1805) 180
Calculus 191
   of probability 190, 192
Calvi, Marco Fabio 28, 29
Calvinism 126
Cambacérès, J-J-R 167
Cambridge 142
   University 108
Cannon, Walter Bradford 243
Cardano, Girolamo 54 n.49, 56 n.67, 57 n.71
Cardiology 290
Carey, Eben 244
Carnot, Paul 269
Carrel, Alexis 269, 272
   L'Homme cet inconnu (1936) 269
Cartesianism 266
Carton Paul 263–4, 270–1
Cartwright, Samuel 225, 226
Case histories 92, 139, 140, 141, 143
Castiglioni, Arturo 267, 280
Castle, George 101
Castro, Roderigo 61
Cathell, D.W. 239, 240, 241
Cathell, William 239
Catholicism, Mystical 272
Cavendish, Margaret (Duchess of Newcastle) 128
Cawadias, Alexandre/Alexander 267–8, 281–3, 287, 288, 289, 290, 291, 293, 294
   The Modern Therapeutics of Internal Diseases (1931) 282
Cellular tissue (in the writings of Bordeu) 161–2

Celsus 54 n.46, 165
Censorship 247
Chaerionia 72, 74, 86 n.81
Chair of Hippocratic medicine, Paris 184
Champier, Symphorien 54 n.49 56 n.68
Chaos (darkness, night) 66, 74
Chapman, Nathaniel 230 n.15
Chaptal, Jean-Antoine 167
Character 268
Charité hospital 182
Charlatan, US concerns about the 216, 233 n.64
Charleton, Walter 60
Chemical
   Philosophy 59, 61, 64–5, 68, 74, 79–80, 83 n.30
   Physicians/Medicine 22, 60, 65, 68, 74, 80, 97–8
Chemistry 38, 102, 193
   Medical 158, 192
Chicken-pox 110
Chinese medicine 266
Chirac, Pierre 165, 174 n.16
Chiracians 166
Chiracisme 165
Chiron 23
Chlorosis 57 n.72
Chomel 219
Christ the healer/Christus medicus 24, 43, 55 n.53
Christian
   Faith 315
   Humanism 43, 271
Civilisation 284, 292, 304, 307, 309 *see also* Crisis
Clairvoyance 264
Classical learning 137, 293–4
Clericuzio, Antonio 81 n.11
Clifton, Francis 137, 139, 140, 141, 142, 143, 144, 145, 149
   Tabular Observations (1731) 139, 140
   The State of Physic (1732) 140
Climate 136, 137, 140, 145, 146, 147
Clinic, The 179, 268, 290
Clinical *see also* Paris
   Elite (in Britain) 283
   Ideals 193
   Medicine 179, 189
   Practice 280–1
Clinicians, Paris 193
Collège de France 182

Columbo, Realdo 117
Commercialisation 302
Communists 284
Computer games 1, 8
Conceptualism 287–8
Condillac, Etienne Bonnot de 179
Confidence man, US concerns about 214
Constantine the African 21
Constitution 122, 129–31, 140, 147, 268, 311
Constitutional
    Medicine 280, 282, 294
    Outlook 290
Conway, Anne 125–6
Cook, Harold J. 84 n.44, 91, 92, 124
Cookeism 208, 211
Cooper, Anthony Ashley 122
Copenhagen 85 n.54
Copenhagen, University of 69
Corde, Maurice de la 30
Cornarius, Janus 56 n.66
Cornil, Lucien 268, 269
Coronis 23
Corvisart, Jean-Nicolas 179, 182, 183, 185, 190
Cos 8, 24, 25, 32, 242
    Oracle of 188
Cotes, Roger 142
Council of 500 179
Coxe, John Redman 201, 202, 229 n.4
Creator, The 65
Crisis
    Economic 304
    Of Civilization 272
    Of illness (Critical days) 164, 165
    Of medicine, debate in interwar Germany 302, 304, 309
Crombie, Alistair 37
Cronin, A.J. 249
Crookshank, Francis 283, 286, 287, 288, 290, 291
Cross, Stephen 243
Crow, Thomas 18 n.44, 32
Crowd mentality 286
Cullen 226
Cullenism 208, 211
Culpepper, Nicholas 119, 121, 124, 130, 131
Cuninghame 95
Cunningham, Andrew 30, 124, 139
Cutting the bladder stone 57 n.74

Dachau concentration camp 315
Dante's Hell 1
Daremberg, Charles 194, 260, 273
Darier, Jean 269
Davidson, William 84 n.40
Davis, Lincoln 245
Dawson, Lord Bertrand 283
Day, William 120–1
De Beauvais, Vincent 56 n.68
De Bordeu, Théophile 158, 159, 160–6, 169
    'Crise' (1754) 164, 166
    Recherchessur le tissue muqueux (1767) 161, 169
De Chauliac, Guy 42
De Liuzzi, Mondino 128
De Mercy, François 259, 260
De Mondeville, Henri 42
De Romanis, Giovanni 57 n.74
De Sauvages, François Boissier 160, 174 n.16 174–5 n.20, 175 n.34
Deception, US concerns about 214–18
Degeneration, Medieval and Renaissance theory of 42, 43
Deidier, Antoine 175 n.34
Delore, Pierre 268, 269, 270
Demagogues 281, 284
Democracy
    Liberal 272
    Social 309
Democratic duty 207
Democritus 25, 48, 117, 180
Demosthenes 282
Denmark 69, 79, 85 n.54
Departmentality 288
Dermatology 290
Desbois de Rochefort 182
Descartes, René 37, 45, 117, 119, 186
Desfosses, Paul 268
Despotism 208
Deutsche Medizinische Wochenschrift 309
Dewhurst, Kenneth 159
Di Santo, Mariano 57 n.74
Diagnosis 259, 280
Dictators 281, 284
Diderot, Denis 160, 176 n.45 *Rêve de d'Alembert* 160
Diepgen, Paul 313
Diet/Dietetics 181, 265
Disease 158–9, 162, 169, 170, 203, 206

see also Fictions, Hippocrates as (Historian of disease), Natural (History of disease)
  Aetiology/Causes of disease 106–7, 118, 122, 159
  And locality 94
  Epidemic disease 182
  'New' diseases 5, 12, 63, 98, 140
  Southern diseases (USA) 224
Disintegration 285
Disruptions economic and social of 1920s & 1930s 13–14, 243, 270, 284, 302, 304
Dissociation 285
Dittler, Edgar 247–9
  The Hippocratic Oath (1938) 247–9
Divine revelation 62
Don Quixot 91–2
Dordrecht 48
Douglas, Lloyd 252–3
  Green Light – the movie 253
  Green Light – the novel (1935) 252–3
  Magnificent Obsession 252
Dr. Hippocrates, the swordfish 1, 8
Dubois, Jacques 43–44, 51 n.36
  Vaesani depulsio 43–44
Duffin, Jacalyn 184
Durham 282
Dynameis 71–2, 74, 79, 86 n.81

Easlea, Brian 27
Eberle, John 203
Eclectic 188, 189, 192
  Eclectic physicians 217
Ecole de Santé 182
Eddy, Mary Baker 273
Edelstein, Ludwig 92, 273
Edinburgh 93–7, 226
  Town Council of 93–5
Efficient agent or cause 65
  Inner efficient, craftsman 71, 74
Egypt, in the writings of Hans Much 306
Egyptian medicine 267
Embryology 74, 84 n.49
Emerton, Norma 83 n.34
Empiric 216, 233 n.64 *see also* Quacks
Empiricism/empirical medicine 27, 63–4, 68, 82 n.26, 124–7, 129, 169, 180, 189, 203, 205, 206, 209, 210–20 *see also* Hippocrates as (empiricist)
Endocrinology 263, 282, 287, 290
England/English 60
  Authentic (& Britain) 293
  Gentlemanly culture 282
  Physiologists 282
English Hippocrates, The (i.e. Thomas Sydenham) 59, 104, 121, 158
Enlightenment, The 179, 182, 183, 204
Ent, George 101, 102
Entities 285, 288
Environmental medicine 136, 179
Epicurian atomism 119
Epicurus 180
Epistemology 181
Eppendorf Hospital 306
Erasistratus of Ceos 47
Erastus, Thomas 65, 88 n.125
Eristratus 117, 118
Estes, John Worth 7
Ethics 4, 31 *see also* Hippocrates (moral qualities), Hippocratic Writings (the *Oath*, *Decorum* and *The Physician*)
  In popular American Culture 245–53
  Medical 283, 303, 310, 315
Euthanasia 310
Evacuation, the seven Hippocratic kinds 106
Evangelismos Hospital, Medical Clinic 282
Experience 107, 187, 216
Experiential epistemology 139
Experiment/Experimentation 64, 120, 269
  see also Hippocrates as Experimentalist, Laboratory
Experimental
  Method 193
    Malleability of 7
  Philosophy 60
Experimentalist 193

Fabricus of Aquapente 117
Falcucci, Nicolò F. 55 n.61
Fallibility 45
Family 22
Fascists 284
Fazio/Facio, Bartolomeo 128
Fee-splitting 248
Female Medical College of Pennsylvania 219
Femininity 21
Fenner, Erasmus Darwin 225
Ferments/Fermentation 74
Fernel, Daniel 117

Fernel, Jean 51 n.36
Fevers 122
  Essay on 184
Ficino, Marsilio 62
Fictions 280, 281, 285, 287, 290
Fiolle, Jean 269, 271
Fischer, Fritz 314
Fishbein, Morris 246
Flatus vocis 287–8
Fleck, Ludwig 130
Flint, Austin 208
Flint, Joshua 221–2
Florentine Art Plaster Company of Philadelphia 241
Fludd, Robert 77, 87 n.109, 120
Flynn, Errol 253
Formalism 280
Fortier-Beronville 267, 268
Fragmentation 284
France 61, 79, *see also* America, Hippocratism/Neo-Hippocratism, Montpellier, Paris, Revolution
Frank, Robert 117, 125
Frederik II, King of Denmark 85 n.52
Freiburg 88 n.124
French, Roger 5
Freud, Sigmund 273
Friend, John 105–7
  Emmenologia (1703) 105
Fuchs, Leonhart 57 n.73
Fundamentalism 303, 310

Gale, Thomas 21, 31
Galen 5, 6, 21, 22, 25, 27, 28, 30, 31, 38–9, 42–4, 46, 48, 59–60, 63, 65, 68–71, 73, 76, 78–9, 82 n.22 & 23, 85 n.53, 88 n.123, 91, 92, 98, 105, 107, 117–19, 120, 123, 124, 128, 139, 141, 164, 165, 181, 185, 186, 227, 240, 241, 259, 266, 270, 285 *see also* Galen's works, Galenic medicine, and Hippocrates (and Galen)
  As evil genie 266
  As 'father of medicine' 21
  As prince of physicians 22, 27–8
  As the great corrupter 99
  As usurper, 22, 98–9
Galen's works
  De locis affectis 29
  De uteri dissectione 52 n.31
  On the usefulness of parts 22
Galenic medicine, Galenist, Galenism 28, 29, 61, 63, 67–8, 70, 72, 74, 77, 80–2, 84–5, 87, 128, 211, 261
Galilei, Galileo 45
Gardeil, Jean Baptiste 260, 264
Gaskell, Walter Holbrook 287
Gassendi, Pierre 117, 119
Gastroenterology 290
General public 281
Generalist(s) 284, 292
Genesis 65, 83, 87 n.116
Genoa 282
German
  Army helmet 306
  College of Physical Education 311
Germany 61, 69, 73, 79, 302–24 *see also* Hippocratism/Neo-Hippocratism, Revolution, Crisis
  Conservative Revolution 309
  Culture, conflict with civilisation 304
  Decadence, fin de siecle in 304
  Elitism in, 305–10
  Imperial Health Council 312
  Insurance system 309
  Middle class, old and new 309
  Music 286
  National People's Party 306
  Pharmaceutical companies 286
  Political commitments of Hippocratists 304
  Sickness insurance in 309
  To British neo-Hippocratists 285–7
  Trade unions in 309
  Volk, concept of 14, 302, 310–11, 312–13
  Welfare state in 304, 308
Gesner, Konrad 56 n.68
Gießen, University of 304
Giroudet 18 n.44
  Hippocrates Refusing the Gifts of Artaxerxes (1792), 18 n.44, 32
Glisson, Francis 101, 102, 117
Goodwin, George 244
  Minute Men of Life (1929) 244
Graham, Peter 22
Graunt, John 98
Grawitz, Ernst Robert von 312
  The Doctor's Eternal Mission 312
Greece 62, 178, 180
Greek *see also* Ancient
  Compulsory learning of language in Britain 293–4

Medicine 188, 194, 267
Myth 23, 24
Names 293
Reading of 28, 293
Republic 282
Revival medicine in the US 222–7
Royal Family 282
Green, Anne 120
Greifswald, University of 306
Gresham College 106
Grmek, Mirki 185
Groenevelt, Johannes 84 n.44
Gross, R.E. 240
Gruner, Christian Gottfried 48
Guelac Henry 173 n.15
Guiart, Jules 269
Günther of Andernach 51 n.24
Gymnastics 311
Gynaecology 28–9

Haematology 192
Haen, Anton de 182
Hahnemann Days Conference (1935) 267
Hahnemann Medical College, Philadelphia 201
Hahnemann, Samuel 24, 222–3, 267
Hales, Stephen 146, 148
Halttunen, Karen 214
Hardwick, Earl of 108
  Athenian Letters (1741) 108
Harley St. 282, 292
Hartmann, Hans 312
Harvey, William 22, 38, 40–1, 47–8, 101, 102, 117–18, 120, 126, 129, 162, 174 n.19, 240
  De Motu Cordis 22, 40, 117, 129
  Epistola de calculo renum et vesicae 48
  Exercitationes de generatione animalium 40
  Lectures on anatomy 40
Hauksbee, Francis 142
Hawthorne, Nathaniel 241
  Dr Heidegger's Experiment (1837) 241
  The Haunted Quack (1831) 241
Health education 282
Health, inequalities of 183
Hearst's International-Cosmopolitan 249, 252
Heberden, William (the elder) 107–11

Hellenists 193
Helmont, Jan Baptist van 60–1, 80–1 n.11
Helmontian chemical medicine 97–8
Helmontian(s) 60, 80–1 n.11
Henderson, John 5
Henderson, Lawrence J. 243
Henricus 117
Heraclitus of Ephesus 267, 306
Hermetic 62, 81 n.18, 87 n.109
Hermeticism 266
Herophilus 47
Herrick, James B. 245
Hieronymus 44
Hierophilus 118
Highmore, Nathaniel 102
Himmler, Heinrich 312
Hippocrate 261, 266–7
Hippocrates
  Ambulance 1
  And Galen 4–5, 10 , 11, 28, 29, 92–111 *passim*, 124–32, 139
  Being Hippocrates 8
  Busts of 157–8, 239, 241, 246, 282
  Circle, 1
  French language works on 257–62
  General Hospital 248
  In computer games 1
  Moral qualities of 31, 97, 283 *see also* Ethics
  On epidemics 209 *see also* Hippocratic writings
  Popularity in websites 15 n.3
  Survivalist accounts of 2
  Visual images of 30–1
Hippocrates as
  Advocate of a focus on the collective 7, 14, 302–24 *passim*
  Advocate of a focus on the individual patient 7, 13–14 *see also* Patient
  Alternative to mainstream medicine 261 *see also* Alternative medicine
  Archetype of Southern US physician 226–7
  Baconian investigator 142 *see also* Bacon/Baconianism
  Clinical physician 109
  Coan Sage 201,
  Cognitive authority 117–19, 121, 123, 131–2
  Compiler of medical details 91
  Compiler of natural histories 142

Divine 25
Empiricist 109, 138, 139, 179, 181, 189–90, 200–28 *see also* Empiricism
Experimentalist 192 *see also* Experiment
Father of holistic medicine 23
Father of medicine 10, 21–36 *passim*, 181, 201, 202
First discoverer 54 n.46
Founder of clinical medicine 7
Founder of experimental medicine 7
God 10, 30
Historian of nature 209 *see also* Natural
Historian of diseases 102 *see also* Natural
Humanist 54 n.45
Iatrochemist 7, 59–87 *passim see also* Iatrochemistry
Iatromechanist 7 *see also* Iatromechanism
Inductivist 91
Initiator of the dosimetric method 261
Médecin-philosophe 179–81
Observer 6, 7, 139 142, 159 *see also* Observation
New Hippocrates, The 46
Paracelsian 11, 59–87 *passim see also* Germany, Paracelsus
Parisian 212
Pathological Anatomist 179, 182
Patron of Nazi's national revolution 312
Precursor of anatomo-pathological method 259
Precursor of the antiseptic method 261
Rational and empirical 100
Renaissance physician 56–7 n.68
Romulus of Medicine 102
Sagacious old man 146
Sceptic of Enlightenment values 179, 182
Source of method 6, 11, 181–2
Source of substantive explanations of disease 6, 11
System-maker 111 *see also* System
True or honest physician 218
Vitalist, 192 *see also* Vitalism
Voice of Nature 168
Warrantor of progress 10, 37–58 *passim*

Young (Eternally) 56 n.66
Hippocrates' genealogy and life 8–10, 260 *see also Pseudoepigrapha, Vita*
Biography by Soranus 28
Biography of 265
Burns library at Cos 8, 32
Cures Athenian plague 8, 25
Cures King Perdiccas 8, 244
Dies in Larissa 8
Disdain for money 31
Genuineness of stories about 9–10
Hippocrates Refusing the Gifts of Artaxerxes (1792), 18 n.44, 32
In fiction 10
Life as a means of discussing social order 9
Patriotism 8, 31
Reading and 7
Refuses gold of Artaxerxes 8, 18 n.49, 32
Sources on 8
Hippocratic
As synonym for medical 269
Doctrine, 181, 184, 188, 194
Medical education 96
Method 181, 182, 184, 188, 190, 191
As Baconian method 12, 138, 139, 140, 147, 149
Methods/Doctrines
Contraries contrariis (method of contraries) 74, 76 , 261, 261
Experiment 7
Healing power of nature 168–9, 183, 261, 267, 270, 283
Similia similibus (method of similars) 75–6, 262
Natural methods 259
Observation 96, 139, 259, 261
Vis medicatrix naturae 181, 243, 292
Revival, Britain C20th 280–301
Revival, Seventeenth century (France)159
Spirit 181, 265
Tradition 190, 191, 193
As invented tradition 3
Values 185
Hippocratic *Corpus* 53 n.42, 181, 270, 273 307
Authenticity of 8, 25
Authorship 8, 25, 229 n.4

INDEX 333

Genuine texts 8, 25
Nature of 6, 23, 24–5
Reading of 7–8, 23
Translations of 5, 28, 258, 259, 260, 261, 264, 265, 273
Hippocratic Writings *see also* Historiography of Hippocrates,
Hippocratic *Corpus*
 Affections 70, 72, 84 n.50, 192
 Airs, Waters and Places 9, 57, 84 n.50, 94, 104, 118, 127, 137, 140, 148, 168, 179, 182
 Ancient medicine 55 n.63, 60, 69–72, 76, 79, 82 n.20, 84 n.50, 85 n.55, 184, 213
 Aphorisms 27, 39, 51 n.31 52 n.35, 70, 74, 84 n.50, 85 n.72, 100, 107, 162, 164, 168, 258
 Breaths 72, 76–7, 84 n.50
 Coan Praenotions 100
 Coan prognostications 64, 83 n.31, 162, 164, 168
 De victu 39
 De victu in morbis acutis 39
 Decorum 4, 96
 Diseases 70-2, 84 n.50
 Diseases of Women 28, 29, 30
 Dreams (Regimen IV) 76, 84 n.50
 Epidemics 4, 31, 52 n.35, 60, 64, 77, 83 n.31, 84 n.50, 103, 104, 105, 107, 110, 118, 127, 137, 140, 144, 147, 148, 162, 164
 Fevers 118
 Fleshes 71, 84 n.50, 101
 Heart 40, 52 n.35, 101
 Humors 77, 84 n.50, 87 n.112
 Law 96
 Letters 53–4 n.45, 56 n.65, 96
 Nature of Man 70–2, 74, 84 n.50, 85 n.69
 Nature of the Child 52 n.38, 71, 74, 84 n.50
 Nature of Woman 28
 Nutriment 78, 84 n.50, 86 n.93
 Oath 4, 13, 14, 23, 31, 43–4, 47, 53 n.45, 96, 157, 183, 219, 240, 244–53, 264, 282, 283, 312
 On Birth 84 n.50
 On Decorum 31
 On Diet (Regimen I) 11, 69–71, 74, 76, 84 n.50, 85 n.56, 86 n.91, 87 n.108

On Generation/Nature of the Child 29
On Head Wounds 52 n.35
On Joints 52 n.35, 55 n.63
On Sacred Diseases 84 n.50
On Sterile Women 28
On the Diseases of Virgins 29
On the Places in Man 73, 84 n.50
Prognostic 39, 52 n.35, 99, 100, 107
Regimen in Health 84 n.50
Seed 101
The Physician 4
Hippocratise 178, 194
Hippocratism/Neo-Hippocratism
 American 12–13
  Nineteenth-Century 201–36
  Twentieth-Century 239–56
 And language 280–301 *see also* Reading
 British
  Seventeenth-Century 11, 91–115, 116–35
  Eighteenth-Century 11–12, 136–53
  Twentieth-Century 13–14, 280–301
 French
  Eighteenth/Nineteenth Centuries 12, 157–77, 178–99
  Twentieth-Century 13, 257–79
  Montpellier 12, 157–77, 190–3
  Paris 12, 178–99
 German
  Eighteenth-Century 6
  Twentieth-Century 14, 301–24
 Material 241–5
 Natural 8
 Nazi 312–16
 Patristic 54–5 n.51
 Renaissance 5–6, 10–11, 21–88
Hippokrates 304, 313
Historiography of Hippocrates (Traditional) 1–4, 157–8, 181, 302
History of Medicine 201–2, 205, 273, 282, 283
 Academic discipline of in Germany 305, 306, 313
 Berlin Institute for 306
 Historical story-telling and medical culture 200–1
History, cyclical concept of 42–3 *see also* History of Medicine
Hitler, Adolf 306, 312, 315
Hoche, Alfred 310

The Permission to Destroy Life Unworthy of Life (1920) 310
Hodder, Reginald 283
Hoffman, Friedrich 165, 174 n.17
Holcombe, William H. 222
Holism 13, 187, 242, 257–74, 302
   Ideological 262, 262
   Pragmatic 262–3
Holistic revival, of the Twentieth Century 262
Hollywood Production Code Administration 247
Homeopathy 201, 218, 222–3, 261, 266, 267, 268, 280, 282, 305, 306 *see also* Hahnemann
   As German mysticism 218
Honest Physician, The 218–20
Honigmann, Georg 304
Hooghelande 117
Hooke, Robert 137
Hooke, William 117
Horder, Lord Thomas 283, 286
Horn of Africa, Hippocratic medicine in 2
Hospital medicine 302
Hospitals 144, 145, 189
Hugo, Victor 18 n.44
Human
   Dissection 47–8, 118
   Experiments 311–12, 314–16
Humanism 271, 280
   Christian 43, 271
   Medical 193, 267
   Melanchthonian 69
Humanist
   Definition of 53 n.43
   Scholars 5, 59
Humbug, concerns about in the US 214
Humoral medicine/pathology 59–60, 68, 70, 85 n.69, 193, 209, 265
Humoralism/ists 119, 161, 192, 193
Humours 192, 193
   Concept of the Four 38, 46
Hunter, John 200, 204
Hunter, William 124
Hutchison, Sir Robert 283, 289, 290, 291
Huxham, John 137, 145, 147, 148, 149
   Observations of the Air and Epidemic Diseases (1739) 147
Hven 87 n.112
Hydropathy 201
Hygiene 183

Hyginus 23
Hypothesis 207, 212

Iapetros 23
Iatrochemistry 123, 145, 159, 162, 174 n.16 *see also* Hippocrates as Iatrochemist
Iatrophysics/iatromechanism 105, 140, 145, 147, 159, 160, 161, 162, 170, 174 n.16 & 17, 174–5 n.20 *see also* Hippocrates as Iatromechanist
Ideologue (s) 179, 181
Ideology 303
   Ideological toolkit 303, 314
Iliadus 74
Iliaster 74
Illness 266, 270
Images 200 *see also* Hippocrates (busts of and visual images)
Immunology 263
Imperial Health Council, Germany 312
Imponderables 271
Improvement 140, 208
Incommunicable
   Judgment 207
   Knowledge 281
India, in the writings of Hans Much 307
Indian Medicine 266
Individualism 280
Inductivism 191
Inductivist philosophers 265
Infection 311
Influenza pandemic (1918) 291
Ingolstadt 88 n.124
International Congress on Neo-Hippocratism
   (1937) 268, 282
   (1939) 268
International Society of Neo-Hippocratic Medicine 282
Intuition 272, 291–2, 308
Isidor de Sevilla 56 n.68
Italy 61, 79

Jaccoud *De l'humorisme ancien et moderne* (1859) 194
Jackson Jr, James 218
Jacquelin, André 269
Jardin Royal, Paris 94
Jefferson Medical College 203
Jenner, Edward 247

Jewish influence on German medicine,
    British concern about 286
Jewson, Nicolas 130
Jousset, Pierre 261
Jurin, James 137, 138, 142, 143, 144,
    145, 147, 149
Jutland 69
Juvenal 39

Kater, Michael 316
Kavvadias, Professor P. 281
Keen, William Williams 242
Keil, James 129
Keith, Arthur 289
Kelly, Howard A. 241
Kempf, E.J. 31, 32
King of Greece 282
King, Helen 138
Kingsley, Sidney 245–7
    Men in White – the movie 247
    Men in White – the play (1933) 245–7
Køning, Mauritz 84 n.40

La press médicale 268–9
La Roche, René 203
Laboratories 291
Laboratory *see also* Experiment
    Experimentation 269
    Medicine 286, 287
    Scientists 280, 281, 284, 285, 289
    Tests 171
    The Laboratory 268, 290, 302
Laennec, René-Théophile 182, 184,
    187–90, 193, 200, 209, 212, 221, 259,
    262, 274
    Thesis of 184
    Treatise on Diseases of the Chest 185
Laignel-Lavastine, Maxime 266, 267,
    268, 269, 271, 282
Lambert, Samuel 244
    Minute Men of Life (1929) 244
Langdon-Brown, Sir Walter 283, 284, 292
Lange, Johannes 29
Langholf, Volker 4, 24
Langley John Newport 287
Larissa 8
Laroche, Guy 269
Latin 293
Latin America, Hippocratic medicine in 2
Latitudinarians 131
Lauderdale, Duke/Earl of 92–3, 95

Laurentius, Andrea 117
Laurie, Joseph 222
Lawrence, Christopher 283
Lebensreform 311
LeClerc, Daniel 173–4 n.15
Legion of Decency 247
Leibbrandt, Werner 302
Leiden/Leyden 94, 138, 140, 142, 159
Leo X (Pope) 53 n.42
Leopold-Bellan Hospital 267
Leriche, René 269
Levy, K. 307
Lewis, Sinclair 249–52
    Arrowsmith (1925) 249, 253
    The Hippocratic Oath (1935) 249–52
Lewis, Thomas 292
L'Homéopathie Moderne 267
Libraries 291
Liébault, Jean 28–9
Liek, Erwin 304
Lifton, Robert Jay 302
Lining, John 146, 147, 148, 149
Linnean Society 282
Littré, Emile 7, 213, 258, 260, 264, 265,
    273
Lloyd, Geoffrey 3–4
Localism 171, 259, 260
Locality and Disease *see* Disease
Locke, John 104, 122–3, 131, 159
    Essay on Human Understanding
    (1692) 123
Loeb Classical Library 242, 285
Loeper, Maurice 269
Logan, Joseph P. 219–20
Lonie, Iain 60
Louis XV 160
Louis, Pierre 207, 209, 211, 212, 218–19,
    221–2, 224
Louisville Medical Institute 221
Lower, Richard 117
Lumière, Auguste 269
Luther, Martin 79

Machaon 39, 81 n.16
Mackenzie, Sir James 283, 289
Maclean, Ian 30
Madrid 282
Magendie, François 193
Major, Ralph 242
Malpighi, Marcello 117
Manichæan 84 n.43

Mannheim, Karl 302
Marseilles Faculty of Medicine 268, 269
Martiny, Marcel 267, 268, 270
Marty, Martin E. 303
  Fundamentalism Observed (1991) 303
Masculinity 21, 26, 27
Mass
  Hypnosis 286
  Medicine 292, 302
  Mind 286
Materialism 265, 273, 280, 287
Mathematics 165
Matrix 66, 72
Maty, Matthew 137, 138
Mayow, John 117
McDowell, Ephraim 26
Means, Alexander 225
Mechanical
  Knowledge (*scientia mechanica*) 66, 73
  Liturgy (*lithurgia/liturgia mechanica*) 66, 83–4 n.40
  Philosophy 66, 138, 146, 148
  Spirits (*spiritus mechanici*) 66, 71, 73, 83 n 37, 86 n.87
Mechanisation 284
Mechanism 273, 287, 293, 308
Medical
  Imagery 42
  Nomenclature 193
  Science 308, 311
  Science of Man 181, 187
  Statistics 191
  Systems 179
  Textbooks 290, 291
  Theses, Antebellum (US) 207
Medicine, Art of 191, 308
Mediterranean medicine 267, 282
Meier, Christian 41
Melanchthon, Philip 51 n.13, 54 n.49 56 n.65 *see also* Humanism
Mendel, Gregor 26
Meng, Heinrich 304
Menstruation 29, 30
Mentality 303
  Of the Herd 284
Mentel, Jacques 48
Ménuret de Chambaud, Jean-Joseph 160, 166, 174 n.19
Mercurialis 85 n.55
Mercurius Britannicus (1643) 97

Mercurius Politicus (1650) 97
Mercurius Pragmaticus (1647) 97
Mercy killings 310
Metchnikoff, Elie 247
Meteorological instruments 137, 142, 144, 146
  Barometer 137, 142, 146
  Hygroscope 137, 144, 146
  Rain gauge 137, 144
  Thermometer 142, 146
  Wind gauge 137, 144
Meteorology 12, 136–53 *passim*, 182
Methodists 43
Miasmas 265
Microscopy 171, 192–3
Mielke, Fred 316
Mind, The Public 285
Minds, Limited/ Narrow, concern about in Britain 288–91
Mineral waters 262
Mitscherlich, Alexander 316
Modern spirit 188
Modernisation 303, 304
Modernity 13–14, 292–3
Moffet, Thomas 79
Moll, Albert 315
Money 31–2
Montpellier 94, 157–77, 181, 186, 190–3
  see also Hippocratism/Neo-Hippocratism
  Faculty of Medicine 264
  Vitalist school 157–77 *passim*, 259, 263
Moravia, Sergio 174 n.15
More, Thomas
  Utopia (1516) 119
Morgagni, G.B. 190, 204, 221
Mortimer, Cromwell 137, 138, 139, 140, 141, 142, 143, 149
Moses 65
Moses, Julius 316
Much, Hans 306–12
  Hippocrates the Great (1926) 307
Murray, Gilbert 294
Mysticism 206
Myth 178, 188, 303, 310 *see also* Greek myth

Naming, concern about in Britain 281
Narbonne 167, 171
Nashville, Tennessee 202

National Institute for the Sciences and Arts 180
Natural 191 *see also* Hippocratic/Neo-Hippocratic and Hippocratism
  Gifts 291
  Healing 305
  History method 91, 123, 124
  History of disease 140, 142, 143, 145, 147, 149, 283
  Laws 308
  Magicians 120
  Method 169
  Perfection 183
  Philosophy 116–35
  Therapies 263
Naturalism
  Attack against 308
  Renaissance 79
Nature, 158, 160, 163–6, 167, 168, 183, 217, 263, 270, 291
  As abyss of cause 130
  Beneficence of, 183
  Book of 45
  Healing power of *see* Hippocratic Methods/Doctrines
  Language of 163
  Rules of 308
  Uniformity of, 183
Naturopathy 263, 268, 316
Naturphilosophie, German 308
Nazi doctors 302, 303, 312–15
Nazi Germany 14, 303–4, 314 *see also* Hippocratism/Neo-Hippocratism
Nedham, Marchamont 22, 97–101
  Medela Medicinae (1665) 97–8
Neisser, Albert 315
Neo-Galenism 158
Neo-Hippocratic Conference (1928) 282
Neo-Hippocratism *see* Hippocratism/Neo-Hippocratism
Neo-Humoralism 280
Neo-Scholasticism 288
Neo-Vitalism/ist *see* Vitalism
Nerve-strain 284
Neurasthenia 285
Neurology 290
New Diseases *see* Diseases
Newman, George 288
Newtonian natural philosophy 142
Nicholas of Cusa 66
Nihell, James 166

Observations Nouvelles (1748) 166
Nin, Anaïs 266
Nisbet, Robert 37
Nivision, Samantha S 219
Nominalism 287–8
North American Homeopathic Journal 222
North-Western German Society of Laryngologists 311
Nosology 141, 143, 184, 259
Nott, Josiah Clark 211, 225
Nova scientia 49
Nudism 264, 311
Numbers 165
Numerical method/system 191, 192, 221–2
Numerists 190, 191
Nuremberg Doctors' Trials 302, 314, 316
Nutton Vivian 4, 28, 60, 80 n.6, 88 n.124

Oath-taking, abandonment of in Germany 304
Observation 4, 7, 123, 138, 159, 165, 166, 168, 170, 174 n.16, 179, 180, 182, 186, 192, 203, 205, 206, 207, 209, 219, 265 283 *see also* Hippocrates as Observer
Occult 264
O'Malley, Charles 39
O'Meara, Edmund 119, 121
Openheimer, Robert 27
Opifex 44, 120
Organicism 193, 302
Orpheus 69, 74, 77
Osborne, Michael 7, 260
Osler, William 108, 242
Oxford
  Physiologists 117–32
  University 105, 117–19, 130

Padua 39
Pagel, Walter 39, 61, 78, 80 n.10
Paine, Martin
  Medical and Physiological Commentaries (1840) 222
Painted woman, US concern about 214
Pantheism 160
Paracelsian medicine 59–87 *passim*
Paracelsus, Theophrastus 27, 38–9, 41, 47, 48, 51 n.13, 60–1, 63, 65–6, 72–81, 83 n.32, 91, 129, 273
  And interwar Germany 303, 304, 305
  And Nazi Germany 312–13

As German Hippocrates 312
Chemical philosophy 11
Commentary on the Hippocratic Aphorisms 39
Labyrinthus 39
Paragranum 47, 58 n.77
Philosophy to the Athenians 74
Severinus view of 11, 59–87 *passim*
Paris 39, 43, 94, 158, 160 *see also* Academy of Medicine, Hippocratism/ Neo-Hippocratism
   Clinical school, American views of 204–10
   Faculty of Medicine 188, 258–9, 264–5, 266
   Medicine 178, 179, 184, 185, 187, 188, 189, 190, 192
   School 178, 179, 184, 187, 188, 189, 192, 193, 260
Pasteur, Louis 200, 240, 274
Pasteurism 261–2, 272
Paternity 21–36
Pathological
   Anatomy 179, 184, 185, 186, 187, 189, 193
   Haematology, 192
   Physiology 189
Patient,
   As a whole 290
   As individual 7, 13–14, 159, 283, 290, 291, 302
   As part of a mass 290
   Rights 316
Patrician values 283
Patronage 93–4
Paul, Elfriede 308
Peisse, Louis 178, 186, 187, 188, 194
   La Médecine et les médecins (1857) 178
Penfield, Wilder 10
People, The 163
Perdiccas 8, 244
Perth, Earl of 93–4, 95, 96
Petrarch 37
Petrequin, J.C. 261
Petty, William 117, 120
Phenomena 104
Philanthropy 220
Philology 42, 305
Philosophers/Philosophy 64, 159, 165, 203, 212 *see also* Systems

Philosophical Transactions 136, 142, 145
Physic gardens, Edinburgh 94
Physical
   Education 311
   Medicine 280, 282, 294
   Sciences 193
Physics 271, 272–3
Physiological medicine 185, 189, 260
Physiology 38, 184, 189 *see also* English, Oxford, Pathological,
   Of the central nervous system 263
Pickering, Roger 144, 145
Pinel, Philippe 179, 181–9, 191, 209
   The Clinical Training Of Doctors: An Essay of 1793 181
Piorry, Pierre-Adolphe 193
Pitcairne, Archibald 105, 129
Pittion, Jean-Paul 39
Plain Man, The 292–3, 294
Plato 4, 8, 24, 25, 42, 96, 117, 282
   Republic 119
Platonic duality of body and soul 265
Pliny 5, 54 n.46, 65
Podaleirios /Podalyrius 39, 81 n.16
Politics, Early Modern (English) 129–32
Positive knowledge 187
Positivism/ists 185, 316
Poucel, Joseph 268
Pox, French 98
Poynter, F.N.L. 172 n.3
Practitioner, individual 291
Predestination(s) 65–7, 77, 79, 83 n.38
Press barons 284
Prince of Physicians 22, 27–8
Profession, medical 31
Professionalism 280
Progress 10, 22, 37–8, 41, 45–9 50 n.6, 181, 182, 202, 210, 221, 267
Prometheus 24
Providence 126
Prussia 312, 315
Pseudoepigrapha 8, 25, 56 n.68
Psychological medicine 280, 287, 294
Pulte, Joseph H 222
Puritan Reformers 131
Pythagoras 117, 180
Pythagoreans/ianism 165, 269

Quacks 215, 233 n.64 *see also* Empiric
Quantification 179
Queen Olga 282

INDEX

Race, Nordic 306, 307
Radcliffe, John 129–30
Rational
  Medicine 27
  Treatment as natural treatment 268
Rationalism 204, 220
  Versus empiricism/mysticism 126
Rationes seminales (seminal reasons) 65, 74, 83 n.33
Rattansi, Piyo 93
Ravensbrück concentration camp 314
Ray, Matthew 283
Rayer, Pierre 192
Reading 7–10, 29, 103
  And British Neo-Hippocratists 290, 291, 293
  Of Greek 28, 293
  Severinus of Hippocrates 68–74
Reagan, Leslie 246
Realism/ist 183, 287
Reason 107
Reductivism 287, 293
Reed, Walter 200
Reification 287
Reinhold, Meyer 227
Religion 124–7
Relollaceum 72, 86 n.81
Republican virtue 214
Restoration, France 260
Revelation 42–3
Revolution *see also* Germany
  French 180, 183, 167
  Germany (1918) 304
  In French Medicine 186, 187, 189
Rey, Roselyne 179, 181, 187
Rhetoric 22, 178, 179
Ribe Latin School (Ribe, Denmark) 69
Riolan, Jean R. the Younger 58 n.81, 117
Risueño d' Amador 190–2
Robert Koch Institute 314
Roger, Henri 265, 273
Roger, Jacques 174 n.15
Rolfinck, Werner 48
Rome 28, 32
Root Doctors 217
Rose, Gerhard 314
Rothschuh, Karl 313
Roux, Augustin 176 n.45
Royal College of Physicians of Edinburgh 95, 96
Royal College of Physicians of London 88 n.124, 92, 97, 100, 101, 104, 105, 106, 107, 124, 139, 140, 283
Royal Physicians (Britain) 283
Royal Society of London 7, 104, 106, 136, 137, 138, 139, 140, 142, 144, 145, 146, 147, 148, 149
Royal Society of Medicine
  Medical history Section 282, 283
Rudolph II, Emperor 81 n.15
Rush, Benjamin 202, 216
Rushism 211
Rushmore, Stephen 244–5
Rusnock, Andrea 129
Russell, James Rutherfurd 9
Rütten, Thomas 3
Rutty, William 137
Ryle, John 283, 288

S.S. 312, 315
Salvation 50 n.6
Santorio, Santorio (Sanctorius) 146, 147, 148
Sapp, Jan 26
Sargent, Émile 269
Saturn 23
Sauter, W. 307
Sawday, Jonathan 21, 26, 29
Schulz, Hugo 306
Science
  Language of 285
  Of numbers 191
Scientia 92
Scientific therapeutics 181
Scotland 93–7
Scurvy 98
Second Coming 44
Sectarians 217
Seed(s) *see also semina*
  In Hippocratic gynaecology 29
  Of diseases (*semina morborum*) 67, 74–5
Self-help books 119
Semina 65–6, 71–2, 74, 77, 83 n.38, 87 n.106
Semina theory defined 65–6
  As chemical philosophy 68
Seneca 25
Sensualist philosophy 179
Serums 271
Severinus, Marcus Aurelius 48
Severinus, Petrus 11, 59–88 *passim*

Idea Medicinae (1571) 59–88 *passim*
Shattuck Jr, George C. 211, 215, 217
Sheldon, Archbishop 130
Shell-shock 285
Sherrington, Charles 287
Shock 271
Sibbald, Sir Robert 94–7
  Commentaries on the Law of Hippocrates (1706) 96
Sigerist, Henry E. 266, 273, 304, 305
Signatures 68, 71, 75
Silvius, Jean 117
Simple/Simplicity 191, 181, 264
Simplest Method of Physick 94
Simpsons, The (1995) 4
Singer, Charles 31
Siraisi, Nancy 128
Sloane, Hans 140, 147
Smallpox 106–7
Smith, Dale 245
Smith, Wesley D. 2, 8, 25, 39, 59–60, 91, 173–4 n.15
Social
  Class 92–3
  Medicine 280, 294
Society of Antiquaries 137
Socrates 109, 282
Soemmerring, Samuel Thomas von 108
Solidism 161, 192, 287
Sophocles
  Antigone 56 n.63
Soranus 28
South Asia, Hippocratic medicine in 2
Southern
  Diseases (USA) *see* Diseases
  Nationalism (USA) 223–7
Sparta 310
Specialists/Specialisation 280, 281, 284, 285, 286, 288, 289, 290, 291, 294, 302, 308
  Specialist terminology 291
Species 122, 143, 170
Speculation 204, 208, 212
Spengler, Oswald 304, 307
Spiritualist(s) 265, 273
Split personality 285
Sprackling, Robert 100
  Medula Ignorantiae (1665) 100
Squier, J. Bentley 243
St. Louis Medical and Surgical Society 202

Standardisation 292
Standesehre 309, 316
Starkey, George 127
Starling Ernest Henry 287
Starr, Paul 171
State
  Ideal, The 310
  Medicine 294
  Officials 280, 281, 286, 288
  Platonic, The 310
  The State 286, 289, 302
Statistics 171
Stethoscope 184
Still, Andrew Taylor 241
Stillé, Alfred 206–7, 211, 215, 216, 217
  Elements of General Pathology (1848) 206, 216
Succussion 185
Supreme Artificer 121
Surgeon-apothecaries of Edinburgh 95
Surgical techniques 46
Switzerland 61, 79
Sydenham, Thomas 6, 11, 59–60, 64, 82 n.28, 91, 92, 102–4, 107, 109, 111, 121–3, 130, 131, 140, 146, 158–9, 172 n.3, 181, 182, 190, 191, 204, 221 *see also* English Hippocrates
  Methodus Curandi Febres (1666) 103, 104, 121, 122
  Observationes Medicae (1676) 103, 104
  View of Hippocrates 102–4
Sylvius, Jacobus *see* Dubois
Syncretism 265–6, 267
Synthesis/Synthetic medicine 13, 263, 266, 270, 280
System 159, 165, 166, 168, 210, 280 *see also* Numerical method/system and Systems
  Building/ers 162, 170, 208, 215
  Spirit of 204, 209
Systems 189
  Philosophical 179

Tables 140, 141, 142, 143, 144, 145
Tachenius, Otto 60
Taste 239
Technê 23–4
Techoueyres, J 269
Temkin, Owsei 30, 39, 59–60, 79–80
Temperament 263, 268

Concept of the four Temperaments 46
Terrain 263
Terrestrial
   Astronomy 87 n.112
   Philosophy 64
The Chymical Galenist (1667) 101
The Method of Chemical Philosophy and Physic (1664) 126
The Moral Responsibility and the Proper Qualifications of the Physician (1844) 220
Theology 159
Theophrastus 65, 73
Theory/*Theoria* 92, 104
Therapeutic procedures 46
Thessalus (Hippocrates's son) 96
Third Reich 312, 313, 316
Thomson, Samuel 216, 240
   New Guide to Health (1822) 240
Thomson, Samuel 7
Thomsonianism 211, 217, 240
Thouret, Michel-Auguste 184, 259
Thucydides 25
Timme, Johannes 48
Tincture(s) 66–7, 71–2, 76
Topography 182
Translation 5, 21, 28, 29, 291
Transplantation(s) 66–8, 76, 84 n.46
Transylvania 207
   Medical College 219
   University 220
True Physician, The 218–20
Tuberculosis sanatorium movement 263
Tzetzes, Johannes 24

Unity of the organism 287
Urban-industrial transformation (C19th) 284

Van Foreest, Pieter 40
Van Helmont J.B. 91, 97–9, 120
Vannier, Léon 269
Varenius, Bernhard 142
Vegetarianism 264
Vernacular medicine 128
Verney, Pierre 56 n.68
Vesalius, Andreas 30, 38–41, 43–4, 47, 48, 63, 117, 204
   Consilium 40
   Fabrica 40, 47, 52 n.52
Virchow, Rudolf 287
Vis medicatrix naturae see Hippocratic doctrine/methods
Vita 8
Vitalism 158, 159, 161, 166, 169, 170, 192–4, 260, 261, 266, 267, 269, 270, 273, 280, 302
Vivisection 47–8
Volk see Germany
Voltaire 247
Von Haller, Albrecht 174 n.18
Von Staden, Heinrich 23

Wagner, Richard 286
Warbasse, James 244
Ward, Seth 119, 120, 125
   Vindicae academarium (1654) 119
Warden, Archibald Adam 283
Warner, John Harley 3, 240
Webster, Charles 88 n.125, 93, 103
Webster, John 119, 120
   Academiarum examen (1654) 119
Weimar Republic/Germany 14, 309, 315
Weindling, Paul 310
Weir, Sir John 283
Weisz, George 185
Westfall, Richard 127
Wharton, Thomas 101, 102, 117
Whiston, William 142
Wilkins, John 119, 127, 131
Williams, Elizabeth 194
Williams, Francis H. 26
Willis, Thomas 102, 117–19, 125–6, 129–30
   Cerebri anatome (1664) 117, 121
   Rational Therapeutics (1674/5) 119
Winthrop, John 126
Wittenberg 69
Women's Medical College of Pennsylvania 245
Wood, Anthony à 97
Woodward, John 106–7
   An Essay toward a Natural History of the Earth (1695) 106
World War I 284, 286, 304, 310
Worm, Ole 85 n.54, 87 n.118
Wren, Christopher 137

Young, Hugh 242

Zeigelstrasse clinic, Berlin 305
Zeus 23, 24, 25
Zootomy 48
Zwinger, Theodor 79, 88 n.125

DATE DUE